AF841978

Historicising the People's Health Movement in West Bengal, India

Nataraj Malakar

Historicising the People's Health Movement in West Bengal, India

palgrave
macmillan

Nataraj Malakar
Department of History
University of Kalyani
Kalyani, West Bengal, India

ISBN 978-3-032-02695-8 ISBN 978-3-032-02696-5 (eBook)
https://doi.org/10.1007/978-3-032-02696-5

© The Editor(s) (if applicable) and The Author(s), under exclusive license to Springer Nature Switzerland AG 2025

This work is subject to copyright. All rights are solely and exclusively licensed by the Publisher, whether the whole or part of the material is concerned, specifically the rights of translation, reprinting, reuse of illustrations, recitation, broadcasting, reproduction on microfilms or in any other physical way, and transmission or information storage and retrieval, electronic adaptation, computer software, or by similar or dissimilar methodology now known or hereafter developed.
The use of general descriptive names, registered names, trademarks, service marks, etc. in this publication does not imply, even in the absence of a specific statement, that such names are exempt from the relevant protective laws and regulations and therefore free for general use.
The publisher, the authors and the editors are safe to assume that the advice and information in this book are believed to be true and accurate at the date of publication. Neither the publisher nor the authors or the editors give a warranty, expressed or implied, with respect to the material contained herein or for any errors or omissions that may have been made. The publisher remains neutral with regard to jurisdictional claims in published maps and institutional affiliations.

This Palgrave Macmillan imprint is published by the registered company Springer Nature Switzerland AG.
The registered company address is: Gewerbestrasse 11, 6330 Cham, Switzerland

If disposing of this product, please recycle the paper.

This book is dedicated to my respected teacher Professor Sabyasachi Chatterjee, from whom I learnt my first lesson in the history of medicine and who has always stood by me in my journey.

Acknowledgements

Before lighting the lamp, the story of making the wick should be told. My research journey began in 2016, when I started to investigate the history of the blood donation movement in West Bengal as a significant aspect of the broader health movement. On the basis of my study I presented a paper on the history of the blood donation movement at the annual conference of the *Paschimbanga Itihas Samsad*. The paper was well received and later selected for publication in *Itihas Anusandhan*.

That marked just the beginning. My formal doctoral research commenced in early 2018, when I was selected as a University Research Scholar (URS) at the University of Kalyani. Without the support of this scholarship, it would not have been possible for me to dedicate myself fully to this work. The work which has been done is obviously the fruit of full-time research. I am indebted to the University of Kalyani, my alma-mater, for providing me the scholarship. This book is the outcome of my PhD dissertation.

The role played by my teacher and mentor, Professor Sabyasachi Chatterjee, has been invaluable. I extend my heartfelt gratitude to him for his unwavering support and guidance throughout this journey. Pursuing research in such a maiden area would not have been possible without his insightful direction. Professor Chatterjee taught me the fundamentals of research methodology with patience and affection, and he played a pivotal role in shaping my academic ideas. Despite his demanding schedule, he took the time to regularly review my writings and offer thoughtful feedback throughout the entire course of my research. It was he who encouraged me to publish my thesis as a monograph with an international publisher for both national and global readers—a suggestion that ultimately led to the publication of this book. He remained closely involved in every stage of the publication process. He is not only my PhD supervisor but also my guardian in every sense of the term.

I would also like to take this opportunity to express my sincere thanks to my teacher, Professor Manosanta Biswas, who introduced me to many new ideas and offered valuable guidance at various stages of my research. I also acknowledge the encouragement from my teacher Dr. Subrata Roy of Santipur College.

I would like to put on record my respect for my teachers at the University of Kalyani. They have enriched me with their precious comments on my research. Among these, Professor Sutapa Sengupta deserves special mention as she was always by my side during the days of my doctoral research. I express my heartfelt gratitude for their thoughtful suggestions to a number of people: Professor Nirban Basu, formerly of the University of Calcutta; Professor Arabinda Samanta, formerly of the University of Burdwan; Dr. Soumitra Srimani of Netaji Subhash Open University; Vice-Chancellor Professor Rup Kumar Barman of Bankura University; Professor Kausik Bandyopadhyay of West Bengal State University; Professor Hitendra Kumar Patel of Rabindra Bharati University; Professor Indranil Mukhopadhyay of O.P. Jindal Global University; and Professor Chandan Basu of Netaji Subhash Open University.

I wish to place on record my deep respect for the octogenarian health activist Dr. Jnanabrata Sil, conversation with whom has enriched my understanding of various issues related to the health movement.

I am also grateful to Dr. Sankar Kumar Nath, a historian of medicine, for his kind and thoughtful suggestions on my writings concerning the history of the junior doctors' movement.

My sincere thanks go to Kumar Rana, who studied public health at Harvard University, for helping me conceptualize the theoretical framework of my study.

I am especially thankful to health activist Dr. Punyabrata Goon, an ardent supporter of my work, for generously sharing rare documents that were crucial in substantiating several of my arguments.

Interaction with health activists, of whom the majority was medical practitioners, were of great assistance in granting me a proper understanding of recent developments. In this respect I would like to express my deep appreciation to Dr. Hiralal Konar and the late Dr. Smarajit Jana. I would also like to thank Ashok Choudhury, Dr. Amitabha Bhattacharya, Binay Basu Mallik and Raghunath Mitra of *Janaswasthya Committee* for their kind cooperation. I am indebted to Dr. Prodyut Sur of the *Association of Health Service Doctors, West Bengal* for his help. Activists such as Naba Dutta of *Nagarik Mancha* and Srijan Sen of *Dr. Dwarkanath Kotnis Memorial Committee* extended their co-operation by providing relevant documents as well as both support and encouragement. I have also been enlightened by writings of health activists.

I will never forget the help I got from Deepak Kumar Dan of *Gobardanga Gabeshana Parishat.* He allowed me to access important documents kept in the institute. I had the opportunity to use many archival documents of the Department of Health and Family Welfare, West Bengal and the Proceedings of the West Bengal Legislative Assembly, most of which were accessed online during the time of lockdown. I used the resources of several libraries, including the National Library, Kolkata, Bangiya Sahitya Parishat Library, the Library of Institute of Development Studies, Kolkata (IDSK), the Central Library of Kalyani University, the Krishnagar Public Library and the Nadia District Library. I am grateful to the staff of those libraries for their kind cooperation. I have also accessed the archives of people's health organizations and the personal archives of health activists, to whom I am grateful.

I am deeply grateful to my fellow researchers at the University of Kalyani, with whom I exchanged ideas and insights throughout the course of my work. Dr. Sujit Rajbanshi (Sujitda), and my dear friend Sukalyan Gain provided valuable support in enhancing my technical skills. Our discussions also helped me gain a deeper understanding of research methodology. Here I must mention the name of Prasenjit Mukherjee (Prasenjitda), who was always ready to lend a helping hand whenever I encountered difficulties. I owe heartfelt thanks to my brother Apurba Ghosh, who assisted me in translating several Bengali quotations into English. He also read draft chapters of this book carefully and offered numerous suggestions that significantly improved the final work. I remain indebted to Shreya Roy, Dr. Milan Roy, Dr. Ujjaini Samanta Roy, Dr. Arunima Roychowdhury, Dr. Asim Mandal, Dr. Samir Mandal, Dr. Shipra Sarkar, Dr. Malyaban Chattopadhyay, Tanmoy Bhattacharjee, Koushik Chakraborty, Sudip Mandal, Manami Mandal, Abhishek Datta, Subhendu Biswas and Sanchalita Bhattacharyya for their support and encouragement.

Like an elder brother, Subhabrota Chakraborty has always inspired me to strive for excellence in my research. His constant encouragement and appreciation played a vital role in motivating me to publish this book.

I would like to pay heartfelt tribute to my late maternal grandmother, whose blessings and memories continue to inspire me. It was her unwavering support that made it possible for me to pursue higher studies. I also express deep respect to my late father, who would have been immensely proud to witness this achievement of his son. The loving support of my maternal uncle and aunt will always be remembered with gratitude. Most importantly, this work would not have been possible without the unconditional love, emotional strength, and quiet sacrifices of my mother and brother. Their presence gave me the peace of mind and support I needed to devote myself fully to my research.

Finally, I would like to express my sincere thanks to the editorial team at Palgrave Macmillan for giving me the opportunity to publish my work. I am especially grateful to Lucy Kidwell for her cooperation throughout the publication process. I have also greatly benefited from the insightful and constructive feedback provided by the anonymous reviewers of the manuscript. Their suggestions played a vital role in shaping and strengthening this book, and I extend my heartfelt thanks to them for guiding me toward improvement. My heartfelt thanks also go to Arun Prasath for his kind assistance during this journey.

About This Book

The book explores the history of the people's health movement in West Bengal, India. It critically evaluates the policy related to health in a historical context. It looks at the dual process of degradation of the public health system and elevation of the private health sector. This process resulted in the deprivation of the right to health of commoners which necessitated the emergence and development of the health movement. The book investigates efforts to heal the health system. It unearths the unethical practice related to medicine and analyses the movement for essential and rational drugs in a detailed manner that was a major part of the health movement. Basically, the health movement is a right movement. It is the right of the people to get the health service as well as to have a living condition where physical, mental and social well-being can be ensured. The health movement is working to make this dream real. It is a significant movement to ensure equity and equality. It can be termed an important addition to the genre of new social movement. The book adds a new perspective to the contemporary social history of India.

Contents

About the Author

Nataraj Malakar specializes in history of the health movement. He undertook his doctoral research in University of Kalyani with a full-time Research Fellowship. His research interest focuses on the social history of health & medicine and the history of the rights movement. He has already published a book (with Sabyasachi Chattopadhyay) on the commercialization of health in Bengali (*Prasanga Swasthya: Pariseba theke Panya*, Kolkata: Sampark, 2025). In addition, he has published a large number of research papers in UGC-Care listed journals which include the *Journal of the Asiatic Society*, *Science and Culture*, the *Journal of People's History and Culture*, *Itikotha* etc. He is a regular contributor on his subject to the editorial pages in the leading Bengali dailies published in Kolkata, India. He is teaching as visiting faculty in the PG Department of History, Vivekananda College, Thakurpukur and in the Department of History (UG and PG), Berhampore Girls' College.

CHAPTER 1

Introducing People's Health

Health is a social, economic and political issue and, above all, a fundamental human right. Inequality, poverty, exploitation, violence and injustice are at the root of ill-health and the deaths of poor and marginalised people. Health for All means that powerful interests have to be challenged…and that political and economic priorities have to be drastically changed.[1]

I

Medicine has evolved through various stages, such as bedside medicine, library medicine, hospital medicine, and laboratory medicine. The Hippocratic approach to medicine was holistic, emphasizing the whole patient within their social and environmental context. The Hippocratic doctor needed to possess an in-depth understanding of their patient, including their social, economic, and familial background, daily habits, diet, travel history, and so on. Ancient Greeks and Indian medicine also shared the idea of 'humors.' In ayurveda, man was viewed as part of nature, a microcosm of the universe, comprised of like matter (rasa) existing in five forms: earth, water, fire, air, and sky. The diagnosis of the patient involved a process known as *bhumi-pariksa*: the examination of the patient in relation to his surroundings.[2] The modern categories of hospital, community, and laboratory medicine took shape in their current forms during

© The Author(s), under exclusive license to Springer Nature Switzerland AG 2025
N. Malakar, *Historicising the People's Health Movement in West Bengal, India*, https://doi.org/10.1007/978-3-032-02696-5_1

the nineteenth century. Hospital medicine represented an expanded form of bedside medicine, characterized by the introduction of innovative diagnostic and therapeutic instruments, along with enhanced medical expertise. Community medicine includes the essential environmental infrastructures such as access to clean water, effective waste management, vaccination initiatives, and health and safety in workplaces. It also involves the analysis of disease patterns and their connections to diet, habits, or exposure to agents in the environment. In contrast, laboratory medicine primarily occurs within laboratory settings, and may be translated into better drugs, and the understanding of bodily mechanisms that can improve diagnosis or treatment.[3]

Hospital medicine was systematically introduced following the French Revolution of 1789. In hospital medicine, patients are removed from their homes and localities, and transferred to hospitals under medical control and observation. In the nineteenth century, certain medical and surgical needs began to influence various elements of hospital architecture. During this period, the development of germ theory meant that advanced hospitals required special laboratories for the cultivation of sputum, blood, urine, and stool samples. The main objective of hospital medicine is to remove the disease from the patient.

The concept of modern public health developed through a number of significant and fundamental shifts. The early concept was influenced by the 'filth' theory, which believed that the improvement of public health depends on the cleanliness and sanitation of the community, an undoubtedly liberal concept. This concept has been shifted by the 'epoch-making' discoveries of 'germ theory' by Louis Pasteur (1822–1895) and Robert Koch (1843–1910), which ushered in a new era. Many historians assume that the rise of germ theory in the late 1800s led to a sudden and radical transformation in medicine—what is often called the "Bacteriological Revolution." However, Worboys argues that the concept of such an abrupt shift is overstated. According to him, "there was no Bacteriological Revolution in nineteenth-century medicine."[4] Instead of a sudden, radical transformation, he suggests that the shift from miasmatic to bacteriological explanations of disease was gradual, uneven, and context-dependent. While the discovery of specific pathogens was significant, practices in public health, medicine, and sanitation did not immediately or uniformly change. Many older practices, such as quarantine, continued even after germ theory gained widespread acceptance. Shifts in medical thinking were not only limited to scientific discovery; they were also influenced by political, economic, and social contexts. Moreover, it soon became evident to many health reformers that community sanitation and medical measures alone would not be sufficient to combat a disease such as tuberculosis since other socio-economic and environmental factors also had a big role to play in its spread. Therefore, the concept of the scope of public health expanded to include issues like new-born mortality, malnutrition, occupational health, and mental hygiene.[5] Accordingly, disease should not be regarded merely as a biomedical issue.

Thus, a concept of 'social medicine' developed. The two main principles of social medicine are: first, health of the people is an issue of direct social concern, meaning that society has an obligation to safeguard and ensure the health of its members; second, health and disease are influenced by social and economic factors. That is why social as well as medical measures must be taken to promote health and to combat diseases.[6] The idea of medicine as a social science emerged in nineteenth-century Europe. During this period, health and social reformers had been concerned with developing the political role of medicine in creating egalitarian societies.[7] However, their idea was significantly ahead of their era. The advancement of the germ theory of disease and discoveries in microbiology hindered the development of that idea. Pratik Chakrabarti has pointed out that social medicine developed in Europe and the USA during the 1930s among physicians who sought to connect the epidemiological challenges of the twentieth century with contemporary economic and social conditions. This era was marked by labour movements, suffragette campaigns, and anti-imperial and liberation movements across Africa, Asia, Europe, and Latin America, all of which recognized public health as an important agenda. Consequently, social medicine during the interwar period became intertwined with political activism and social reform.[8] In 1978, the Alma-Ata Conference placed a focus on social medicine by emphasizing health as a fundamental human right and the importance of community participation in health care. In 1948, the World Health Organization (WHO) defined health as "a state of complete physical, mental and social well-being and not merely an absence of disease or infirmity."[9] In 1978, this statement was amplified to include the ability to lead a "socially and economically productive life."[10]

Modern medicine has been subjected to many critiques in different times. In the 1970s, the book *Where There is No Doctor*, written by David Werner, suggested that people could take care of their health needs without the presence of doctors. Similarly, Ivan Illich's book *Medical Nemesis*, published in 1975, denounced medical practice and the 'medicalization' of life. Illich also pointed to the negative consequences of 'medicalization.' Like Werner, Illich argued that medical care and technology should be placed in the hands of the common people. In a similar vein, Thomas McKeown's book *The Modern Rise of Population* questioned the contribution of medicine and public health to the reduction of mortality and population growth. McKeown argued that improvements in the overall standards of living conditions, especially in respect of diet and nutritional status, that resulted from better economic conditions accounted for these demographic changes. The book also supported the arguments of those who believed that efforts to improve people's health needed to address the social and economic determinants of health.[11]

Modern medicine is often accused of focusing on the study of disease and neglecting the study of health. In Park's *Text Book of Preventive and Social Medicine*, for instance, it was stated that over the past century, a tremendous growth of specialization has taken place in response to advances in medical technology as the result of changes in the nature and distribution of health and disease patterns in the community. Specialization has undoubtedly raised the standards of medical care, but it has also escalated the costs of treatment, placing specialist medical care beyond the means of the average citizen. This has infringed upon the basic tenets of socialism.[12] The combination of hospital medicine and laboratory medicine constitutes what has been referred to as 'techno medicine.' Herbert L. Fred has argued that ties between patients and their doctors remained strong until the early 1970s, when high-tech medicine began replacing the so-called 'high-touch,' i.e., bedside-based, medicine. The past five decades have witnessed a progressive demise of such personal care. An over-reliance on technology has crippled physicians' use of the mind and the five sensory faculties to make diagnoses.[13] In clinical medicine, doctors are also unhappy. Based on her observations and conversations with hundreds of doctors conducted over a twenty-year period, Caroline Elton, a UK psychologist, has written a book titled *Also Human: The Inner Lives of Doctors.*[14] She has said "I saw how medical training often fails to acknowledge that doctors are people too, with their own thoughts, feelings, fantasies, and desires."[15] She has focused on the stresses and struggles of doctors, observing that doctors were suffering from anxiety and depression caused by a variety of issues. Depressed doctors made more medical errors than non-depressed doctors. Doctor burnout caused decreased patient satisfaction. In an article entitled "Doctors can't care for patients if the system doesn't care for them,"[16] Elton stated that "physician burnout is a global phenomenon; worldwide, we need to think more carefully about the human cost to doctors of providing patient care."[17]

Modern medicine has enhanced longevity and life expectancy; however, it has not necessarily improved the quality of end-of-life care. Atul Gawande,[18] an American surgeon and writer, noted that "scientific advances have turned the processes of aging and dying into medical experiences, matters to be managed by health care professionals. And we in the medical world have proved alarmingly unprepared for it."[19] Medical science and medical education emphasized how to treat a disease and how to ensure that a person lives a long life. In this medical system doctors are not taught to deal with death in a better and more meaningful way. That is why the more intensive and extended treatment that is given to patients causes a lot of suffering. Gawande has said "our reluctance to honestly examine the experience of aging and dying has increased the harm we inflict on people and denied them the basic comforts they most need (human company and love). Lacking a coherent view of how people might live successfully all the way to their very end, we have allowed our fates to be controlled by the imperatives of medicine, technology, and strangers."[20] Gawande recommends that doctors should focus on well-being rather than survival.

As mentioned earlier, the rise of modern medicine, or so-called "Medicine 2.0," is often traced to the advent of germ theory in the mid-nineteenth century, which marked a decisive break from the observational and largely speculative practices of the Hippocratic era, or "Medicine 1.0." While germ theory laid the conceptual groundwork for a scientific understanding of disease causation, it was not until the mid-twentieth century—with the introduction of antibiotics—that biomedicine gained the practical tools to manage many acute and life-threatening conditions effectively. This treatment-based and increasingly specialized form of medicine has achieved remarkable successes, including the almost total eradication of polio and smallpox, the containment of HIV/AIDS, and the cure of hepatitis C. However, Medicine 2.0 remains limited in its capacity to prevent and manage life-threatening diseases such as cancer. Its orientation toward intervention rather than prevention often leads to an extended lifespan without corresponding gains in quality of life. This paradox—of longer lives accompanied by prolonged morbidity—reveals a structural weakness in the biomedical model, particularly its insufficient attention to the social, behavioral, and environmental determinants of health. In his book titled

Outlive,[21] Peter Attia, a noted doctor, coined the term 'Medicine 3.0,' which emphasizes a focus on the prevention of ailments such as cancer and heart disease rather than merely their treatment. The goal of this new medicine, according to Attia "is not to patch people up and get them out the door, removing their tumors and hoping for the best, but rather to prevent the tumors from appearing and spreading in the first place; or to avoid that first heart attack; or to divert someone from the path to Alzheimer's disease. Our treatments, and our prevention and detection strategies, need to change to fit the nature of these diseases, with their long, slow prologues."[22] Medicine 3.0 is a proposed future of medicine, which includes four key characteristics: an emphasis on prevention rather than treatment; considering the patient as a unique individual; honest assessment and acceptance of risk; maintaining health-span, the quality of life.

II

Prevention is always better than cure. However, Medicine 3.0 cannot take the place of Medicine 2.0. Hospitals still play a crucial role in the treatment of acute illness. That is why the state should play a crucial role in the health system. In this context, it is worth mentioning here that the authors Vicente Navarro and Leiyu Shi asserted that political variables have a significant impact on a country's social inequality and health indicators.[23] The term 'socialized medicine' has been widely used in history and sociology. In their book *Health Communism*,[24] Beatrice Adler-Bolton and Artie Vierkant listed some common characteristics of socialized medicine: first, socialized medicine is principally understood as a more 'equitable distribution of healthcare,' where access to healthcare is no longer determined by an individual's socio-economic status, financial resources, ethnicity, physical ability, or gender; second, socialized medicine is perceived as a program implemented by the state, aimed at providing care to its citizens; third, socialized medicine is often thought of as a state welfare program that can effectively coexist within a predominantly capitalist framework. The term 'socialized medicine' was subsequently popularized by leftist intellectuals. In 1937, the medical historian Henry E. Sigerist published *Socialized Medicine in the Soviet Union*. He was an admirer of the Soviet system of state-run health services and a leading figure in left-wing and progressive groups.

However, the concept of socialized medicine, which was committed to securing justice for all people, has faced significant challenges during the period of neo-liberal economic policies. The world is facing a crisis in health with the coming of neo-liberalism. Margaret Thatcher, the UK prime minister from 1979 to 1990, stated, "There is no alternative (TINA)" to capitalism. In the developed world, 'Reaganism'[25] and 'Thatcherism'[26] were the most effective policies in tearing down the welfare states. According to Francis Fukuyama, humanity had arrived at the "end of history"[27] following the fall of the Berlin Wall and it was no longer possible to conceive of a world outside of Western liberal capitalism. In the words of Vicente Navarro, "capitalism without borders became the name of the game in world affairs, reproducing a narrative that became known as neo-liberalism adding the neo prefix to indicate that this was indeed a new, broader, more advanced form of the old-liberalism." Neoliberal ideology holds that the state's role in various aspects of economic and social life should be minimized in order to unleash the enormous potential of market forces. 'Neo-liberalism' is the ideology and practice of the dominant classes in both the developed and the developing worlds. The application of neo-liberal policies within the international economic order became known as 'globalization.' These related terms, 'neo-liberalism' and 'globalization.' are two sides of the same coin. The neo-liberal administrations of the United States pushed for the privatization and commodification of medicine. This model of health care has become dominant across the world. However, Navarro mentioned that while managed competition, privatization, and for-profit medicine is a fashionable doctrine with the U.S. establishment, they are not popular at the street level in the United States. The majority of people have a profound distrust of insurance companies.[28] In contrast, the UK, one of the pioneer neo-liberal countries, retained a largely public health system, with only partial market-oriented reforms. Benjamin Goodair[29] has pointed out that "England's National Health Service has observed a 20-year period of privatisation through increases in outsourcing of clinical healthcare provision to the private sector. Services are still funded by the NHS, paid largely out of general taxation and, mostly, free at the point of use—but delivered by a private company. Consecutive UK Governments have introduced national regulation to significantly empower private companies to deliver treatments instead of NHS providers." As a result of neo-liberal policy, inequities were baked in both within and between nations. Health was turned into a commodity to be purchased and sold in the marketplace. Meri Koivusalo[30] has argued that the process of economic globalization presents a common challenge for global health systems. Health inequalities are closely linked to social inequalities. Consequently, the reduction of health inequalities through a health system becomes increasingly challenging if social inequalities are being exacerbated by globalization. National health policies have thus been influenced by economic globalization. In many countries, the World Bank and the International Monetary Fund (IMF) have played an important role in the health care reform processes, both directly, through sectoral health care reforms, and indirectly, by limiting public investments and budgets, and broader public sector reforms.

The impact of economic globalization on health has been debated amongst scholars. Richard G. A. Feachem, in an article entitled 'Globalisation is good for your health, mostly,'[31] published in the *British Medical Journal* (BMJ), defining globalization as openness to trade, to ideas, to investment, to people, and to culture has argued that globalization brings benefits today, as it has for centuries and continues to bring benefits to the incomes and health of the poor. In response to this article, Andrew Porter, a consultant pediatrician at William Harvey Hospital in the UK, addressed the editor of the *BMJ*, stating that while the slave trade had brought great benefits to the American plantation owners it did little for the millions of Africans who were unwillingly globalized. Similarly, today, access to world markets brings ever-increasing benefits to the large multinational companies and their stockholders, who are overwhelmingly based in the richest countries, but not to the poorest people in the countries being opened up to trade. Porter cited the example of Hyderabad, India, where modern motorways, palatial residential areas and hotels, and increasing numbers of sophisticated private hospitals exist yet the public Nilufar Children's Hospital, once the pride of the region, now stands neglected and in disrepair.[32] These offer clear indications of why the impact of economic globalization on health policy cannot be comprehended within the framework of traditional approaches to the mobility of goods across borders.

Mackintosh and Koivusalo have pointed out that, since the 1970s, the commercialization of health care has been integrated into wider trends of economic liberalization in both developing and transitional countries. (In this context a transitional country refers to a country that is in the process of shifting its economic structure from a state-run system to one that is driven by market forces.) In the 1980s, many countries faced powerful pressures, especially from multilateral agencies, to shift toward the establishment of commercialized health systems amid poverty-stricken and informalized economies. This led to the implementation of out-of-pocket (OOP) payments for public health services, as well as the establishment or growth of private health insurance in areas where income levels were sufficiently high. They define the term 'commercialized health care' as follows: "the provision of health care services through market relationships to those able to pay; investment in, and production of, those services, and of inputs to them, for cash income or profit, including private contracting and supply to publicly financed health care; and health care finance derived from individual payment and private insurance."[33] Mackintosh has similarly argued that commercialized health care acts to embed inequality in societies in new and often more extreme forms. Her view is against the prevailing policy assumption that health systems can derive benefits from liberalization in the same manner as other commodities. According to her, "highly regressive fee payment systems that push households into poverty, particularly through forced asset sales and loss of income-earners because of exclusion from care." Cross-country comparative data showed that the commercialization of health care does not positively influence access to health care services and health outcomes. Nevertheless, commercialization has increasingly become the prevailing model in primary care across many low-income countries. Mackintosh holds the view that "the poorer the country, the more dominant out-of-pocket spending on health care is likely to be." In developing countries, commercialized health systems are generally unregulated, because, in liberalized markets, 'formal regulation is very hard to achieve.' In low-income developing countries, particularly in Sub-Saharan Africa, where widespread poverty prevails, the liberalization of predominantly unregulated clinical services has led to "a substantially informalised, fee-for-service primary health sector which is exclusionary, low quality and under stress'."[34]

In response to an article titled 'Private Health Care in Developing Countries'[35] published in the *BMJ*, Philip Crowley from Durham addressed the editor, stating he had spent five years in northern Nicaragua, from 1989 to 1994. During that period, he had observed the strengths of the primary health care system developed by the Sandinista government in partnership with powerful community and social organizations. He also witnessed the involvement of the World Bank and the International Monetary Fund in Nicaragua and the subsequent effects on health and health care. One key principle enforced by these organizations was the requirement for local residents to pay user fees for their health and education services. During this period, public sector funding was significantly curtailed, leading to the transformation of free-state healthcare into a private, 'pay-as-you-go' model administered by the state. This had serious implications, for instance, local families were often compelled to sell their only cow, which was their sole source of milk, in order to afford essential medications, resulting in increased malnutrition. In parallel, doctors provided private health care in clinics. The cumulative effect of these changes was to deprive the majority of poor local people of meaningful access to health care. The reductions in public sector funding led to substantial declines in malaria control and other public health initiatives, culminating in a notable rise in cases of both malaria and dengue fever.[36]

Through such measures, health care has been industrialized in much the same way as textile manufacturing was in the nineteenth century. Business groups, with the support of politicians, tried to form only one particular type of economy and one possible mode of production, i.e., capitalist production for the market. That system expanded not to meet human needs but to satisfy profitable consumers and thereby maximize profit. These groups believed that if medical care was a production system, then its products must be commodities. This is how care systems have usefully been measured and evaluated as production systems.[37] Corporate enterprises came forward with capital to enter into the health care sector, developing the multi-institutional and multi-facility systems for profit-making. This led to an 'explosive growth' of the 'healthcare industry,' which comprises hospitals, diagnostic centers, pharmaceutical manufacturers, medical equipment and device manufacturers, the health insurance industry and so on. Arnold S. Relman, the editor of *The New England Journal of Medicine*, wrote that the "'New medical-industrial complex' is a large and growing network of private corporations engaged in business of supplying health-care services to patients for a profit—services heretofore provided by non-profit institutions or individual practitioners…It is the most important recent development in America."[38] As noted above, this trend was a global phenomenon not only in developed countries. It has been reported in *The Economic Times* that the Indian health care sector is one of the fastest-growing sectors of the economy. It has also been stated that, according to the Department of Industrial Policy and Promotion (DIPP), the hospital and diagnostics sector attracted $6.8 billion in foreign direct investment (FDI) between April 2000 and June 2020.[39]

Health care reforms in India commenced in the 1970s, but gained momentum particularly after the 1990s. During the 1970s and 1980s, the sector experienced significant privatization, which led to escalating costs and rendered health care increasingly unattainable for a substantial segment of the population. Today, a considerable portion of India's populace continues to face inadequate or nonexistent access to basic health services. Over the past three decades, health inequalities have increased rapidly. Although health inequalities did exist in India even in the 1950s and 1960s, there was a focused effort during these decades to tackle these issues through public investment and state intervention aimed at diminishing such inequalities. The government's commitment to health care intervention was rooted in the Nehruvian development discourse, which advocated for a government-led health care system that would progressively alleviate health inequities and improve overall health outcomes.[40] Purendra Prasad has observed three prominent recent trends within the Indian health system: first, the role of state has significantly changed in the way the state has allowed private capital to enter the health care industry; second, the market has had increasing influence in the development of health care; third, individual patients have been transformed into consumers under medical neo-liberalism.

Over the past three decades, corporate hospitals have established an increasingly prominent role in India's health care sector. According to Indira Chakravarthi, corporate medical care providers are not limited to major metropolitan cities; they also operate through regional networks, offering a range of medical services, including certain kinds of education and training. As stated by the president and CEO of GE Healthcare India, "India is the first country to have a large number of multinational health care providers. There are seven–eight very active MNCs." Chakravarthi has argued that there is strong advocacy and promotion by the industry of the idea that "Health care infrastructure should not just be viewed as a social good but also as a viable economic venture with productivity." The Federation of Indian Chambers of Commerce and Industry (FICCI) Health Services Division has called on the government to attract private health care investment to supplement the public funding deficit in health care allocations, by offering various fiscal and non-fiscal incentives. The International Finance Corporation (IFC), part of the World Bank group, has been facilitating loans to assist private providers in their attempts to enter new markets. During the IFC's International Private Health Conference held in May 2011, for example, one IFC functionary stated that "Health care has become a major global industry, growing faster than GDP in most countries...as the world recovers from the international financial crisis, the expansion of the private health sector continues rapidly across emerging markets." According to Chakravarthi, India has historically maintained a significant private sector within its health care system; this primarily includes individual practitioners (both qualified and unqualified), charitable hospitals, and nursing homes owned by doctors. The health sector reforms initiated in the 1990s under the country's neo-liberal regime explicitly encouraged the private sector to act as a collaborator and solution to the challenges faced by the public sector. Since the early 1990s, a period during which the healthcare sector in India was regarded as a 'sunrise industry,' several major corporate entities, including Fortis Healthcare (backed by Ranbaxy Laboratories), Wockhardt Hospitals (promoted by the pharma company Wockhardt), and Max Healthcare, revealed their intentions to establish hospital chains across the country. However, no regulatory measures were established to oversee this expansion. As a result, the private sector has experienced unchecked growth in its institutions. The India Brand Equity Foundation (IBEF) has stated that "India is one of the world's most lucrative health care markets and is expanding rapidly..."[41]

Therefore, over this period medicine has transformed from an art and science dedicated to saving people's lives into a business run for profit. Accordingly, people have been deprived of the right to health. The achievement of 'health for all' has remained an elusive goal. In this context, we can situate the people's health movement, which emerged in a new form centring on 'alternative approach to health care.' I have used the term *people's health* in the title of the book as I have attempted to trace the history of the 'right to health.' This movement aims for a world in which everyone has access to a healthy life. It is constructed on a belief that health is a social, economic, and political issue.

III

Let us try to elaborate the concept of 'people.' Generally, we use the terms 'public health' and 'people's health' interchangeably to denote the health of the common people in a society. Leftists are in favor of using the term 'people's health' rather than 'public health' as they try to project themselves as the representatives of the 'proletariat'. However, the historian Sabyasachi Bhattacharya offered a different viewpoint. He opined "*people's history* is neither new nor Left necessarily. Likewise, in Indian historiography the term *history of the people* is bandied about right, left and centre."[42] The precise term 'public health' can be used to refer to the government health system. Zafrullah Chowdhury, a noted health activist from Bangladesh, was once asked the reason behind the naming of their organization *Gonoshasthya Kendra* (People's Health Centre), a rural health care organization, instead of *Janaswasthya Kendra* (Public Health Centre). He responded that if it had been named the *Janaswasthya Kendra*, it would have sounded like a government health initiative. The foundational element of Zafarullah's approach was people and communities for their health and development.

The adjective 'people' has become particularly popular in the modern intellectual world since the emergence of Mao Tse-tung, who emphasized people's participation in the Chinese *Cultural Revolution*. The *People's Republic of China* (PRC) had been established in 1949. Thus does not mean, however, that the concept 'people' had not been used before Mao Tse-tung. In 1932, for example, the British Labour Party had published a memorandum titled *The People's Health*,[43] which was based on the discussion by a group of party members particularly interested in public health. The booklet advocated for a system of universal health care. It stated that such a service must be free to all and that there must be no economic barrier between the doctor and his patient. Similarly, a book titled *A People's History of England*"[44] by Arthur Leslie Morton was published in 1938, and in 1943 the British Communist Party (North-East District Branch) published their report of a conference which was titled *The People's Health*.[45] These early ideas and campaigns in Britain fed into the debate which ultimately culminated in the establishment of the National Health Service (NHS) in 1948. The NHS enshrined the principle that health care should be universally accessible, state-funded, and free at the point of use.[46] This development constituted a significant milestone, whereby the principles of people's health were formally integrated into national policy and the state assumed responsibility for the health and welfare of its population.

In India, the concept of *people's*, in respect of health, had its mention in the 1940s (1946). An article titled 'People's Health and State's Responsibilities' had appeared in the October 1946 issue of the renowned journal *Current Science*.[47] Following this, a number of scholars used the term 'people's' to signify a focus on the marginalized poor. Morton traced the people's history of England in general in the 1930s. The history of people's health in particular has been discussed later. However, a book with the specific title of *The People's Health* appeared in the 1950s. The full title was *The People's Health: A History of Public Health in Minnesota to 1948*,[48] by Philip D. Jordan, suggesting that the author has used the terms *People's Health* and *Public Health* synonymously. That problem is still present and it affects us while we try to trace the history of any such movements. But what is more significant in considering Jordan's work is that a full monograph was published on that theme as early as 1953 with a case study of a state of the USA, i.e., Minnesota. It opened up a window to discuss the scope of the study. One reviewer[49] commented that "It is stated that the People's Health is an informal history written for the general reader, emphasizing the social aspects of public health and the roles of persons and organizations in the program." In this book, we can find some outlining of the notion of people's health. The term was used again in the title of the book *The People's Health, 1830–1910*[50] in 1979. That book dealt with different health issues suffered by the people of Britain, such as infants' maladies, smallpox, and the health of people living in the workhouse. Yet, as stated earlier, the country where the word 'people's' had been most popularized in recent decades was undoubtedly China. Recently, Zhou Xun wrote *The People's Health: Health Intervention and Delivery in Mao's China, 1949–1983*.[51] The book provides a critical analysis of public health policies in China during the Mao era. It demonstrates how politics and health are inextricably linked and examines major public health initiatives, including the anti-chistosomiasis campaign and the Barefoot Doctor program.

According to Purendra Prasad, it was civil society activism which first posed serious questions about the changing trajectory of health care that was moving away from a state-directed path of welfare. Health research and policy in India was influenced by two kinds of activism: one, the movement framework; second, academic activists from Jawaharlal Nehru University's (JNU) Centre of Social Medicine and Community Health and other universities produced a counter-narrative, highlighting perspectives of the local communities.[52] The health movement is not a homogenous one. It may be best compared to a part of the *alternative globalization movement*,[53] which, as a major collective force, emerged as a protest against the structural adjustment policies imposed by the *World Bank* and the *International Monetary Fund* (IMF) on the developing world in the 1980s. Members of the *alternative globalization movement* formed the *World Social Forum* in 2001, asserting that "another world is possible."[54] A statement delivered by the *International Forum for the Defense of the Health of People* at the second *World Social Forum*, held in Porto Alegre on January 30, 2002, enunciates that "this second *World Social Forum* begins a new step in the fight for the universalization of social rights, particularly the right to health."[55] A global network of health activists named the *People's Health Movement* (PHM) was also founded in 2000. In other words, the health movement may be regarded as a component of new social movements. Adopting some of this framework, I have attempted to historicize this health movement in the geographical specification of West Bengal, a state of eastern region of Independent India.

In India, the people's health movement (otherwise the health movement) has developed as a multifaceted movement which promotes social justice. It has both socio-economic and political dimensions. The people's health movement is defined as a movement that apparently strives for bettering the health of people and implementing 'universal access to healthcare.' It demands 'equitable public health systems' and that the government should ensure rights to health and the environment. Both those environmental movements which focused on ameliorating people's health, such as fighting against the harmful effects of pollution on health, and the occupational health movement can also be considered health movements. The notion of a health movement includes movements to enhance social services such as rationing, public hygiene etc. Although struggles for better wages may affect health, they cannot be regarded as a component of the health movement. Nonetheless, the efforts of people to promote health determinants, including pure drinking water, may be viewed in such a light, as may campaigns for a rational drug policy and the provision of essential drugs for all. Groups of doctors/medical students have occasionally raised demands for the betterment of health services, in addition to their professional demands. Such activities and their activism also fall into the course of the health movement. Health movements are also linked to people's science movements which engage in health awareness campaigns as part of their science popularization program and are involved in initiatives on specific health-related issues, such as campaigns for the rational treatment of snakebite patients. Such a movement can also encompass campaigns for blood donation, and organ donations following death. Furthermore, the mental health movement is also included in the larger scope of health movement. The health movement demands not only the widespread availability of health services but also radical changes in the current health system. Several health activists and organizations have engaged themselves to build up an alternative health care model to challenge the existing health system. The Indian health movement aims to make people more aware of the growing commercialization of health care and its nature in the country, as well as to create pressure on the government to change the health policies in order to make them more appropriate to people's needs. In summary, the health movement encourages all segments of the population to fight for 'health for all.'

The history of health or public health has received much attention from historians over the last four decades. In India, several studies on the theme of the history of medicine and public health in colonial rule have been conducted. The history of health and medicine in Bengal has also been the subject of research. Research trends in medicine have highlighted colonial intervention in medicine, along with the decline of the traditional medical system. In the context of public health, scholars have argued that public health under British authority only attempted to protect the health of British civilians and military personnel under colonial rule. The theories of Foucault and Gramsci (who has introduced the concept of hegemony) have had a significant influence on scholars studying science and medicine. In his book,[56] Ashis Nandy argues that science has been portrayed as a new 'reason of state.' He explains that the state and its various institutions can "kill, maim or exploit in the name of science." Science itself, as a tool of state power, can be used to justify violence in the name of national security or development. In the field of history of medicine, several scholars have examined how medicine has functioned as a mechanism of power and social control. Within this scholarly landscape, David Arnold makes a significant contribution, preferring the use of the term "state medicine" over "public health" to describe the colonial approach to health in India. Analysing the process of 'colonizing the body,' he says, "Nineteenth-century India presents us with a medical system that attempted not just to function for the benefit of the colonial rulers themselves (though that was undoubtedly one of its priorities) but also, often ineffectually, to straddle the vastness of a peculiarly colonial divide."[57] Arnold argues that Western medicine in colonial India functioned both as an instrument of imperial control and as a medium of cultural hegemony. Initially, it served the British colonial state as a coercive tool to regulate and manage the Indian population, particularly through state-imposed health interventions. Over time, however, Western medicine gained hegemonic power—not merely through force, but by reshaping Indian society's perceptions of health, modernity, and social reform. As Arnold states, "The cultural rhetoric and political authority of Western medicine had by 1914 become too powerful for India's elites to ignore. It represented not only an immediate domain of health but also a wider realm of cultural and political hegemony."[58]

In *Nationalizing the Body*, Projit Bihari Mukharji argues the idea that Western medicine in colonial Bengal was not simply imposed by the British as a tool of control. Instead, he shows that Indian practitioners—known as *daktars*—actively engaged with and adapted Western medicine, integrating it into local social and cultural frameworks. He focuses in particular on the 'vernacularization' of Western medicine. As Mukharji writes, "'Western' medicine…is not always already an imposition. Instead, it might in itself function as a site of 'resistance'. It might also 'produce' new subjectivities, spaces and objects which can be marshalled for the cause of such 'resistance'."[59] Mukharji critiques the concept of 'complete hegemony.' He urges scholars to move beyond the narrow focus on state medicine and instead examine the broader, dynamic medical marketplace, where Indian agency played a critical role. In his words, "It would be wrong to gravitate to the other extreme and contend that 'western' medicine had—in the colonial period—achieved a 'complete hegemony'. The focus on state medicine needs to be supplemented by accounts of the thriving medical market."[60]

However, those studies are confined within pre-independence India. It is pertinent to note that no in-depth historical research has been done on the more recent history of health in West Bengal. Thus, this field is a maiden one. Though the history of public health has been probed by the historians to some extent, the history of the public health movement remains unexplored. I have pointed out earlier in this Introduction that the health movement is classified as a new social movement. While books on social movements have often dealt with the human rights and environmental movements, health movements have received little attention. The activists of the movement had penned their feelings and experiences. However, a full-fledged historical study is yet to be done.

IV

In the present book, I would like to situate the history of the people's health movement in India in general, and West Bengal in particular, in a global context. I have contextualized this development in India after independence against the backdrop of the colonial period. I have presented my findings through the following chapters.

Initially, I have traced the origins of the global health movement with a specific focus on India. The public health movement in England, led by Edwin Chadwick, had emerged in the mid-nineteenth century. The post-industrial revolution in England witnessed a social change that resulted in overcrowding in slums, and an increase of the death rate, especially among women and children, which indicates a deterioration of public health. In this situation, Chadwick emphasized the importance of sanitation in urban settings. The sanitary movement gradually spread from England to other countries such as America, France, Spain, Australia, Germany, Italy etc. After World War II (1939–1945), the process of decolonization began in Asia, Africa, and Latin America. These independent developing countries focused on primary health care for their people and took various initiatives for the development of primary health care. In the 1960s, the doctor David Werner organized a health movement in Mexico; he wrote a book, *There is No Doctor*, to raise awareness of primary health. Developing countries used this book to address the primary health care problem. In this arena, the people's health movement earned a new dimension. In 1972, *Gonoshasthaya Kendra* was founded under the leadership of Zafrullah Chowdhury in Bangladesh just after the successful liberation war in the country. In colonial India, the sanitary movement did not develop as it had done in England. In order to develop health awareness, however, the voluntary initiative was evident in the first half of the twentieth century in colonial Bengal. In the colonial era, several health journals had been published in order to raise public awareness in Bengal. For example, *Swasthya Samachar*, edited by Kartik Chandra Basu, was published between 1910 and 1955. After the Alma-Ata declaration of 1978, however, people's health movement was no longer limited solely to building health awareness; the goal expanded. This movement began to demand health as a 'right' of the people. I have tried to highlight how the concept of 'right to health' was born and spread. It also explains 'social medicine' and its evolution. The Cold War ended with the collapse of the *Union of Soviet Socialist Republics* (USSR) in 1991. Following that, the word globalization had achieved a special height. How did globalization and the liberal economy affect the health movement? The study has tried to address this unanswered question.

In 1946, in the last phase of colonial rule in India, the report of the *Bhore Committee* was published in four parts. The report stated that the country has to take responsibility for the health of its people. However, since this time government expenditure on health care has actually fallen. Private health services took a pivotal role in place of governmental ones. The government of India is now advocating an insurance-centric health care system rather than developing public health institutions. The government is engaged with curative medicine rather than prevention of diseases.

The following chapter tries to identify the reasons for India's inability to achieve the goal of 'Health for All.' In this context, I have referred to the health policy of the union government of India in general, and of the state government of West Bengal in particular. I have tried to undertake a comparative study between the health system of West Bengal and the health system of other states of India.

People's health organizations have played an important role in both the prevention and cure of diseases. Pamphlets, magazines, and leaflets for the prevention of disease had been published to raise people's awareness. In 1983, Norman Bethune *Janaswasthya Andolan* (Norman Bethune People's Health Movement), led by Dr. Sukhamoy Bhattacharya and Dr. Jnanabrata Sil, emphasized the importance of disease prevention. This organization published many booklets. Inspired by Shankar Guha Niyogi's health movement for labor, a number of organizations was formed in West Bengal, including *Belur Shramajibi Haspatal* (1983), *Shramik-Krishak Maitri Swasthya Kendra* (1995), *Shramajibi Swasthya Udyog* (1999) etc. In respect of curing disease, they have tried to offer an alternative model. They proved that it is possible to obtain good-quality medical care at a small cost. These organizations, besides providing health care facilities for preventing and curing disease, exerted pressure on the government to do its duty properly.

The fourth chapter attempted to investigate the history of the movement led by these organizations. In this context, the study has tried to examine the movement of junior doctors, who raised the slogan that, 'health is not a matter of charity, the right to health is one's fundamental right.' In this chapter, I have studied the health journals which were published in the period under review. I have tried to investigate the impact that left ideology had on the people's health movement. At the end of the 1960s and in the early 1970s, West Bengal witnessed a radical movement for social change. That movement did not achieve its goal, but it did play a significant role in socio-cultural aspects of West Bengal. This chapter has tried to find out how that movement affected the people's health movement. I have paid attention to the attitudes of the party in power toward people's health organizations.

Modern medicine is used for the removal of diseases from the patient's body. Curative medicine is thousands of years old, but modern medicine is hardly a hundred years old. The triumph of modern medicine was achieved through an allopathic revolution that occurred in the mid-twentieth century. Modern medicine is significant for the treatment of ailments. Now, however, in the case of treatment of disease, the majority of expenditure is spent on pharmaceuticals. The poor become poorer to spend money on medicine. There are fashionable markets for unnecessary medicines. Poor people are helpless. People's health organizations have spoken about these medicines. They have created pressure on the government to serve its duty in this regard. In this respect, an important role has been played by the *All India Drug Action Network* (1984). In the very same year, the *Drug Action Forum* was established in West Bengal, publishing many booklets to make people conscious of essential drugs.

In the following chapter, I have tried to examine the movement to increase access to essential drugs. In this respect I have also focused government policy on medicine.

After analyzing these issues, this study has tried to show how the march toward a better world has been developed, both quantitatively and qualitatively, in the course of time through this multidimensional health movement. This concluding chapter has tried to bring out a systematic critical analysis of the various Left and other social movements and a discussion on future pathways. It has explored successful attempts from other social movements of other countries and states. Those are fighting for social justice.

It is important to discuss the methodology which the study of the book has followed. Historical research basically involves two forms—the addition of new data and the new interpretation of known data. In what follows I have tried to include new information. In addition, I have also used an analytical approach to synthesize the facts and examine the existing views. This study is basically concerned with contemporary history. There are, however, many obstacles to the writing of contemporary history. To overcome these obstacles, a noted historian, Ramachandra Guha,[61] suggested the use of different types of sources such as official records, private papers, periodicals and daily newspapers, oral history, and the official papers of other countries. This study has depended on such primary sources. As secondary sources, I have cited Bangla and English books and articles.

Let's begin to read the book.

Notes

1. The People's Charter for Health – People's Health Movement, People's Health Assembly held at Dhaka, Bangladesh in December 2000, p. 2.
2. Mark Harrison, "Tropical Medicine in Nineteenth-Century India", *The British Journal for the History of Science*, Vol. 25, No. 3, Sep., 1992, pp. 299–318.
3. William Bynum, *The History of Medicine: A Very Short Introduction*, Oxford University Press, 2008.
4. Michael Worboys, "Was there a Bacteriological Revolution in Late Nineteenth-century Medicine?", *Studies in History and Philosophy of Science Part C: Studies in History and Philosophy of Biological and Biomedical Sciences*, Vol. 38, No. 1, 2007, pp. 20–42.

5. Edgar Sydenstricker, "The Changing Concept of Public Health", *The Milbank Memorial Fund Quarterly*, Vol. 13, No. 4, October 1935, pp. 301–310.
6. George Rosen "Approaches to a Concept of Social Medicine: A Historical Survey", *The Milbank Memorial Fund Quarterly*, Vol. 26, No. 1, January 1948, pp. 7–21.
7. Dorothy Porter, "How Did Social Medicine Evolve, and Where Is It Heading?", *PLoS Medicine*, Vol. 3, No. 10, October 2006, p. e399.
8. Pratik Chakrabarti, "Health as Activism: Rethinking Social Medicine in India", *The Lancet*, Vol. 399, No. 10341, pp. 2096–2097.
9. World Health Organization, Preamble to the Constitution of the World Health Organization as adopted by the International Health Conference, New York, June 19–22, 1946; signed on July 22, 1946 by the representatives of 61 States (Official Records of the World Health Organization, no. 2, p. 100) and entered into force on April 7, 1948, in Basic Documents, 15th ed. Geneva: World Health Organization, 2006.
10. World Health Organization, Declaration of Alma-Ata, International Conference on Primary Health Care, Alma-Ata, USSR, September 6–12, 1978.
11. Randall M. Packard, *A History of Global Health: Interventions into the Lives of Other People*, Baltimore: Johns Hopkins University Press, 2016, pp. 240–241.
12. K Park, *Park's Textbook of Preventive and Social Medicine*, Jabalpur: Banarasidas Bhanot, 2017, p. 7.
13. Herbert L Fred, "The Downside of Medical Progress: The Mourning of a Medical Dinosaur", *Tex Heart Institute Journal*, Vol. 36, No. 1, 2009, pp. 4–7.

    Although Herbert L. Fred emphasizes the persistence of strong patient–doctor relationships until the 1970s, this appears to contrast with Michel Foucault's argument in *The Birth of the Clinic* (1963), where he describes the 'disappearance of the patient' beginning in the late eighteenth century. According to Foucault, with the rise of clinical medicine—especially after the French Revolution—medicine shifted its focus from the patient's subjective narrative to observable, anatomical, and pathological signs. The doctor's role moved away from listening to the patient's experience and toward interpreting visible symptoms and what could be detected through clinical techniques. The patient, as a speaking and feeling subject, began to "disappear," replaced by the body as an object of observation. Foucault introduces the concept of the "clinical gaze," in which doctors were trained to examine the body through a scientific lens, detaching illness from the individual's personal experience. It is important to note, however, that Foucault was concerned with a discursive and epistemological transformation in medical knowledge—not with the development of techno-medicine itself. The development of techno-medicine, characterized by technologies such as MRI and CT scans, occurred in the 1970s. Recognizing this distinction helps reconcile the apparent divergence between Fred's and Foucault's perspectives. Rather than contradicting Foucault, the emergence of techno-medicine can be seen as deepening his concept of the disappearance of the patient: machines now replace even the doctor's senses, and the body becomes a data-producing object subject to technological interpretation. Nowadays, people's lives are constantly under medical surveillance. Routine procedures like blood pressure and sugar checks have become a normal part of everyday life. The use of standard parameters of 'normal ranges' is closely related to Foucault's theory of biopower, the medical gaze and the process of 'othering'. In Foucault's philosophy, those who fall outside these established norms are often excluded or categorized as 'abnormal'.

14. Caroline Elton, *Also Human: The Inner Lives of Doctors*, New York: Basic Books, 2018.
15. Ibid., p. 12.
16. Caroline Elton, "Doctors can't care for patients if the system doesn't care for them", *British Medical Journal*, Vol. 364, No. 1968, March 2019.
17. Ibid.
18. Atul Gawande, *Being Mortal: Medicine and What Matters in the End*, New York: Henry Holt and Company, 2014.
19. Ibid., p. 16.
20. Ibid., p. 19.
21. Peter Attia, *Outlive: The Science and Art of Longevity*, New York: Harmony, 2023.
22. Ibid., p. 29.
23. Vicente Navarro and Leiyu Shi, "The Political Context of Social Inequalities and Health", *International Journal of Health Services*, Vol. 31, No. 1, 2001, pp. 1–21.
24. Beatrice Adler-Bolton and Artie Vierkant, *Health Communism*, London/New York: Verso, 2022.
25. Ronald Wilson Reagan (1911–2004) served as the 40th president of the United States of America from 1981 to 1989. The term *Reaganism* refers to the neoliberal economic policies promoted by Reagan. That economic policy emphasized lower taxes and less spending on public services, and less government control of the economy.
26. Thatcherism is a branch of Conservative ideology that originated from the ideals and teachings of Margaret Thatcher (1925–2013), the Prime Minister of the United Kingdom from 1979 until 1990, who believed in

the primacy of competition and a free market, and possessed a fundamental distrust of the power of government.

27. Francis Fukuyama, *End of History and the Last Man*, New York: Free Press, 1992.
28. Vicente Navarro (ed.), *Neoliberalism, Globalization, and Inequalities: Consequences for Health and Quality of Life*, New York: Routledge, 2017, pp. 1–23, 203–212.
29. Benjamin Goodair, "'Accident and emergency'? Exploring the reasons for increased privatisation in England's NHS", Health policy, Vol. 138, 2023.
30. Meri Koivusalo, "The Impact of Economic Globalisation on Health", *Theoretical Medicine and Bioethics*, Vol. 27, 2006, pp. 13–34.
31. Richard G. A. Feachem, "Globalisation is Good for Your Health, Mostly", *British Medical Journal*, Vol. 323, 1 September 2001, pp. 504–506.
32. Andrew Porter, "Globalisation is Not Good for Your Health", Letter, *British Medical Journal*, Vol. 324, 5 January, 2002, p. 46.
33. Maureen Mackintosh and Meri Koivusalo, "Health Systems and Commercialization: In Search of Good Sense", in Maureen Mackintosh and Meri Koivusalo (eds.), *Commercialization of Health Care: Global and Local Dynamics and Policy Responses*, Basingstoke: Palgrave Macmillan, 2005, p. 3.
34. Maureen Mackintosh and Sergey Kovalev, "Commercialisation, inequality and the limits to transition in health care: a Polanyian framework for policy analysis", Journal of International Development, Vol. 18, No. 2006, pp. 393–406; Maureen Mackintosh and Meri Koivusalo, "Commercialization and Globalization of Health Care: Lessons from UNRISD Research", available: https://www.google.com/url?sa=t&source=web&rct=j&opi=89978449&url=https://www.files.ethz.ch/isn/48350/RPB7e.pdf&ved=2ahUKEwjNu8D46JeJAxX1XWwGHfs0G2IQFnoECBQQBg&usg=AOvVaw0JFrff9yy3SleBqPY83Bf8, retrieved on October 18, 2024.
35. Anthony B Zwi et al., "Private Health Care in Developing Countries", *British Medical Journal*, Vol. 323, 1 September 2001, pp. 463–464.
36. Philip Crowley, "Strong Public Provision is Only Hope for Health Care in Developing Countries", Letter, *British Medical Journal*, Vol. 324, 5 January 2002, p. 47.
37. Julian Tudor Hart, "Health Care or Health Trade? A Historic Moment of Choice", *International Journal of Health Services*, Vol. 34, No. 2, 2004, pp. 245–254.
38. Arnold S Relman, "The new medical industrial complex", *The New England Journal of Medicine*, Vol. 303, No. 17, October 1980, pp. 963–970.

39. Kanika Jain, "The boom in India's healthcare firms isn't showing signs of slowing", *The Economic Times*, January 19, 2022, Available at: https://economictimes.indiatimes.com/industry/healthcare/biotech/healthcare/the-boom-in-indias-healthcare-firms-isnt-showing-signs-of-slowing/articleshow/88966321.cms, retrieved on January 27, 2023.
40. Purendra Prasad, "Introduction: Health Inequalities in India – The Larger Dimensions", in Purendra Prasad and Amar Jesani (ed.), *Equity and Access: Health Care Studies in India*, Oxford University Press, 2018, pp. 1–21.
41. Indira Chakravarthi, "The Emerging 'Health Care Industry' in India: A Public Health Perspective", *Social Change*, Vol. 43, No. 2, 2013, pp. 165–176; Indira Chakravarthi, "Corporate presence in the healthcare sector in India", *Social Medicine*, Vol. 5, No. 4, pp. 192–204.
42. Sabyasachi Bhattacharya, "History from Below", *Social Scientist*, Vol. 11, No. 4, April 1983, p. 5.
43. Somerville Hastings, *The People's Health*, London: Labour Party, 1932.
44. Arthur Leslie Morton, *A People's History of England*, London: Victor Gollancz Ltd, 1938.
45. *The People's Health* published by North-East District Committee, Communist Party, England: Newcastle-on-Tyne, 1943.
46. Charles Webster, *The National Health Service: A Political History*, Oxford: Oxford University Press, 2002.
47. C.S Pichamuthu, "People's Health and State's Responsibilities", *Current Science*, Vol. 15, No. 10, October 1946, pp. 269–272.
48. Philip D. Jordan, *The People's Health: A History of Public Health in Minnesota to 1948*, USA: Minnesota Historical Society, 1953.
49. Robert G. Paterson reviewed that book in *Bulletin of the History of Medicine*, Vol. 29, No. 2, March–April, 1955, p. 190.
50. F. B Smith, *The People's Health, 1830–1910*, New York: Holmes and Meier, 1979.
51. Zhou Xun, *The People's Health: Health Intervention and Delivery in Mao's China, 1949–1983*, Montreal & Kingston, London, Chicago: McGill-Queen's University Press, 2020.
52. Purendra Prasad, "Introduction: Health Inequalities in India – The Larger Dimensions", op cit.
53. Chamsy el-Ojeili and Patrick Hayden, *Critical Theories of Globalization*, Basingstoke, New York: Palgrave Macmillan, 2006, pp. 178–210.
54. Thomas Ponniah and William F. Fisher, "The World Social Forum and the Reinvention of Democracy", in William F. Fisher and Thomas Ponniah (eds.), *Another World is Possible: World Social Forum Proposals for An Alternative Globalization*, London: Zed Books, reprint 2015 (first published 2003), pp. 1–20.

55. International Forum for the Defense of the Health of People, "Health as an Essential Human Need, a Right of Citizenship, and a Public Good: Health For All is Possible and Necessary", *International Journal of Health Services*, Vol. 32, No. 3, 2002, pp. 601–606.
56. Ashis Nandy (ed.), *Science, Hegemony and Violence: A Requiem for Modernity*, Oxford: Oxford University Press, 1988.
57. David Arnold, *Colonizing the Body: State Medicine and Epidemic Disease in Nineteenth-Century India*, California: University of California Press, 1993, p. 7.
58. Ibid., p. 41.
59. Projit Bihari Mukharji, *Nationalizing the Body: The Medical Market, Print and Daktari Medicine*, London: Anthem Press, 2009, p. 12.
60. Ibid., p. 14.
61. Ramachandra Guha, "The Challenge of Contemporary History", *Economic and Political Weekly*, Vol. 43, No. 26/27, June 28–July 11 2008, pp. 192–200.

CHAPTER 2

Tracing the Origins of the Health Movement

In 2020–2021, the global community faced the issues caused by COVID-19. However, this was not the first such public health crisis. Human civilization has evolved through many such problems. Indeed, any contemporary crisis influences a scholar of history to look at its past. While discussing public health, economist Amiya Kumar Bagchi once remarked: "No important contemporary problem can be discussed without historical perspective."[1] Therefore it is pertinent to shed fresh light on the history of public health. The present study's objective is to do so.

Concept of Public Health

Before discussing its history, it is necessary to understand the meaning of the term *public health.* In the broadest sense, public health encompasses a wide range of concepts. Thus, it is a little difficult to define or understand.[2] In 1920, Charles-Edward A. Winslow, an American scholar of public health, defined *public health* as:

> The science and the art of preventing disease, prolonging life, and promoting physical health and efficiency through organized community efforts for the sanitation of the environment, the control of community infections, the education of the individual in principles of personal hygiene, the organization of medical and nursing services for the early diagnosis and preventive

© The Author(s), under exclusive license to Springer Nature Switzerland AG 2025

N. Malakar, *Historicising the People's Health Movement in West Bengal, India*, https://doi.org/10.1007/978-3-032-02696-5_2

> treatment of disease, and the development of the social machinery which will ensure to every individual in the community a standard of living adequate for the maintenance of health.[3]

Later, Winslow altered the term "physical health" to "physical and mental health."[4] Basically, public health is the sum total of certain factors, such as availability of food, clothing, housing, proper sanitation, pure drinking water, education, employment, and pollution-free environment, which prevent the spreading of diseases and improve the quality of life. In spite of the presence of an advanced public health system, diseases can occur and, naturally, treatment may be required. Actually, public health and health care are complementary to each other. It is not possible to have *health for all* when we look at these two things separately.[5] Public health basically means the prevention of diseases. Undoubtedly, 'prevention is better than cure.' While describing public health and people's health, Ernest M. Gruenberg wrote in an article that: "The three main forces affecting the level of a people's health are the natural hazards to survival and their distribution, the level of civilization, and the advance of public health."[6] The concept of public health or disease prevention has been widely implemented through a social movement.[7]

Public health literally translates as the health of the people. This is significant because such a definition shifts the focus of the deliberation on health from the individual person to the group or community. The philosophy of public health aims to put policies in place to promote population health.[8] John Coggon claims that public health is primarily a moral and political issue. He opines that the term "public" in public health refers to a political community's "shared concern." Coggon places a strong focus on collective and group identity, which is based on common interests.[9] According to him, public health is underpinned by a moral mandate, which is typically divided into two distinct, but related parts: first, an obligation to promote population health; and second, a responsibility to alleviate unfair health inequalities.[10]

How did the concept of public health or the public health movement come about? The book titled *The New Public Health* mentions "history provides a background for the development of understanding and coping with health problems of communities…All societies had to face the realities of disease and death, and develop concepts and methods to manage them."[11] Thus, we can investigate the history of public health from the prehistoric age. In the early prehistoric days, people were hunters and food gatherers. Contamination of food was one of the reasons for their short life span. Then people learned to produce food, and began to live in groups. They created an agricultural society and gradually urbanization had also developed. Required foods were available through agriculture, but problems arose in different areas.[12] Earlier, people had been nomads; after the *Neolithic Revolution*,[13] however, when they learned to live in a certain place, they also polluted the environment, which led to regular outbreaks of infectious diseases. According to Dorothy Porter, "human settlements offered greater opportunity for constant contact with intestinal parasites carried through human faeces, whereas a band of hunters constantly on the move were much less at risk from such infections."[14]

At that time the causes of the disease were regarded as curses from god. Some ancient societies (like the Chinese, Egyptian, Hebrew, Indian, and Incan) incorporated preventive health measures such as cleanliness, personal hygiene, sewage, and drainage systems into their religious practice.[15] Hippocrates (c. 460 BC–c. 370 BC), a Greek physician, was one of the first to look beyond the religious and mystical traditions of healing. He focused on science, stating that supernatural forces had nothing to do with the cause of diseases. According to him, environmental causes were at the root of all human illness.[16] Of this development, William Bynum writes "Hippocrates has become the favoured Father for healers of all stripes"[17] because of his lasting influence on Western medical thought. However, this idea has been questioned by other scholars. Giving all the credit to Hippocrates ignores the fact that medical knowledge developed in many parts of the world—not just in Greece. For example, India had developed medical systems long before modern times. Ancient Indian texts such as the *Caraka Samhita* and the *Susruta Samhita* discussed diseases, treatments, surgery, and ethics in great detail. Dr. R.D. Lele, an Indian medical historian, argued that even if there is debate about the exact time when Caraka and Susruta lived, they should be given the same respect and importance as Hippocrates because of their huge contributions to medicine.[18] Another scholar, Debiprasad Chattopadhyaya,[19] contends that Caraka and Susruta were not individual historical figures; rather, they should be considered collective representatives of medical communities and traditions. This interpretation challenges the idea of a singular founding figure in medical history and highlights the collaborative and cumulative nature of ancient knowledge systems. Recognizing multiple contributions from different cultures gives us a more accurate and inclusive understanding of the history of medicine.

Epidemics such as plague, cholera, and smallpox were common incidents in Europe until the eighteenth century. However, the cause of such disease outbreaks was not properly understood. Thus, various theories were prevalent regarding the causes of the diseases. In Europe, the church stated that poor moral and spiritual conditions were responsible for the occurrence of diseases.[20] According to them, prayer and piety were needed to get rid of the epidemics. But the most popular theory at that time was that of the 'miasma.' Miasmists hold the view that contagious disease was caused by harmful vapors generated from filth in the towns. According to them, the main way to prevent contagious diseases was to set up sanitary measures to clean the sewage from the streets.[21]

It was initially believed that diseases spread through interpersonal contact. So, in cases of an epidemic, the only method used was the isolation of the ailing person and the quarantine of the travellers. The popularity of that method had increased since the fourteenth century. That method was used to prevent the spread of plague in Italy. The term quarantine came from the Italian "quaranta," meaning forty.[22] In 1377, quarantine was first introduced in the republic of Ragusa (now Dubrovnik in Croatia) for a period of thirty days, which was increased to forty days in 1397. The quarantine system was followed by Marseilles (1383), Venice (1423), Pisa (1464), and Genoa (1467).[23] When epidemics occurred, people would try to flee from those cities. The state forcibly imposed quarantine and isolation measures on the common people. As a result, the rich suffered economically. But it was the poor that suffered the most. And so, they occasionally became rebellious. The state deployed its troops to put down the rebellion and enacted legislation.[24] That measure was followed to prevent the possibility of further revolts around the world. In later centuries, British America also adopted rules of trade quarantine. For example, in 1701, the colony of Massachusetts passed a law to prevent a small pox epidemic.[25]

Health in the Era of Enlightenment

The world had reached the era of enlightenment in the eighteenth century. That era was the foundation period for the nineteenth century's public health revolution. The French philosophers Diderot, d'Alembert, Voltaire, and Rousseau emphasized the goal of social reformation. The articles contained in the *Encyclopédie des Arts, Sciences et Métiers* revealed the philosophers' thoughts on public health.[26] The 80 years from 1750 to

1830 marked a pivotal period in the evolution of public health. According to George Rosen, "the peculiar interest of these decades derives from the creation during this period of the foundation for the sanitary movement of the nineteenth century, a development fraught with momentous consequences for modern public health."[27] During that period Jeremy Bentham's utilitarian theory focused on "greatest good for the greatest numbers." Drawing on Bentham's idea, Edwin Chadwick organized a sanitary movement in England.[28]

The American Revolution (1775–1783) and the French Revolution (1789) both took place in the late eighteenth century. The principles of Jeffersonian democracy (1790s–1820s) in America emphasized the liberty of the people. Thomas Jefferson stated that states were created to keep people happy. Any regime that could not keep the citizens happy must fall.[29] Jefferson believed that a sick political system gave birth to a sick population. According to him, despotism yields malady, whereas democracy generates good health.[30] "French revolutionaries added health to the rights of man and asserted that health citizenship should be a characteristic of the modern democratic state."[31]

In France, the *National Assembly* came to power in July 1789. The Assembly appointed a "Committee on Mendicity," chaired by François Alexandre Frédéric, duc de la Rochefoucauld-Liancourt for dealing with the problem of 'beggary.'[32] The committee realized that charity would not be an appropriate step for removing poverty from the country because such poverty was the very consequence of the economic system in place. Accordingly, assistance ought to be provided as a 'right' of the people. Leancourt argued that every human being had an important socio-economic right, "le droit à la subsistence," (or "the right to subsistence,") which he called for including in the Declaration of Human Rights.[33] In the case of health care, "the Committee seems to have been influenced by the ideas of pre-revolutionary thinkers like Tenon."[34]

George Rosen wrote "Liancourt recognized fully well the important role of sickness as a cause of indigency, and the first section of the plan deals with assistance to the sick poor in the country and city."[35] The committee proposed that medical care should be given free of cost to the sick poor. Government-paid physicians or surgeons would have delivered medical services to every rural district (canton) and town, and free hospital services would have been provided to all people in France.[36] Another *Health Committee* was also appointed by the *French National Assembly*. In its *Draft Legislation*, this committee noted that: "each canton shall provide for a physician who shall care for poor patients in their homes free of charge…The physicians shall visit the ill in their residencies as soon as informed and treat their infirmities, illnesses."[37]

Although Enlightenment thinkers and revolutionaries in France developed powerful ideas about health being a right of citizens and a duty of the state, these ideals were not put into practice in any real or effective way during this period. Even though Enlightenment-era states failed to act, the hope for health as a citizen's right did not disappear. Real reforms came later, driven not by ideals but by economic necessity in the age of industrialization—when public health became a means of protecting productivity and profit. The idea of health as a right of democratic citizenship—first declared by the French revolutionaries in the 1790s—was gradually realized over time. This transformation was not automatic, but was pushed forward by the harsh consequences of industrialization and urbanization, which exposed the social costs of poor health conditions.[38]

The Sanitary Movement in Europe

The industrial revolution had a bad effect on public health. Post-industrial revolution England witnessed a social change that resulted in overcrowding in slums and increase of death rates, especially among women and children, which indicates a deterioration of public health. A new disease, cholera, spread in industrial cities.[39] In this situation, Edwin Chadwick (1800–1890) had emphasized the importance of sanitary movement. Chadwick's public health movement can be understood from a reading of two excellent monographs written by R. A. Lewis[40] and S. E. Finer,[41] both published in 1952. Chadwick was a lawyer and journalist who became private secretary to the philosopher Jeremy Bentham (1748–1832) for a short time. He was also appointed as the secretary of the new Poor Law Commission. The government had given him the responsibility to investigate sanitary conditions in England. After conducting the survey, he published his 'Report on the Sanitary Conditions of the Labouring Population of Great Britain' in 1842, in which he demonstrated that heaps of garbage, atmospheric impurities, and poor sanitation and drainage systems were the main causes of diseases or ill-health. Therefore, Chadwick proposed for the improvement of the sewage system, water supply, and street cleanness. As a result, in 1848, a public health act was passed. Local boards were formed to deal with the issue of public health in the cities. Before 1848, there had been no public health regulation and no health worker was appointed in England. After the 1848 Act, 11 more regulations were enforced until the 1870s.[42] In 1844, the *Health of Towns Association* was established as a pressure group, with the aim of putting pressure on the government to improve the condition of public health in the towns and cities of England. The Association functioned for only a brief period, i.e., from 1844 to 1849. In order to spread awareness among professional groups and to influence the opinion of leaders, it arranged lectures and published the *Journal of Public Health.* It also helped Chadwick to bring about the *Public Health Act of 1848.*[43]

But there was a counterpoint to Chadwick's arguments at that time by Karl Marx and Frederick Engels. They published *The Condition of the Working Class in England*[44] and the *Communist Manifesto*[45] in 1844 and 1848, respectively. Engels's class study showed that factory workers' poor living and working conditions were related to a number of health problems. In his book, he discussed different issues related to health such as poor diet, alcohol consumption, venereal disease, and chronic physical and mental exhaustion. He also provided evidence of the direct link between chronic lung diseases like tuberculosis and factors such as crowding, inadequate ventilation, and open fires. He wrote:

> In many rooms of the cotton and flax spinning mills, the air is filled with fibrous dust, which produces chest affections, especially among workers in the carding and combing rooms. Some constitutions can bear it, some cannot;...The most common effects of this breathing of dust are blood-spitting, hard, noisy breathing, pains in the chest, coughs, sleeplessness, in short all the symptoms of asthma ending in the worst cases in consumption...Another effect of flax spinning is a peculiar deformity of the shoulder, especially a projection of the right shoulder blade, consequent upon the nature of the work. This sort of spinning and the throttle-spinning of cotton frequently produce diseases of the knee-pan which is used to check the spindle during the joining of broken threads.[46]

Engels expressed the opinion that the capitalist economic system and the exploitation of the working class were the primary causes of 'social inequalities in health.' He held that in order to improve the condition of working men or address poverty and its health effects, political action was necessary.[47] Chadwick placed a greater emphasis on public sanitation, a pure water supply and drainage system than food, work, and wages as a solution for pauperism in general. Chadwick did not believe that poverty itself was one of the causes of illness. "He resented the inclusion by William Farr of the category 'starvation' in the bills of mortality, arguing that it was impossible for a person to starve to death in London."[48]

The medical historian Roy Porter remarked that, "as the salaried secretary of Poor Law Commission, Chadwick became the most hated man in England, detested alike by the poor, by vestrymen, and by local boards of guardians for his 'Prussian' style of operation."[49] In addition, Chadwick did not depart from 'miasma theory.' An English epidemiologist, John Snow, later tried to find an individual cause for the disease. He studied the epidemiology of cholera in London and showed that polluted drinking water was the main cause. In this way 'germ theory' first emerged. John Snow has been called the 'father of public health'.[50]

The concept of public health became clearer in the nineteenth century. Governments of European countries focused on the issue. The sanitary movement gradually spread from England to other countries, such as America, France, Spain, Australia, Germany, Italy etc.[51] As a result, there was a reduction in the mortality rate in Europe. In the early nineteenth century, the French public health movement was an indigenous and urban one, organized by a group of physicians, pharmacists-chemists, engineers, veterinarians and administrators to improve public hygiene and reduce the mortality and morbidity rates. French hygienists convened the government to develop sewerage systems and water supplies and to reform regulations related to housing and factories.[52]

Rights to Health: A Journey Toward 'Health for All'

As we have seen, in the eighteenth-century Enlightenment era, the American Revolution and the French Revolution considered health to be both a social and a political right. As a result of socio-economic inequality, however, the concept of universal health rights had not developed. The people were naturally deprived of their right to food, clothing, shelter, education, and health. Karl Marx then advanced a theory for the liberation of the people from that condition.[53] Marx and Engels referred to the relationship between poverty and disease as being a social phenomenon. According to them, the poor suffered more from diseases and illness than other groups. Therefore, Marxian analysis focused on equity and state intervention in health care.[54] In the German state of Prussia, the pathologist Rudolf Virchow (1821–1902) elaborated the theory of 'social medicine,' as it was analysed by Friedrich Engels (1820–1895).[55] Virchow is now regarded as the founder of social medicine. In Virchow's view, material deprivation caused the diseases in the individuals and transmission in the community. He narrated that malnutrition, inadequate housing, adverse climate, economic insecurity, and political disenfranchisement all contributed to the spread of illness. According to him, "economic stability and active political participation by the poor were necessary for good health."[56] Virchow also focused on the idea of right to health and health care, urging that all people have an equal right to enjoy a healthy life. He believed that the government is responsible for ensuring that right and that a government health service should be provided on the basis of people's needs: "hospital admission must therefore be open to every patient that needs it, irrespective of whether he has money or not, whether he be Jew or heathen."[57] Following the Berlin Revolution of 1848, Virchow joined the Prussian "medical reform" movement and started to publish a journal with the same name. In this he wrote that "Medical organization is to be reformed not so much for the benefit of physicians as for that of the patients...physicians surely are the natural advocates of the poor and the social problem largely falls within their scope."[58] The Marxian theory was first successfully applied by the Union of Soviet Socialist Republics (USSR), which was formed after the Russian Revolution (1917). In 1937, it became the first country to adopt the standard of universal distribution and equity in the field of health[59]

Before the Russian Revolution, however, the German government had been forced to consider the issue of workers' health. The development of capitalism increased insecurity in the life of the working class. Inequality became increasingly acute after the spreading of the industrial revolution in the nineteenth century. Millions of people depended on the labor market for their livelihood. Yet the standard of living of the workers was very low. They had to work long hours for too low wages. They worked at the risk of their lives. Moreover, they were thrown out of work due to disease, accidents, old-age, and periodic economic crises, which were inherent in the capitalist system of production.[60]

In the nineteenth century, the trade union movement was started up in Germany to address the problems caused by inequality, including health. In that situation, then German Chancellor Bismarck (1871–1890) introduced health insurance, which later took the form of Universal Health Care, to alleviate workers' dissatisfaction. Bismarck launched Universal

Health Care primarily in the wake of social unrest. But he also had other considerations: first, he wanted to make sure that trade unions would not become more proactive; secondly, he felt that, in the early stages of the industrial revolution, Germany needed the supply of healthy young people; thirdly, he understood that for expanding the empire, it was necessary to ensure the supply of healthy young people in the army.[61] In 1871, Bismarck wrote a letter to Count Itzenplitz, minister of Commerce, in which he pointed out that the only way to stop the socialist movement was to fulfil the socialist demands as much as possible.[62] As a result, a Health Insurance Law, establishing the world's first social health insurance system, was enacted in Germany on June 15, 1883. Basically, the social policy of Bismarck was a trick to shape society through politics.[63]

Following Germany, a number of other European countries, such as Sweden (1891), Denmark (1892), France (1910), and Switzerland (1912), all started some kind of health insurance programs. However, those programs were not intended to be universal at first and were basically designed to keep workers' earnings stable and buy their political allegiance.[64]

The Tsarist regime in Russia ended in 1917with the Bolshevik Revolution and the establishment of a socialist republican government. Five years later, 16 republics came together to form the USSR, which was a source of renewed hope to the common people.[65] Thereafter, all lands, mineral resources, forests, and reservoirs were recognized as being 'the people's property.' The socialist government led by Vladimir Lenin (1917–1924) had issued various decrees to protect the fundamental rights of the people.[66] The government paid equal attention to both the health of the people and the socio-economic condition of the country. As a result of detailed planning, the USSR witnessed a radical change in a very short period. Rabindranath commented: "Finally, I have come to Russia. What I see is surprising. It is not like any other country. All things are different here. They have awakened all human beings equally…A few years ago, the condition of public health in Russia was very similar to that of India. The situation in Russia has changed rapidly in such a short period. But India has not witnessed any change."[67]

During this period Sir Arthur Newsholme from the United Kingdom and John Adams Kingsbury from the United States also visited the USSR to see the Soviet health system in practice. They wrote of their experiences in a book titled *Red Medicine: Socialized Health in Soviet Russia*.[68] In 1933, in the preface to their book, they wrote that when a Russian got ill the government would take action to help them. Soviet Russia had thus made the decision that the health of the individual was the responsibility of society as a whole. In fact, at this time the Soviet Union was the only country in the world to have designed a comprehensive health system for the prevention and treatment of diseases of every man, woman, and child living within its borders.[69]

Dr. Jnanabrata Sil, who was attached to West Bengal Medical Education Service, visited Russia in 1974. The oral testimony he gave matches the experiences of both Newsholme and Kingsbury. He said that Soviet Russia was like a paradise on earth, with the state overseeing the health of every citizen from birth to death. Food was cheap and the cost of living was very low. If someone had an accident on the street, they received prompt treatment. The ambulance service was also very advanced.[70]

Before the revolution, the state of health care in Russia had been very bad. Hospitals, sanatoria, and asylums were established in many cities, but that was not sufficient. Moreover, it was not possible for ordinary people to spend money on treatment. In Soviet Russia, by contrast, sometimes even unskilled men provided health care. Even ordinary people often had to rely on village priests to cure diseases.[71] Following the revolution, the state acknowledged the people's right to health. An emphasis was placed on preventive medicine. Vaccination against smallpox was introduced in Ukraine in 1920. In 1930, vaccination against diphtheria was made compulsory: There was a rule that no child could enter school without being vaccinated. As a result, infant mortality rates began to decline.[72]

Health education was also provided to raise public awareness about disease prevention. Initiatives were taken to make the citizens aware of the importance of cleanliness in the home and workplace through lectures, exhibits, demonstrations, and discussion groups. People were also made aware of the significance of personal hygiene, women's hygiene, and children's hygiene to prevent infectious diseases and avoid accidents.[73] In the USSR, the whole of the health system was centrally controlled, and there was no longer any recourse to direct financial transactions in the field of medical services.[74] This meant that health expenditure was borne by the state; as afar as the people were concerned, it was completely free of cost. Doctors used to regard their patients as fellows members of society.[75]

After World War I, the spread of communism became a headache for capitalist states like England. In this context, massive public support was needed to deal with the communist forces. At the same time, the Great

Depression of 1929 in the USA led to the spread of extreme unemployment, declining productivity, and social and political turmoil in the whole world. However, Russia was not affected by the Great Depression, leading to an increase in the popularity of socialist ideology. On the other hand, capitalist states were also looking for a way out of the recession. To overcome the ill-effects of the Great Depression, the then US president Franklin Roosevelt (1933–1945) launched the New Deal, a welfare program that expanded spending on social services like health from 1933 onward.[76]

At that time, British economist John Maynard Keynes's theory of welfare also became very relevant. Economic principles based on Keynes's work indicated a more influential role for the state in economic development.[77] Keynesian economics lay at the heart of New Deal policies in the United States.[78] According to this theory, increasing government spending on social services, such as communications, power projects, employment, housing, schools, hospitals, etc., would increase demand for the products in the market. As a result, the recession would subside and the financial situation would improve. Keynesian economic theory also facilitated the post-World War II growth of the welfare state.[79] This was intended to provide welfare for the poor. It emphasized social services, social insurance, and social rights.[80] The institutions of the welfare state protected people against the vagaries of the market economy: inability to earn due to unemployment, ill-health, old age, disability, and other detrimental life events.[81] Following Keynesian economic theory, the capitalist states improved their economic conditions in the post-World War II period. According to the ideals of the welfare state, they look after food, clothing, and shelter as well as the health of the people. For instance, in the UK, the National Health Service (NHS) was introduced. But Keynes's theory was never a leftist model. In fact, it was deployed by the United Kingdom in an effort to placate the pressures from below, which were demanding food, clothing, shelter, and health.[82]

In the UK, the movement demanding health services to the people at the government's expense had begun many decades earlier. Prior to the formation of the NHS, there had been a mixed economy of health care that combined private, public, and voluntary provision. Through the Poor Law, the local state offered institutional care, most often of a basic quality. The growth of the labor movement took shape in the second half of the nineteenth century, and was focused on the issues of the long hours of work, extreme poverty, malnutrition, poor workplace conditions and disease with very little treatment. Robert Owen, Keir Hardie, and many others proposed improvements of the living conditions for the working classes. (Two works of fiction published around this time, *Erewhon* (1872) by Samuel Butler and *Looking Backward* (1888) by Edward Bellamy, also dealt with the politics of health.) However, it was the Fabian socialists who first made health a political issue. The need for a 'State Medical Service' providing early diagnosis and treatment, enforcing a healthy environment and personal hygiene, and preventing the recurrence or spread of disease was first outlined in a so-called 'minority report' on the Poor Law published by Beatrice Webb and George Lansbury in 1909. The political labor movement and the growing influence of trade unions at the beginning of the twentieth century compelled Lloyd George to enact the *National Health Insurance Act* of 1911.[83] The Liberal government passed the act, following German Chancellor Otto von Bismarck's reforms of the 1880s. But there were many limitations in the legislation: it only applied to workers, it instituted insufficient sick pay, and it was financially tied to the workplace. Additionally, it required mandatory contributions for insurance that were too expensive for apprentices and low-wage workers. Some even went on strike in opposition to its passage. The scheme was criticized as being a "porous plaster to cover the disease that poverty causes" by Keir Hardie, the leader of the UK Labour Party at the time. Treatment costs were imposed on patients in hospitals where insurance was not accepted. "Payment often had an impact on treatment, with facilities segregated to privilege those who could contribute most."[84] Fighting for greater access to health care became a top priority for the expanding working-class movement. The *Labour Party* (1900) and the *Trades Union Congress* (TUC) (1868) both adopted policies calling for a national health service as a result, and this argument took on national dimensions. By far the most significant intervention, however, came with the creation of *Friendly Societies*, enormous mutual funds set up in working-class neighborhoods to offer health insurance. One of the most effective of these schemes was located in the Welsh mining community of Tredegar. The *Tredegar Medical Aid Society* was founded in 1890 by the miners and ironworkers, and expanded to become one of the first examples of comprehensive health care provision available in working-class Britain.[85]

Early socialist analysis tended to view the abolition of capitalism as the remedy to all problems, including those pertaining to health. This attitude continued into the twentieth century. By the turn of the this century, it was widely acknowledged that reformation of the existing medical system was of the utmost importance and that "such reconstruction could in itself contribute to the transition to a socialist society." A number of left-wing medical pressure groups were also established in the early 1900s. In 1911 Benjamin Moore, a physician based in Liverpool, published his proposals for medical reform. He was instrumental in founding the *State Medical Service Association* (SMSA), which held its inaugural meeting in July 1912. Demanding universal health care, the British Labour Party called a nation-wide strike in 1912. This pressure spurred efforts at social reform, with health care provision prominent on the agenda. In 1930 Left-leaning doctors of the UK formed an organization named the *Socialist Medical Association* (SMA), which demanded that health care services should be provided in a socialist manner. Many decades later, the Labour Party came to power in 1945. The NHS was launched on July 5, 1948, at the initiative of Aneurin Bevan, minister of Health in the cabinet of Prime Minister Clement Attlee.[86] In terms of medical systems, the policy of equitable distribution was adopted. The benefits of establishing social justice had been found very quickly. The life expectancy of new-borns increased in England and Wales in the 1940s. But sadly, the famine of 1943 occurred in Bengal, part of the British Empire, when England succeeded in solving its public health problems.[87] However, before the NHS was introduced, people in Britain had to spend money on getting medical care. The situation changed dramatically after the NHS had been launched.[88]

We have discussed the evolution of public health in the West, with a particular focus on state intervention in health care and the recognition of health as a fundamental right. The health system in Britain, in particular, has come under critical scrutiny in this context. Given that India remained a British colony for nearly two centuries (1757–1947), it is essential to extend our analysis to the health conditions in colonial India. Following the Battle of Plassey in 1757, India came under the control of the English East India Company, and, after the Revolt of 1857, governance passed directly to the British Crown. Therefore, alongside our discussion of the British health system, special attention must be given to the public health policies and conditions prevailed in colonial India. This is especially important since our primary focus in the rest of the book is on India—and Bengal in particular. With this in mind, we now turn our attention to the Indian context.

Public Health in Colonial India

Before moving on to the colonial context, it can be said at the very outset that in pre-colonial India the concept of public health did exist, albeit in a very rudimentary form. A kind of philanthropic health care model was already present in ancient or medieval India. The second rock edict of the Mauryan emperor Asoka (c. 268 to 232 BCE) referred to the fact that he arranged medical care for human beings and cattle. He built hospitals for the treatment of human beings.[89] In medieval India, charitable hospitals, which were known as *darush-shifa* or *shifakhanas*, were built to treat the poor. Apart from the capital, there were hospitals in other parts of the state. In this regard, the role played by Feroze Shah Tughlaq (1351–1388 AD) was significant in the Sultanate era. During the Mughal period, the construction of a charitable hospital was started on a government initiative during the time of Jahangir (1605–1627 AD).[90]

Western medicine came to India with the arrival of the Europeans, especially through the English East India Company. In 1764, the Company set up the Indian Medical Service (IMS) for the Europeans living in the country. Though it played a key role in shaping health services, the IMS also reflected colonial hierarchies. Indian doctors in the IMS were often expected to adopt British values, leading to criticism. In 1929, Bidhan Chandra Roy, an Indian nationalist politician and a doctor by profession, expressed frustration over the exclusion of highly qualified Indian physicians from top positions simply because they were not part of the IMS. Despite these issues, there were some positive developments most notably the establishment of medical colleges in Calcutta, Bombay, and Madras in 1835, a milestone in India's medical education history.[91] However, in the first half of the nineteenth century, the colonial government in India emphasized the needs of the British military and the white civilian population. While Britain supported sanitation, nutrition, and welfare reforms at home, in India public health efforts were largely limited to military barracks and did not extend to the general population.[92]

After the revolt of 1857, the administrative power of India was shifted from the Company raj to the British Crown. During the mutiny, the main problem of the British troops was epidemic disease, particularly cholera. Therefore, in 1859, a Royal Commission was set up by the new government to inquire into the health of the army in India. The commission's report, which was probably the first document of 'public health policy' in British India, was published in 1863. The commission recommended to improve the health of the British army both sanitation and the prevention of epidemics in distinct areas of European habitation (military cantonment and civil line) needed to be improved.[93] The commission clearly stated that the decrease of the death rate in the corps and the development of its environmental sanitary status would be impossible unless measures were taken for the development of public health in general, and for the prevention of the more clear causes of maladies amongst the community in particular.[94]

The report of the Royal Commission had an immediate effect.[95] In 1864, sanitary boards were formed in each province to enhance civil sanitary conditions, and a public health commissioner was appointed in 1869. But the colonial government was primarily concerned with the health of its own army and civilian personnel, neglecting the health of the indigenous people. The curative health services, which were provided by the IMS, were urban-centric. Indeed, the IMS was a wing of the British Indian Army. Health services and facilities were intended for the ruling class and elites. "A few metropolitan hospitals in the district headquarters were meant for the urban elites and there too, the white ruling class was privileged."[96]

By the mid-nineteenth century, British India's hospital system had developed into a structured network classified into four main types. The foremost were military hospitals, divided into temporary camp hospitals near battlefields and permanent establishments within cantonments, serving the Company's soldiers and sailors. The second category included hospitals dedicated exclusively to European civilians, primarily located in metropolitan centers and district headquarters. The third comprised general hospitals accessible to all, including 'native' Indians, while the fourth category consisted of charitable hospitals and dispensaries for 'natives,' mostly founded and maintained through 'native' initiatives and public subscriptions, with some in receipt of government aid. In addition to these general and military hospitals, the British colonial medical policy established specialized institutions such as lunatic asylums for Europeans, leprosy asylums, tuberculosis sanatoriums, and fever hospitals to address chronic and contagious diseases. Temporary hospitals were also created during epidemics like smallpox, cholera, and plague, with their duration depending on the endemic status of diseases. One particularly exploitative institution was the 'lock hospital' system within European regiments, designed to control venereal diseases by subjecting Indian women to compulsory medical examinations and treatment.[97]

The Dufferin Fund, officially known as the National Association for Supplying Female Medical Aid to the Women of India, was established in 1885 by Lady Dufferin, the wife of the then Viceroy of India. It represented one of the earliest formal efforts by the British colonial administration to improve medical care for Indian women, particularly through promoting the training and employment of female medical professionals. The Fund aimed to provide medical education for women—training female doctors, hospital assistants, nurses, and midwives—and to expand access to health care through the establishment of dispensaries, women's hospitals, female wards, and the deployment of female doctors. It also emphasized the importance of training nurses and midwives to serve the needs of Indian women more effectively.[98] However, such efforts were often limited in scope, fragmented, and insufficient to meet the broader health needs of the population, particularly in rural areas. Moreover, racial discrimination was a pervasive feature of colonial hospitals, evident in the segregation of wards into 'European' and 'Native,' differentiated dietary regimens, and unequal access to medical treatments.[99]

The British health services were essentially based on curative measures; preventive and sanitary measures were not properly addressed. The imperial government largely neglected public health before 1919. The Government of India Act, 1919, commonly known as the *Montagu-Chelmsford Reform Act*, emphasized the necessity for a proper water supply, sanitation, and a public health infrastructure. The public health sphere of government passed into the hands of provincial ministers. In spite of great hope and expectation, however, that act could not bring any key change in government health policy. Therefore, the mortality rate of people in British India was very high.[100] But the mortality rate in the army reduced dramatically due to development of a health system targeted at this group.[101]

The Indian subcontinent was imagined by the Europeans to be a quagmire of lethal epidemics and decimating diseases.[102] There was racial discrimination in colonial India; Europeans feared indigenous people as carriers of all kinds of infectious diseases. White towns were separated from black towns. In the case of sexual diseases, they blamed indigenous prostitutes and segregated them. Moreover, segregation was the watchword of imperial medicine.[103]

India was considered to be the source of cholera which had spread across Europe since 1830. Quarantine was imposed in India for the interest of colonial power after the Sanitary Conference in Constantinople in

1866. This had a considerable impact on Haj pilgrims. As a community, Muslims were blamed for the spread of the epidemic. Despite the advent of germ theory in the late nineteenth century, a quarantine policy was imposed.[104] The colonial government tried to bind the bodies of the people through public health-centric "laws, proclamations, decrees and legislations." That policy might be branded as either 'biological imperialism' or 'Ecological Imperialism.'[105] Alfred W. Crosby coined the latter term, 'Ecological Imperialism,' while discussing the success of European imperialists in founding settler societies in different regions across the globe. Arabinda Samanta then contextualized it in the light of the Bombay plague in 1896.[106] To curb the outbreak of the deadly bubonic plague, the Epidemics Disease Act of 1897 was enacted. This act empowered sanitary officials to enter houses, detain, segregate, and quarantine those who were suspected of having the disease. Villages were burnt down and over 100,000 people were left homeless. As a result, discontent was generated among the local population.[107] David Arnold expressed that "the colonial government and colonial medicine attempted such forceful and far-reaching controls those were indicative of the interventionist ambitions and capacity of India's mature colonial state."[108] Under colonial rule, if anyone was suspected to be suffering from a disease in this country, he was forcibly taken to a hospital and kept in hospital to separate him from the society.[109]

It was alleged that the imposition of quarantine would deny the philosophy of the American Revolution and the French Revolution, which upheld the ideal of the liberty of individuals. Mark Harrison wrote "Quarantine had always had its critics. Quarantine seemed like a vestige of a less enlightened era: it encouraged corruption, despotism and economic stagnation at a time when the wealth of nations depended on liberty and free trade."[110] Post-modernists also criticized the quarantine and isolation system.[111] They said that through this system individuals' bodies had been brought under the surveillance of the state.

The noted Bengali novelist Sarat Chandra Chattopadhyay (1876–1938) wrote about the torment of quarantined life. He remarked that the pain of quarantine was mainly experienced by lower-class people.[112] Quarantine is still harmful to the poor. The mass quarantine system daily wage earners from earning a living. They cannot afford nutritious food. As a result, they become weak, and are more susceptible to attacks from germs. In the absence of an adequate government health system, people have to suffer more.[113]

However, government policy was not monolithic. Historians suggest that colonial government vigilance primarily peaked during specific crises—such as the plague years—while broader public health measures were often neglected both before and after these periods. Arabinda Samanta offers a striking comparison between the government's vigorous response to the bubonic plague and its relatively passive approach to outbreaks of malarial fever in Bengal. When plague broke out in Bombay in September 1896, 'contagion-ism' had become the dominant medical theory and was firmly guiding colonial health policy. The plague, believed to have been imported from Hong Kong, was viewed as an invasive disease threatening the commercial viability of India's second-largest port and manufacturing hub. As Samanta notes, this triggered an urgent official reaction. Mass inoculation also became central to the anti-plague campaign. By contrast, the government's approach to malaria in Bengal was marked by inertia. Although malaria was a major killer, its effects were less immediate and visually dramatic than those of either plague or cholera. Crucially, it was not contagious—a fact conclusively established in the 1890s—, making it less alarming within the colonial medical framework. According to Samanta, this lack of urgency explains why the anti-malaria programme in Bengal remained limited and half-hearted, highlighting how colonial medical intervention was often shaped by economic, political, and perceptual factors rather than by the severity of disease alone.[114]

The colonial state's neglect of sustained public health intervention is further evident in its handling of *kala-azar* in Bengal. As Achintya Kumar Dutta notes, the overall medical response was grossly inadequate. After 1920, responsibility was largely devolved to local bodies like District Boards, which struggled with insufficient funding and lacked the capacity to manage the crisis. Kala-azar centres were too few, poorly equipped, and often staffed by unqualified personnel. Even senior officials such as Sir Arthur Dash acknowledged the dire state of these facilities. As a result, many patients had to travel to Calcutta for treatment, but hospitals were overcrowded and could not admit everyone. Overwhelmed by patient inflows, institutions such as the School of Tropical Medicine in Calcutta turned many sufferers away. In rural areas, inadequate diagnostic facilities meant kala-azar was frequently misidentified as malaria, leading to mistreatment and preventable deaths.[115]

Poonam Bala has asserted that Western medicine was introduced in India as part of the bureaucratic machinery, whereas in Britain it was part of a broader social and economic movement.[116] The colonial state gave little importance to preventive and social medicine. That is why colonial India witnessed the regular outbreak of epidemics like malaria, cholera, and so on. But the role of the colonial government to combat epidemic diseases was not commendable. Due to inadequate and unsatisfactory anti-malarial measures, 100 million people suffered from this disease, with 20 million dying every year even in the 1930s. C.A. Bentley observed that only a very small proportion of the malaria-affected people of Bengal received adequate medical care.[117] Roger Jeffery wrote that "public health in India thus has to be seen as a qualified failure. Even in the towns most directly amenable to British influence and action the conditions of life of most inhabitants remained appalling, with very high mortality and morbidity rates in the worst areas. Only European areas enjoyed the benefits of civic concern."[118] In India, the imperial government was willing to develop a public health and medical system for people to a limited extent. Indeed, in British public health policy, 'native' people could not get proper health facilities. The ruler had no concern for the health and suffering of the indigenous population. Though hospital and dispensary networks were established, these were not for the masses. At the end of the period of British rule, only the ruling and the elite classes could access proper medical services. At this time the common people accounted for more than 90 per cent of the population and only a few of them were able to receive small amounts of medical care from hospitals and dispensaries run by government agencies, missionaries, philanthropic institutions, and private practitioners. Medical colleges were established by British rulers to train Indians (the first medical college in India was established in Calcutta in 1835). But only elites or the privileged section of the society had the opportunities to study in these institutions.[119]

The Public Health Movement in Bengal: The Formative Years

We have seen from the above analysis that the colonial government had hardly paid any attention to the poor condition of public health in this country. The indigenous people were also severely unaware of public hygiene. Thus, suffering from diseases was a common matter. British health officers stated that 'ignorant Indians' lacked sanitary awareness. A portrait of filth, clogged drains, refuse-filled courtyards, and excreta left unattended in Indian neighborhoods was depicted in health reports.

Health officers persistently described that the unhealthy habits of Indians and uncleanliness of their houses caused disease.[120] In 1888, while speaking at a dinner hosted by the Scottish residents of Calcutta in celebration of St. Andrews Day, Lord Dufferin, the then Viceroy of India, stated:

> Where is there a more crying need for sanitary reform than among those who take bathing in the same pond from which they get their drinking water, and where millions of men, women, and children die yearly, or what is even worse become the victims of chronic debility, disease, and racial deterioration, from the preventable cause? (Lord Dufferin's speech, November 30, 1888)[121]

But it is found that before the sanitary reformation in nineteenth-century Europe, there was no proper concept of public health. Sanitary conditions in England had improved only after the emergence of the sanitary movement launched by Chadwick. Yet no figure of the stature of either Chadwick (1800–1890) or John Snow (1813–1858) was born in India. Dhrub Kumar Singh wrote: "In contrast to the absence of any sanitary movement in India England saw a full-fledged movement led by Chadwick, Snow and John Simon…In India the 'dynamism' of the colonial government did not produce any Chadwicks and Simons."[122] The colonial government's reluctance to invest in public health created a vacuum that was increasingly filled by voluntary and civil society initiatives. Initially, Christian missionaries played a leading role in promoting health services; over time, however, Indian middle-class reformers emerged as prominent actors in advancing new ideas about health, hygiene, and social reform. New norms of healthy behavior circulated widely through the growing print culture—especially journals and periodicals—within the limited but significant public sphere that developed across India in the late nineteenth century.[123] Although the British colonial state remained largely indifferent, Indian thinkers and reformers did not remain passive. They took independent initiatives to raise health awareness among the population. As a result, a public health movement began to gain momentum in Bengal during the last decade of the nineteenth century and into the early twentieth. According to Kabita Ray, voluntary associations worked better than the colonial government in solving the problems of public health in the twentieth century.[124]

One of the most striking examples of early voluntary initiatives in colonial Bengal was the formation of the *Bharat-Samskar Sabha* in 1870 by the influential Brahmo reformer Keshabchandra Sen. The *Sabha* had five aims, one of which was to improve public health. To fulfill this aim, it designated Bijoykrishna Goswami, a high-caste Brahmin and graduate of Calcutta Medical College, to serve in the malarial suburb of Behala. Despite his elite background, Goswami chose to work among low-caste, poor communities suffering from malaria. He would rise very early each morning and, after washing and meditating, he would set out for his samskar work, carrying a bag filled with essential medicines and dietary supplements. Until 11 a.m., he worked among the sick in the malarial suburb of Behala. Returning by noon, he would take a quick lunch before hurrying off to teach at an adult education center—also established under the guidance of Keshabchandra Sen.[125]

The Ramakrishna Mission (established in 1897) played a major role in battling against the plague which hit in Calcutta in 1898–1899. During that epidemic, Swami Vivekananda made an appeal on behalf of Ramakrishna Mission for public awareness in Bengali and Hindi, which was widely circulated in Calcutta.[126] Swamiji said, "If we have to sell the land of our new monastery to serve the people, to give medicine, to treat them, we will do it."[127] Vivekananda also emphasized the need for cleanliness. He wrote, "Unclean water and unclean food are the cause of maladies."[128] Another medical pioneer, Sister Nivedita (1867–1911), a disciple of Swami Vivekananda, played the leading role in the anti-plague activities organized by the *Ramakrishna Mission* (RKM). In order to organize relief work, a committee was set up under the auspices of RKM in 1899, with Nivedita as the secretary. Without considering the risk to her own health, she actively participated in the anti-plague activities. Nivedita appealed for funds through newspapers. She also gave lectures on 'Plague and the Duty of Students' at the Classic Lecture Auditorium in an effort to encourage the students to participate in the anti-plague operations. Immediately, 15 students stepped forward and signed up to be volunteers. As part of the measures, she cleaned up the waste in Baghbazar with a broomstick and a basket. She also distributed leaflets containing instructions and safety measures on the plague.[129] In 1901, the disease reappeared in Calcutta, causing people to flee the city in fear. Rabindranath was in Shilaidaha (an area of present-day Bangladesh) at that time. Despite his sickness, he returned to Calcutta after hearing the news of the outbreak of plague there, intending to stand with the people.[130] In his book titled *Jorasankor Dhare*, Abanindranath Tagore, a nephew of Rabindranath, wrote that "at that time plague broke out in Calcutta. Epidemics were going on all around;

people were dying from house to house. Rabikaka [Rabi Uncle] and all of us in this house collectively opened a plague hospital by collecting subscriptions, and we started distributing lime. Rabikaka and Sister Nivedita used to go from one neighbourhood to another for inspection. Nurses and doctors were all employed by us."[131] Rabindranath was well aware of the inadequacy of medical services in this country. There was a lack of sufficient doctors in the country. Moreover, there was a need to secure money to provide modern medicine that it was virtually impossible for the common people to acquire. The rural people used to go to the unqualified 'quack' practitioners to get treatment. Therefore, Rabindranath paid more attention to prevention of disease than to its cure.[132]

Aaj Mongalbar. Parar jungle saf karar din (Today is Tuesday. It is the day for cleaning the jungle of the neighborhood) he wrote in *Sahaj Path*[133] in order to develop the concept of rural reconstruction and co-operative disease prevention among the children. A team, named *Brati-Balak*, was also formed. Boys from the team used to go to the villages to try to improve the health and education system there. News of the boys' works, along with reports of various ailments in the villages, were published in a monthly mouthpiece, also called *Brati-Balak*, edited by Satish Chandra Roy and Dhirananda Roy from 1929.[134] Rabindranath wrote the regulations for the village society, which had a total of 15 objectives, most of which were health-related.[135] In 1933, a two-day fair was organized at Binuniya Health Center near Santiniketan. At the fair, in addition to other activities, initiatives were taken to create public awareness about health, with a model of the ideal maternity home being among the exhibits. Rebecca Timbers, the wife of Dr. Harry Timbers, and Sudhamay Mukherjee gave an explanation of the science of obstetrics to local girls. Public health-related educational films were also shown at night.[136] On the advice of Rabindranath, Dr. Pashupati Bhattacharya wrote a book titled *Bharatiya Byadhi Ebong Adhunik Chikitsa* (Indian Diseases and Modern Medicine) in order to acquaint poor people with the issue so that they could easily deal with the diseases.[137] In introducing the book Rabindranath wrote:

> I have been working in the village for some time; I have seen that the most serious problem is the lack of healing...Rural people of this country should have been taught in various ways how to prevent the disease. For this purpose, we should have a state health department. The responsibility of the mass healing campaign should have been placed on it. I have seen in Russia

> how extensively this type of work was being carried out throughout the country. Our country needs the same more than there. But there is no such arrangement in our country...This book written by Dr. Pashupati will be useful to them...If there are a few philanthropic educated people in the villages, they could serve people using this book.[138]

There were some similarities between Gandhi's and Rabindranath's philosophy with regard to sanitary reform; both of them placed an emphasis on the issue of rural reconstruction. The *Akhil Bharatiya Gramin Udyog Sangha* was formed for the purposes of rural reconstruction. According to Gandhi, it was the duty of the Sangha's workers to take measures to stop the spread of diseases in their areas. He stated that they would tell people about the causes of the diseases and advise the patients of the process necessary to prevent the diseases. As a result, people could gain knowledge regarding the prevention of disease by staying clean. His argument was that by following some simple general rules of hygiene, people could get rid of most diseases without giving any other effort or paying extra expense.[139] In relation to Gandhian philosophy, Debabar Banerji wrote that "During the freedom struggle, Mahatma Gandhi had (as had Mao Tse Tung during the Long March) acknowledged that the needy people of this country have very bounded access to health services. In his programme of 'constructive work', Gandhi had comprised simple but effective methods of rural sanitation and the use of naturopathy to protect and promote the rural people's health."[140]

During the influenza epidemic of 1918–1919, members of the middle class also stepped forward to help the sick.[141] In the words of a report of the British Government in India: "Never before, perhaps, in the history of India, have the educated and more fortunately placed members of the community, come forward in such large numbers to help their poorer brethren in time of distress."[142]

The contribution of missionaries to public health movement in India should also be acknowledged. Dr. Ida Sophia Scudder (1870–1960), a third-generation American medical missionary in India, was one of the leading figures. She had been born in India but had moved to America as an eight-year-old child. Later, she returned to India. Seeing the poor health condition of women and the lack of female doctors in India she decided to become a medical practitioner. In 1900, she started a dispensary in Vellore (a city of Tamil Nadu) which later became a medical college named the *Christian Medical College* (CMC). She served Indian women and took initiatives to train them as compounders and nurses.[143] The efforts of the medical missionaries were observed not only in southern India, but also in Bengal. Partha Dutta observes that "the Christian medical mission was organized purely by strong belief in the sanctity of life and universal access to healthcare."[144] During the smallpox epidemic, missionaries visited and treated the people. Nuns gave medicine to the sick and also baptized several people. The Loreto nuns went around villages to teach men, women, and children about Christianity and to visit the sick.[145] Medical missionaries also made significant contributions to healthcare, particularly for women.[146]

In the second half of the nineteenth century, books on general hygiene in Bengali language were published on the initiative of indigenous intellectuals in Bengal. In 1851, Akshaykumar Dutta wrote *Bahya Bastur Sahit Manab Prakritir Sambandha Bichar*[147] (A Consideration of the Relationship between Human Nature and External Matter), which was published in two volumes. The general proposition of the first part of the book was that good health and living a life free of disease results from compliance with the natural laws of the universe and rules of health, whereas suffering results from transgression of those laws. It became one of Dutta's most-read books. In 1856, Akshaykumar published a book entitled *Dharmaneeti*[148] (Principles of Morals). In the seventh chapter of this volume, he discusses child health and the duties of parents toward their children. According to him, it is the primary responsibility of parents to ensure that their babies are born healthy and without deformities. They must also ensure that the rules of health are followed in rearing children from their infancy. In order to accomplish this, both parents must become educated and become familiar with these rules. However, "he stresses the role of society and specifically of the government in preventing child mortality and does not leave the question of children's health to their parents alone. This awareness of the larger socio-political perspective of the problem is unique for any writer in Bengal in the 19th century."[149] In 1885, another early contributor, Dharmadas Basu, had published *Swasthya Raksha O Sadharan Swasthya Tattwa* (Hygiene and Public Health, Vol. 1).[150] In that text, it was stated that by adopting general rules of hygiene, the same benefits could be achieved in India as in other countries.[151] In addition, a guide book on midwifery was written in the Bengali language: In 1867, Jadunath Mukhopadhyay authored *Dhatrishiksha Ebang Prasutishiksha*[152] (Guide to 'Native' Midwives and to Mothers) in two parts in order to teach 'practical midwifery' to illiterate midwives. In describing the background of writing this book, he states, "My first child died as a result of the ignorance and negligence of *dhai* (midwife). I made the decision to write this kind of book in the hope that no one from this nation would experience such unfortunate circumstances and suffer as a result of intolerable mental anguish."

Dr. Pashupati Bhattacharya then wrote another book in Bengali, *Ahar O Aharya* (Food and Diet).[153] The foreword to that book was again written by Rabindranath. In another contribution, Chunilal Basu wrote *Palli Swasthya* (Village Sanitation),[154] which was a compilation of two lectures on health given by Chunilal Bose at the Rammohun Library in 1917.[155] At the beginning of that book, the author said that "cholera, smallpox, etc. have emerged as epidemics that have caused many deaths. But these diseases are preventable. These diseases can be prevented by taking a little precaution and following certain rules of public hygiene."[156] A second book by Chunilal Basu was titled *Sharir Swasthya-bidhan* (*Personal Hygiene*).[157]

Besides publishing books, health periodicals also began to appear as in the late nineteenth and the early twentieth centuries. While elaborating on that endeavor we would have to mention *Swasthya Samachar*, which was published by Kartik Chandra Bose (1873–1955 AD). A doctor by profession, Bose's mother had died without treatment due to a lack of money. As a result, he decided to become a doctor and treat the poor. Until his death, he continued to serve the poor, charging low fees as a so-called 'Bazar Doctor.' He also built the first sanatorium for tuberculosis patients in Deoghar (a city in Jharkhand).[158] Simultaneously a doctor, researcher, pharmacist, and writer of different aspects on health, Bose also published the health magazine *Swasthya Samachar* in Bengali.[159] *Swasthya Samachar*[160] was first published in 1912, and its publication lasted until his death in 1955. His main purpose was to make people aware of preventive medicine. Following the same mission, *Swasthya* (*Health*),[161] a monthly health magazine, was published in 1329 BS (1922 AD) under the editorship of Dr. Brajendranath Ganguly. This journal was the mouthpiece of the *Anti-Malaria Society* for a considerable period In the second year, on the cover page of the magazine it was identified as the "organ of the Central Co-operative Anti-Malaria Society Ltd."[162] It should be mentioned here that from 1304 BS to 1308 BS (1897 AD–1901 AD), another monthly called *Swasthya*, this one edited by Durgadas Gupta, had been published from Madan Mitra Lane in Kolkata. That latter periodical campaigned against the weakness of the government health system.[163] In

1900, a long editorial in the journal explained that the government could not prevent the spread of plague, even if its intentions were good. As long as people remained unaware of the disease, the epidemic would continue. The article criticized the government for not providing basic information on important questions like: "What is plague? How can it be cured? What steps can people take to stay safe?" It stated that the available information was either too hard to access or that it had not been preserved. The editors recommended that the government should disseminate free pamphlets in order to educate the public. Since the government did not do this, the editors decided to take on the task themselves.[164] There were also a few other periodicals related to health in the nineteenth century. Of these, mention may be made of *Anubikshan* (*Microscope*)[165] (editor: Dr Harish Chandra Shanna), *Chikitsa Sammilani* (*Medical Collective*),[166] and *Chikitsak o Samalochak* (*Physician and Critique*)[167] (editor: Dr Satya Krishna Ray).

The establishment of the *Anti-Malaria Society* on the initiative of Dr. Gopal Chandra Chattopadhyay marked the first organized public health movement to be started in Bengal. On August 13, 1908, at a conference organized by the *Calcutta Medical Club*, Gopal Chandra presented a paper on 'The Preventable Diseases of Lower Bengal, Their Effect on the Population and Measures for Their Prevention.' He proposed the establishment of anti-malaria leagues in India like those found in Greece and Italy, stating that "Pamphlets written in vernacular should be widely distributed, conferences should be held to discuss anti-malaria measures and demonstrations with lantern slides on the life cycle of malaria parasite and mosquitoes should also be showed."[168] In response to Gopal Chandra's speech, Dr. Chunilal Basu said that the "Cooperation of the people is solicited as it is essentially needed for the successful application of preventive measures against any disease, but unless the people are sufficiently educated, they could hardly expect their help and support in works of sanitation."[169]

In 1914, a large number of people had died due to an outbreak of malaria at Panihati (an area of North 24 Parganas District, WB), Gopal Chandra's own village. He realized that it was impossible to get rid of the epidemic just by simply relying on the municipality. He held the view that public health would have improved if the villagers had only worked together to deal with the disease. In 1914, inspired by the ideals of Gopal Chandra, some young men from Panihati started a campaign to eradicate malaria. They explained to the villagers that malaria could be eradicated from the village if they worked together in a scientific way. In 1918, Gopal Chandra was able to convince the people through a lecture at Panihati School that malaria could be prevented. In an effort to organize concerted action, the Panihati Cooperative Anti-Malaria Society was established on March 24, 1918 with 27 members.[170]

The Society started its work on April 3, 1918. In 1919, Gopal Chandra organized a meeting at the Rammohan Library in Calcutta, at which the *Central Co-operative Anti-Malaria Society* was formed.[171] Many became interested in such associations. Under the supervision of the Central Society, several branch societies were formed in different villages of Bengal,[172] which led to the beginning of a massive public health movement. The news of the society's work was published in a periodical called *Sonar Bangla*, which also played an important role in making people aware of matters relating to health.[173] Rabindranath praised Gopal Chandra's work in his writings.[174] The Central Society functioned as an advisory body and assisted rural societies with financial help. Qualified medical practitioners and senior medical students, who not only treated the case of illness but also provided instructions about preventive methods to people, engaged themselves in the Society's work. In addition to malaria, the Society combated ***kala-azar*** (a kind of fever), cholera, and other preventable diseases. By publishing leaflets and monthly journals, and organizing magic-lantern lectures, the Central Society wanted to encourage people to form rural public health societies and to educate their members.[175]

Admiring the work of the *Anti-Malarial Co-operative Society*, Surendranath Banerjee, who was the then minister of Education and Health in the Government of Bengal, stated that "they [the Anti-Malarial Co-operative Societies] have provided a field of beneficent activity to our village population, which will not only improve their health, but strengthen their public spirit and stimulate their civic life."[176]

The *Bengal Health Association* and the *Central Co-operative Anti-Malaria Society* set up a number of kala-azar centers. For instance, the large kala-azar centre at Dogachia in 24-Parganas run by the *Bengal Health Association* provided relief to hundreds of sufferers. The volunteers of that center diagnosed patients by blood examination and Aldehyde test and offered free treatment. However, the government offered them very small grants as assistance. The *Bengal Health Association* and the *Central Co-operative Anti-Malaria Society* also played key roles in the anti-cholera campaign. They formed cholera brigades. The *Anti-Malaria Society* was successful in spreading awareness for the utility of deep tube wells as a safe and cost-effective source of providing clean drinking water for preventing cholera in rural Bengal. Additionally, thanks to the Society's efforts, anti-cholera preventive inoculation was first tried on a large scale in Swarupnagar (24-Parganas) in order to prevent the high incidence of cholera epidemics. That method of preventive inoculation against cholera was also popularized by the Society in the province. When cholera broke out in Birbhum in 1924 due to a severe lack of drinking water, the leader of the *Bengal Health Association*, A. C. Banerji, came up with a novel plan. He formed a *Kodali Brigade* composed of some students of Calcutta, who went to one of the worst cholera-affected areas in Birbhum. The Brigade was able to relieve the circumstance by digging up *katcha* wells in beds of dried-up tanks.[177]

In a similar development, an association named *Palli Mandali* inaugurated anti-malaria operations at Birnagar (Ula) in October 1923.[178] In 1925, Gurusaday Dutt founded the *Soroj Nalini Dutta Memorial Association* following the death of his wife Soroj Nalini Dutta; it was intended to promote the welfare of women through the formation of *Mahila Samitis* in rural and urban areas.[179] Under this association, in addition to their other work, *Mahila Samitis* launched campaigns to make village women familiar with the up-to-date ideas related to sanitation, hygiene, and public health.[180] The *Bengal Social Service League*, which was founded by Dr Dwijendranath Maitra in 1915, organized relief work at the time of floods, famines and epidemics.[181]

Tuberculosis (TB) was another disease to cause concern in colonial India.[182] In the early twentieth century, extensive initiatives had been taken in America and European countries to eradicate tuberculosis. Many state and local TB associations were formed in the USA in the period from 1900 to 1917.[183] The national anti-tuberculosis societies of those countries worked at a rapid pace; consequently, the death rate on account of tuberculosis was greatly reduced. The anti-TB movement in India started comparatively late, however. Furthermore, the Indian government was not concerned about this.[184] On June 15, 1929, the *Tuberculosis Association of Bengal* was set up by a group of Englishmen and women and Indians, comprised of doctors, social workers, and common people who sympathized with tuberculosis patients. They tried to help the needy people who were going to perish owing to lack of treatment and nourishment.[185]

The volunteer doctors of the Society provided free treatment to the people. Trained health inspectors from the Society made regular visits to the homes of the patients and offered them advice regarding the prevention of TB. The Society campaigned for the prevention of the disease among school children and the common people in various ways. The number of beds in tuberculosis hospitals in India was very low, making it impossible to treat a huge number of patients. Therefore, patients who did not get the opportunity to be treated in the sanatorium were advised by the Society to stay at home and to follow the rules of the sanatorium.[186] In 1939, the *Tuberculosis Association of Bengal* was renamed as the *Bengal Tuberculosis Association* (BTA).[187] It offered various services seeking to control tuberculosis. The BTA waged a war against the disease through its Children's Chest Clinic, which started in 1961. This was the first of its kind, where children up to 14 years of age enjoyed free diagnostic and treatment facilities. BTA also undertook health education visits to educational institutions to inform pupils through the use of lectures and audio-visual methods. It launched its first TB seal Sale Campaign in 1950, and has been staging similar campaigns on since then. They proved an important means of raising funds and creating awareness. It also started a mass BCG campaign in 1949.[188]

One of the partners in the public health movement was the *People's Relief Committee* (*PRC*), which was established in 1943 under the initiative of various people's organizations. This organization had an inseparable relationship with the movement of *Bangiya Pradeshik Kisan Sabha* (1946). During the riots in Noakhali in 1946, the PRC took part in medical and other relief work with the *Kisan Sabha*.[189] It had associations with many doctors, including Dr. Bijay Basu, Dr. Bimal Bagchi, Dr. Amiya Banerjee, Dr. Anil Banerjee, and Dr. Samar Roy.[190] A hospital, called the Red Aid Cure Home, was built on Boubazar Street (now BB Ganguly Street) in Kolkata to treat sick members of the Communist Party. The PRC served not only party members, but also members of the general public.[191] During the famine of 1943, the members of the PRC stood by the people. At this time many people fell ill due to the lack of proper food, clothing, and shelter and also the lack of pure drinking water. The famine resulted in an epidemic, involving outbreaks of cholera, malaria, tuberculosis, pneumonia, and smallpox.[192] At this point, the *All Calcutta Teachers and Students United Relief Committee* was formed to fight against the epidemic, with Dr. Bidhanchandra Roy, the then Vice-Chancellor of Calcutta University, as the president. This body started to send medical squads to epidemic affected districts.[193] The book *Socialised Medicine in the Soviet Union*,[194] written by Dr. Henry E. Sigerist, first arrived in Kolkata at that time. It had a significant impact on the *People's Relief Committee.* The PRC tried to open medical camps akin to the field hospitals of the USSR to serve victims of flood and famine.[195] It also decided to form a medical board. On 26 February 1944, the *Bengal Medical Relief Coordination Committee* (BMRCC) was formed, including representatives of 18 relief organizations. Dr. Roy was also the president of that committee. In 1944, the committee sent 55 medical squads to different parts of Bengal and treated a total of 6 lakh people. Under the organizational umbrella of the BMRCC, other relief committees sent 150 medical teams to different regions and saved the lives of 19 lakh people. PRC had sent a demand letter to the then Governor-General Wavell to protect the people from epidemic.[196]

After India achieved independence in 1947, voluntary initiatives were decreased. Activists believed that the works which had been carried out by the voluntary organizations would now be done by an independent Indian government.[197] The medical institutions that were set up by the indigenous people during the freedom struggle were unable to survive. Kolkata-based institutions like Carmichael Medical College (which was renamed R. G. Kar Medical College and Hospital in 1948) and Jadavpur TB Hospital (1938) were taken over by the government. The Upendranath Mukherjee Hospital in Beliaghata was closed. But the government was unable to meet the needs of the people.[198] In this situation, the movement for *Students Health Home* (1951) began. The purpose of that movement was to make students aware of their own health matters. Initiatives were taken to build students' own institutions for the treatment of students on the same lines as had been established in Poland, Switzerland, and France. Dr. Arun Sen played a pivotal role in that movement.[199]

It is pertinent to note that this last movement, which has been elaborated here, may be marked as an awareness campaign and social service for public health. Some dedicated doctors provided free health care to people or facilities at low cost. Even though organizations like PRC focused on providing relief to people, there have been instances of raising political demands for health and also being part of a larger political movement. The consciousness of the political movement must have shaped the agenda of both the PRC and others.

Toward Alma-Ata

Through the establishment of the World Health Organization (WHO), the 'right to health' concept appeared on the international stage. After the end of World War II, initiatives were taken to establish peace in the world, and activities concerning health began at the international level. As a result, when diplomats assembled in San Francisco in 1945 to establish the United Nations, they also decided to form a global health organization. This is how, in 1948, the *World Health Organization* (WHO) was formed.[200] Before 1945, on the international stage, health was a "forgotten" matter. K. Evang noted, for example, that "Only at the last moment was world health brought in, producing the Health Section of the League of Nations, one of the forerunners of the present FAO, as well as of WHO."[201]

An international conference was organized in New York in 1946 at the initiative of the United Nations. On June 19, the first meeting of the *International Health Conference* was held at the Henry Hudson Hotel in New York City, chaired by Sir Ramaswamy Mudaliar (India), president of the *Economic and Social Council.* At the end of the conference, on 22 July, the WHO's constitution was drafted by a consensus of representatives from 61 countries around the world, and the first universally accepted definition of health was determined.[202] The definition of health given in the document stated that "Health is a state of complete physical, mental and social well-being and not merely the absence of disease or infirmity."[203] It was also stated that "Irrespective of race, religion, political belief, and financial or social condition, each human being has the rights to get the highest attainable standard of health. To provide adequate health services to people is the governments' responsibility."[204] The constitution of WHO came into effect on April 7, 1948.[205]

The third United Nations General Assembly, which took place in Paris in December 1948, saw the adoption the Universal Declaration of Human Rights. People's right to health was also included in human rights. India was one of the 48 countries supporting the Charter,[206] Article 25 of which stated that "Everyone has the right to a standard of living adequate for the health and well-being of himself and of his family…"[207]

After World War II, medical science began to make great strides, especially in the 1950s–1970s. That period saw the development of medical technology as well as the discovery of new antibiotics. Vaccines for various infectious diseases were made available to people. That level of development was unprecedented.[208] Yet the development of medical science had not greatly improved the public health of the newly independent countries of Asia, Africa, and Latin America, as it had not been possible for the governments of those countries to provide advanced medical services to all citizens. Moreover, the primary health care system in those countries was also underdeveloped. As a result, developing countries such as China, Cuba, Venezuela, and Tanzania used their limited resources to fight hunger and disease and tried to solve primary health problems in their own way.[209]

However, the Western healthcare model, to which there had been no real alternative until World War II, was also prevalent in these developing countries. This healthcare model had been developed in Europe and North America, and was subsequently imported into their colonies like India, which had their own distinctive characteristics. It was highly centralized, urban-oriented and institution-based. Such a model suited the needs of the industrially developed West but was obviously ill-suited to the needs of predominantly rural and agricultural society-based colonies such as India. The so-called Third World continued to rely on the infrastructure created by the colonial powers, long after independence. Some of the earliest attempts to break from this structure were seen in the People's Republic of China. After the successful outbreak of the Revolution of 1949, the Chinese Communist Party came to power in China. Realizing the inadequacy of the Western model of healthcare delivery, the Chinese, after their revolution, embarked on a major program of the decentralization of health services.[210] Four key guidelines for the organization of their healthcare system were declared at the first National Health Congress of China, held in August 1950: health services should be delivered to the peasants, workers, and soldiers; preventive medicine rather than curative medicine should be emphasized; integration should be made between Chinese traditional medicine and Western scientific medicine; and healthcare should be integrated with the mass movement.[211]

In 1952 a 'patriotic health movement' was launched in China.[212] Initially, urban development was prioritized, but gradually the emphasis was placed on village construction. As a result, crude death rates, child mortality rates, and infectious disease rates were also reduced.[213] On June 26, 1966, prior to the Cultural Revolution (1966–1976), Mao Tse Tung (1896–1976) sharply criticized the country's urban-based health system.[214] One of the main pillars in the Chinese new healthcare model was 'barefoot doctors,' who were employed to meet the shortage of doctors at a village level.[215] International organizations such as the WHO followed the Chinese development model. In the 1970s, the slogan "Lessons learned from China's healthcare system" was raised in the West.[216]

After assuming power in Cuba in 1959, Fidel Castro sought to establish a socialist government in the country, along similar lines to those seen in the Soviet Union and China. The new government took steps to eradicate the socio-economic causes of the disease. Che Guevara, a revolutionary physician and Cuban minister, said: "Now the work of the Ministry of Health and similar organizations is to provide health services to the greatest possible number of people, to carry out disease prevention programs, to educate the people in hygienic practices."[217]

Cuba achieved great success with the adoption of the Family Doctor program. After the country's revolution, there was an emphasis on creating a sufficient number of doctors and nurses in the country to fill the shortage of health professionals. There was also an emphasis on health education. The government bore all expenditure on health care. Every component of health care for the people (with the exception of a few medicines) was provided free of cost from government hospitals/polyclinics.[218] Adopting that kind of policy radically changed the Cuban health system. That change would be visualized when we look at the indicators of changes in Cuba's health care system from 1957–1958 to 2007–2008.[219] The *New England Journal of Medicine* praised Cuba's healthcare system. Two doctors from the USA wrote in this journal that "there were plenty of doctors in Cuba. Every family had a family physician. Treatment was completely free. The whole system was well organized, with much emphasis on disease prevention. Cuba had solved the public health problem well with limited resources but America had not been able to do that."[220]

There are some common features in these socialist countries such as the Soviet Union, China, and Cuba. According to Imrana Qadeer, these countries did strive to produce a surplus, but this was owned by the state, and the distribution of that surplus was certainly less inequitable. This new socio-economic framework gave the health service system a distinct character. It was, to a large extent, a package of food, housing, clothing, clean drinking water, education, and employment for all.[221] It is noteworthy that the implementation of Universal Health Care had been made possible in those countries in the wake of the efforts made for elimination of social inequality.

There was actually another universal health care model before the Alma-Ata conference, which was known as the *Tommy Douglas model.*

While health services were provided by the private sector in that model, they were paid through a government-run insurance scheme to which all citizens contributed through taxes.[222] After much controversy, Tommy Douglas, a leader of the socialist political party *Co-operative Commonwealth Federation* (CCF), introduced a universal health insurance plan in Saskatchewan province, Canada, in the early 1960s.[223]

In addition, in the 1960s–1970s, David Werner's grassroots community-based health care project at Piaxtla in Mexico,[224] the comprehensive rural health project at Jamkhed (Maharashtra) in India,[225] and the Zafrullah Chowdhury-led *Gonoshasthaya Kendra* in Bangladesh[226] set a model of people-based primary health care. Drawing on the experiences of the *Piaxtla* project, Werner wrote a book titled *Donde No Hay Doctor* (*Where There is No Doctor*)[227] for primary health awareness, which very quickly became popular around the globe. Werner wrote, "My own involvement with the struggle for health and justice began in Piaxtla." The works of the Piaxtla project included medical service, preventive measures, and social and political action.[228] In 1972, *Gonoshasthaya Kendra* (*GK*) was founded under the leadership of Zafarullah Choudhury in Bangladesh just after the successful liberation war of the country. That organization tried to improve the condition of rural health. It also translated *Where There is No Doctor* into Bengali.[229]

Dr. Zafrullah Chowdhury said that the *Gonoshasthaya Kendra* (*GK*) was one of the experiment centers of the primary health care system. GK emphasized community participation in the health system. Women, who had not received formal education, were trained in preventive and curative medicine. It may be stated that GK wanted to follow the socialistic path in the health system. Dr. Chowdhury said, "By participating in the liberation war, we have learned how to get people involved in the primary health care system."[230]

Meanwhile, in the wake of the Cold War, the USSR and China began to pressurize the WHO to expand the primary health care system.[231]

Alma-Ata and After

An international conference to develop a primary healthcare strategy was held in Alma-Ata, the capital of the Kazakh Soviet Socialist Republic from September 6 to September 12, 1978. The conference was attended by delegates from 134 countries and by representatives of 67 non-governmental organizations. J, Prasad Yadav was the representative of the

Government of India and became one of the five vice-presidents elected at the conference.[232]

The conference declared that "health is a fundamental human right"; and asserted that the right to health of all people in the world would be guaranteed by the year 2000. The report of the conference noted that the health condition of billions of people on this planet was poor; more than half of the world's population lacked access to adequate healthcare; the situation in developing countries, in particular, was bleak; although most people in the developed countries had access to health care, no one would have received proper health care, with the exception of rich people in developing countries. As a result, recognizing the global situation, the Alma-Ata Declaration stated that inequality in human health status "between developed and developing countries as well as within the country was politically, socially and economically unacceptable." So, it was decided that to deal with this acute health problem, the disparities in health status between developed and developing countries must be removed.[233]

The organizers of the conference realized that in order to meet the goal of "Health for All by 2000 AD," it was necessary to focus on primary health care. Therefore, this declaration gave a clear idea about the objectives and meaning of primary health care. It was said that providing primary health care was the responsibility of every government. It was also stated that in order to make the primary health care system effective "it will be necessary to exercise political will, to mobilize the country's resources and to use available external resources rationally."[234] It outlined important elements of primary health care: health education; the adoption of policies for the supply of essential nutritious food; the adoption of a requisite water and sanitation system; the arrangement for the formulation of a preventive medicare system to prevent major local infectious diseases; the prevention and control of local diseases; immunization against major infectious diseases; arrangement for the treatment of general diseases and accidental and emergency medical facilities; and the supply of essential medicines. India, along with the other countries in attendance, committed to achieving this.[235]

In 1978, the Alma-Ata Conference strengthened the foundations of the people's health movement in the world. Countries pledged to achieve the goal of "Health for All by 2000". The Alma-Ata Declaration was a significant point in the history of the people's health movement. However, one year before the Alma- Ata meeting a rough plan was drawn up for the goal of "Health for All by 2000 AD" in the 30th session of the World Health Organization (WHO) held in Geneva in 1977.[236] At the heart of that plan was the philosophy of the then director-general of the World Health Organization, Halfdan Mahler (1973–1983). In 1981, he highlighted some major points about 'Health for All':

- Health for All eliminates barriers to health like "malnutrition, lack of pure drinking water, lack of unhygienic housing and lack of medical care."
- Health for All depends on the continued progress of medical services and public health. Medical services should be extended to all people through primary health care so that basic medical care would be available in every village.
- Health for All is actually a holistic concept, which includes the improvement of medical services and public health as well as agriculture, industry, education, housing, and communication. Medical services alone cannot get health to the hut. So people need high-quality living opportunities for their health.[237]

Following the Alma-Ata conference, the comprehensive primary health care approach was attacked as too costly and unrealistic. The PHC approach was replaced by the selective primary health care (SPHC) approach, which gave the highest priority to the control of major diseases. The SPHC approach defined health as the absence of disease. According to Susan B. Rifkin and Gill Walt, the SPHC approach not only failed to address equity but also consolidated health provision in the hands of the professionals and gave high credence to the importance of medical technology without sufficient recognition of the importance of infrastructure, attitudes, and perceptions.[238]

The Alma-Ata Declaration stressed the importance of social medicine, covering adequate food, pure drinking water, housing, and sanitation. We know that one of the root causes of diseases is malnutrition, which results from poor people's inability to procure food. There is an interrelationship between malnutrition and disease. On the one hand, malnutrition led to the suffering of people from various contagious diseases; on the other, infectious diseases caused malnutrition.[239] That is why famine was one of the primary causes of death in colonial India. In the early twentieth century, one deadly epidemic disease was influenza, which, according to Kingsley Davis, killed 20 million people or some 5 per cent of the total population in 1918–1919. Lack of medical treatment, as well as the generally poor physical health of Indians, was responsible for the deaths because it was relatively easy for the disease to take root in the bodies of poor Indians.[240]

However, in addition to malnutrition, the lack of pure drinking water, a poor environment and a patchy public health system also all caused diseases. Additionally, parental illiteracy could lead to poor health among their children. As a result, there was a need to improve these social determinants of health such as pure drinking water, sufficient food, clothing, housing, education, gender awareness, employment, personal income, etc. Despite the improvement in social determinants, however, a proper health care service is greatly needed when people are subject to diseases. In this case, if the patient is deprived of proper medical care, then there is no way open for them except death. Therefore, to implement the goal of "Health for All," it is necessary to improve the health service of the country as well as the condition of the social determinants of health.[241]

According to the Preston Curve,[242] life expectancy depends on the per capita growth in gross domestic product (GDP). Thus, it is assumed that a country with high GDP is likely to have a better health care system.[243] According to economists like Wilkinson and Pickett, however, the health index of a country's citizens does not depend solely on per capita GDP. To them, it depended on social policy. It is argued that greater equality in the society led to a better health index for people in a country.[244] Equality is the basis of universal health care. Therefore, in order to implement the goal of 'Health for All,' a more equal society must be established. This is what was indicated in the Alma-Ata Declaration.

As we have outlined, there are a number of different health care models in the world. The Marxist and socialistic health care model was a state-owned model where the responsibility to provide the highest acquirable standard of health to the people, irrespective of religion, race, caste and socio-economic status, fell to the state. There was no role for the market in these models. There was also a paternalistic model, a "market minus and state plus" model, which was prevalent in countries such as Greece, Italy, Germany, Spain, Sweden, Finland, and Norway. The Alma-Ata Declaration focused on such models.

In the 1970s, neo-liberalism began to take control of political and economic decision-making. Neo-liberalism is characterized by free markets, sovereign individuals, free trade, rigorous property rights, and less government intervention. The crisis of the 1970s triggered economic and social reforms that overturned planned welfare expansion and replaced it with restrictive monetary policies. In the late 1970s, Latin America was the first region to be affected by the new economic policies; this was followed by African economies and, in the late 1980s and early 1990s, much of Asia. By the early 1980s, most governments in Europe had opened up their services to market competition.[245]

The neo-liberal model was a "state minus and market plus" model. Liberals believed that the state should have no responsibility in providing health to the people; being a consumer commodity, it could be sold or bought like other consumer goods in the market.[246] In the 1980s, the UK, the USA, and New Zealand welcomed the introduction of neo-liberal ideology. The United Kingdom had the earliest and most advanced privatization programs in Western Europe, probably because of its particularly close political, economic, and cultural relationship with the United States. The UK and the USA also persuaded other countries to adopt similar policies. However, countries like France, Germany, and Sweden did not change their policy despite being placed under considerable pressure.[247]

Since the early 1980s, in different parts of the world, even though the infant mortality rate decreased and life expectancy increased, in terms of mortality the gap between poor and rich, both between and within the countries, also significantly increased. In Sub-Saharan African (SSA) countries, the impact of economic recession, neo-liberal policy, drought, war and civil unrest, and the spread of HIV/AIDS also increased child mortality in the 1980s. In developing countries, the main cause of death under 5 years of age was acute respiratory infection (ARI) and diarrheal diseases. There was also a resurgence and spread of several old diseases, such as cholera, malaria, tuberculosis, yellow fever, etc. with HIV/AIDS.[248] David Werner pointed to a four-pronged attack on primary health care: these were "selective primary health care introduced in the late 70s in lieu of comprehensive primary health care; Structural Adjustment Programs (SAP) introduced in the early 1980s; World Bank's takeover of Third World Health Policy in the 1990s; [and] partnerships by UNICEF and WHO with transnational corporations in the 2000s."[249] He also wrote

> …the year 2000 has come and gone, and the goal of Health for All in some ways seems farther than ever from being reached…While a few health indicators have improved decently since 1978, for billions of the poorest people, health and quality of life have actually deteriorated. This is partly because of the decreasing access to costly health services. But it is also because the

world's neediest people have been increasingly marginalized by the dominant model of economic development.[250]

The development of the market economy and the decline of the WHO's authority jointly led to the failure to achieve the goal of 'Health for All by 2000 AD'. As a result, people increasingly had to depend on the private health sector.[251] Corporate power has been mobilized over the past few decades. The neo-liberal healthcare agenda had facilitated the commercialization of health care services around the globe. The World Bank had put pressure on low-income countries to impose "user fees" on poor people for their access to healthcare services: "Nations in both the developing and developed world were taking steps towards health system privatization in ways that sometimes threatened the right to healthcare for their citizens."[252] "Rising out-of-pocket spending on public and private healthcare services was driving many families into poverty and exacerbating the poverty of those who were already poor. The magnitude of this situation is known as 'the medical poverty trap'."[253]

In 2005, at the 58th Conference of the *World Health Organization*, *Universal Health Coverage* (UHC) was declared as a strategy to address health problems in the age of globalization.[254] The strategy was to protect people from financial loss for receiving health care. In the definition of UHC, it was stated that "ensuring that all people and communities can use the promotive, preventive, curative, rehabilitative and palliative health services they need,...also ensuring that the use of these services does not expose the user to financial hardship."[255] Indranil Mukhopadhyay argues that "UHC and health for all mean entirely different things...Under UHC, governments are being seen as a major purchaser of health services (and not the only provider) and different forms of purchasing mechanisms are proposed including tax financed health insurance, mandatory social insurance and managed care models."[256] In 2015, the *United Nations* adopted *Sustainable Development Goals* (SDGs) as a global call to action to eradicate poverty, safeguard the environment, and ensure that everyone lives in peace and prosperity by 2030. In a related development, one of the 17 Sustainable Development Goals set by the United Nations was SDG 3 (or Global Goal 3), which focused on "Good Health and Well-Being." Its aim is: "To ensure healthy lives and promote well-being for all people of all ages," the official statement read.[257]

International People's Health Council and Its Follow-Up

The goal of *Health for All*, or UHC, has not been achieved in most of the countries of the world, including India. As a result, the people's health movement has expanded. Attempts have also been made to develop people's health movement from a global perspective. In December 1991, the *International People's Health Council* (IPHC), "an informal network of socially progressive groups and movements committed to work for the health and rights of disadvantaged people, and, ultimately, of all people," was conceived in a meeting on 'Health Care in Societies in Transition' held in Managua, Nicaragua, which was attended by health rights activists from South Africa, Zimbabwe, India, Bangladesh, El Salvador, Guatemala, Panama, Mexico, the United States, and other countries. Participants in the meeting stressed health politics, connecting the extensive health and social well-being crisis to the global economic downturn and, more particularly, to the broadening gap between rich and poor, both within and between countries. Members of the IPHC asserted that a global grassroots movement was needed to promote a healthier world order.[258] It was also assumed that "the struggle for health is a struggle for liberation from poverty, hunger, and unfair socio-economic structures."[259] After discussions about the people's health movement for more than a decade, in 1998, a number of organizations began the process of developing a *People's Health Assembly* (PHA) and planned to hold large international conferences. In December 2000, the first international conference of people's health organizations was held in *Gonoshasthaya Kendra* (1972) in Savar, Bangladesh, drawing representatives from 92 countries. In that five-day conference, the total number of participants was 1453. People from different countries exposed the failures of the respective governments and international organizations. The Assembly emphasized five main themes: "Health, Life and Well-Being; Inequality, Poverty and Health; Health Care and Health Services; Environment and Survival; and The Ways Forward." It resulted in the publication of a *People's Charter for Health*.[260] The Charter stated that: The negative effects of globalization aggravated inequality within and between the countries, leading to a health crisis for the people. Failure to implement the principles of primary health care adopted in Alma Ata had exacerbated the global health crisis. Governments and international organizations were entirely responsible for that failure. "That is why several international organizations, civil society movements,

NGOs, women's organizations have come under one umbrella to work for achieving the goal of Health for All."[261]

The People's Health Assembly pledged to strengthen the people's health movement to fight against the global health crisis. The people's health charter urged the people of the world to:

- Demand that all governments and international organizations must restructure and implement their policies and actions in a way that respects the right to health.
- Organize broad-based people's health movements and pressure on the governments so that they include health and human rights into national constitutions and legislation.
- Demand changes in the World Trade Organization (WTO) and the global trading system in order that it stops violating the social, environmental, economic, and health rights of people and work in the interests of the southern countries.
- Demand effective management so that the multinational corporations could not adversely affect the people's health and environment.
- Demand that governments stand against the privatization of public healthcare and regulate the private health sector effectively.[262]

Through the first PHA at Savar, a network named *People's Health Movement (PHM)* was formed to get people's health activists and civil society organizations around the globe together. The Savar assembly was followed by the 2nd PHA in Cuenca, Ecuador in 2005, the 3rd PHA in Cape Town in 2012, and the 4th PHA in Bangladesh in 2018. PHM had many country circles.[263] Every three to four years, PHM, in collaboration with other organizations, used to publish an alternative global health report entitled the *Global Health Watch* (GHW) to highlight the worldwide health crisis. GHW1 was published in 2005, followed by GHW2 (2008), GHW3 (2011), GHW4 (2014), and GHW5 (2017).[264] *Jan Swasthya Abhiyan* (JSA), the Indian chapter of PHM, began its journey in 2000, and was formally started in 2001. In 2003, it began the right to health campaign. The first phase of the campaign documented denial of the health care system.[265] A detailed study of the activities of the *Jan Swasthya Abhiyan* is given in Chap. 3 of this book.

The PHM in different countries vehemently opposed the idea of privatization in the health sector. In this respect we may study the happenings of El Salvador, where the government chose privatization in health care in the 1990s. In the 2000s, privatization adversely affected health services. As a result, the people of El Salvador started a movement to stall the government's attempt of privatization. In 2002–2003, protests and strikes by health workers against the privatization of health care in El Salvador sparked a social movement, with strikes by health workers lasting nine months. There were also outbreaks in Central American countries such as Nicaragua and Guatemala against the growing presence of privatization in health. Yet the health movement of Salvadorians was different in nature. On this occasion activists had organized a wider and deeper mass movement, one involving more than just a workers' strike in just one sector.[266] Howard Waitzkin wrote "Efforts to resist privatization of health services and the public health system in El Salvador emerged as a model for analogous social movements elsewhere in Latin America. The example of El Salvador also illustrated similar processes that were to occur in many other countries throughout the world during the early twenty-first century, as imperial policies met with sustained resistance."[267] Against that backdrop *Frente Farabundo Marti para la Liberacion Nacional* (FMLN), a left-wing political party assumed power in June 2009. The new government adopted a health system reform policy titled 'Building Hope' that considered health to be a public good and a fundamental right of people, to be guaranteed by the government. In 2010, the National Health Forum (NHF) emerged. This worked as a pressure group, which sought to ensure community participation in health care.[268]

The neo-liberal economy also had an adverse impact on people's lives in many parts of Europe. As a result, there was an intensification of the protests and resistance movements against the policies imposed by neo-liberal governments in European countries.[269] In Spain, health professionals (doctors, nurses, health workers) and civil society organized a movement, known as 'marea blanca' (white tide), against the privatization of the country's health care services. Agitators held a prolonged strike and massive street protests; as a result, in January 2014 the government in Madrid cancelled its plan to privatize health services in six local public hospitals. In Italy, health professionals' trade unions launched the 'Save our NHS' campaign in 2013. The Italian 'anti-Mafia' group launched another campaign, which was supported by the people. There were also several public campaigns in the UK, led by an organization named 'Keep Our NHS Public.' To challenge the reform of the NHS made by the Conservative government in 2012, the *National Health Action Party* was created by a group of health professionals in the UK. Belgium, Germany,

Greece and Portugal all also witnessed agitations against privatization in health care.[270]

Although it is widely acknowledged that the principles of the Alma-Ata Conference are still relevant today, regrettably many countries have failed to fulfil their commitment. In this scenario, a global conference on 'Primary Health Care: From Alma-Ata to Universal Health Coverage and the Sustainable Development Goals' was held in Astana, Kazakhstan in October 2018, with 2000 delegates from over 120 countries in attendance. Its intention was to renew the political commitment to comprehensive primary health care for all from governments, global health and development organizations, and other stakeholders. The Astana declaration affirmed the "commitment to the fundamental right of every human being to the enjoyment of the highest attainable standard of health without distinction of any kind."[271] In the midst of the worldwide health crisis, in November 2018, more than 1400 health activists from 73 nations across the globe gathered in Savar, Bangladesh for the 4th People's Health Assembly, where they reaffirmed their commitment to the struggle for health. Participants at the assembly joined in with the chanted: "The Struggle for Health is the Struggle for a More Equitable, Just and Caring World."[272]

Notes

1. Krishna Soman and Subharanjan Dasgupta, "Public Health: Historical Experience", *Economic and Political Weekly*, Vol. 38, No. 47, November 22–28, 2003, pp. 4942–4944.
2. Mary-Jane Schneider, *Introduction to Public Health,* United States of America: Jones & Bartlett Learning, Fifth edition 2017, pp. 4–5.
3. C.E.A. Winslow, "The Untilled Fields of Public Health", in *Science* (published by American Association for the Advancement of Science), New Series, Vol. 51, No. 1306, January 9, 1920, p. 30.
4. Milton Terris, "Epidemiology and the Public Health Movement", *Journal of Public Health Policy*, Autumn 1987, Vol. 8, No. 3, p. 317.
5. Sabyasachi Chattopadhyay & Nataraj Malakar, "Shudhui Cikitsa Ebang Bima, Rog Pratirodh Jaruri Nay?", *Ei Samay*, Kolkata, 06.05.2019, p. 8.
6. Ernest M. Gruenberg, "Public Health and the People's Health", *Public Health Reports* (1896–1970), Vol. 72, No. 1, January 1957, pp. 47–50, available at: https://www.jstor.org/stable/4589684.
7. Ibid.

8. Awanish Kumar, "Caste and Public Health", Frontline, https://frontline.thehindu.com/cover-story/article31525708.ece, retrieved on December 28, 2021.
9. John Coggon, *What Makes Health Public: A Critical Evaluation of Moral, Legal, and Political Claims in Public Health*, Cambridge: Cambridge University Press, 2012.
10. John Coggon & Lawrence O. Gostin, "The Two Most Important Questions for Ethical Public Health", *Journal of Public Health*, Vol. 42, No. 1, pp. 198–202.
11. Theodore H. Tulchinsky and Elena A. Varavikova, *The New Public Health*, Amsterdam: Elsevier, 2014 (third edition), p. 1.
12. Upinder Singh, *A History of Ancient and Early Medieval India: For the Stone Age to the 12th Century*, Delhi: Pearson, second impression 2012, pp. 59–131.
13. V. Gordon Childe, *Man Makes Himself*, New York: New American Library, 1951 (Originally published in England in 1936).
14. Dorothy Porter, *Health, Civilization and the State: A history of public health from ancient to modern times*, London and New York: Routledge, First Published 1999, pp. 11–12.
15. Theodore H. Tulchinsky and Elena A. Varavikova, op. cit., pp. 2–4.
16. Dorothy Porter, op. cit., pp. 13–16.
17. William Bynum, *The History of Medicine: A Very Short Introduction*, New York: Oxford University Press, 2008, p. 5.
18. R.D. Lele, *Ayurveda and Modern Medicine*, Bombay: Bharatiya Vidya Bhavan, 1986, p. 1.
19. Debiprasad Chattopadhyaya, *Science and Society in Ancient India*, Kolkata: Research India Publications, 1977; Debiprasad Chattopadhyaya, *Prachin Bharate Chikitsabijnan*, Kolkata: Paschimbanga Bangla Academy, 1992.
20. "A History of The Public Health System", in *The Future of Public Health*, Committee for the Study of the Future of Public Health, Division of Health Care Services, Institute of Medicine, US: National Academies Press, twelfth printing 1997, pp. 56–72.
21. Theodore H. Tulchinsky and Elena A. Varavikova, op. cit., p. 16.
22. Eugenia Tognotti, "Lessons from the History of Quarantine, rom Plague to Influenza A", *Emerging Infectious Diseases*, Vol. 19, No. 2, February 2013, pp. 254–259.
23. Mark Harrison, *Disease and Modern World: 1500 to the present day*, Cambridge: Polity Press, 2004, p. 38.
24. Dorothy Porter, op. cit., pp. 30–36.
25. "A History of The Public Health System", op. cit.

26. George Rosen, *A History of Public Health*, Baltimore: Johns Hopkins University Press, first published 1958, reprint 2015, pp. 68–105.
27. Ibid.
28. Ibid.
29. Allan Nevins, *A Pocket History of the United States*, USA: Pocket Books, 1990, chapter IV.
30. Dorothy Porter, op. cit., pp. 56–57.
31. Ibid.
32. Adam Gaffney, *To Heal Humankind: the Right to Health in History*, New York: Routledge, 2018, pp. 43–44.
33. Ibid.
34. Ibid.
35. George Rosen, "Hospitals, Medical Care and Social Policy in the French Revolution", *Bulletin of the History of Medicine*, Vol. 30, No. 2, March–April, 1956, pp. 124–149.
36. Ibid.
37. Adam Gaffney, *To Heal Humankind the Right to Health in History*, op. cit., pp. 44–45.
38. Dorothy Porter, *Health, Civilization and the State: A history of public health from ancient to modern times*, op. cit., p. 57; Dorothy Porter, "Introduction", in Dorothy Porter (ed.), *The History of Public Health and the Modern State*, Amsterdam: Rodopi, 1994.
39. George Rosen, *A History of Public Health*, op. cit., pp. 106–168; Mark Harrison, *Disease and Modern World: 1500 to the present day*, op. cit., pp. 133–134.
40. R. A. Lewis, *Edwin Chadwick and Public Health Movement 1832–1854*, London: Longmans, Green and Co., 1952.
41. S.E. Finer, *The Life and Times of Sir Edwin Chadwick*, UK: The British Book Centre, Inc., 1952.
42. Dharmadas Basu, *Swasthya-Raksha O Sadharan Swasthya-Tatwa*, Vol. 1, Calcutta: H. M. Mookerjea & Co, 1885, pp. 2–3.
43. Glenn Laverack, *Health Activism: Foundations and Strategies*, London, New Delhi, Singapore: SAGE Publications, 2013, p. 9.
44. Frederick Engels, *The Condition of the Working Class in England in 1944* (translated by Florence Kelley Wiscunewetzky), New York: John W. Lovell Company, 1887.
45. Karl Marx and Frederick Engels, *Communist Manifesto*, Chicago: Charles H. Kerr & Company, 1906.
46. Frederick Engels, *The Condition of the Working Class in England in 1944*, op. cit., pp. 109–110.

47. Anne-Emanuelle Birn et al., *Textbook of International Health: Global Health in Dynamic World*, New York & Oxford: Oxford University Press, 2009 (third edition), pp. 34–35, 342.
48. Stephen Corbett, "Review Work" (of *Public Health and Social Justice in the Age of Chadwick Britain 1800–1854* by Christopher Hamlin), *Health Promotion International*, Volume 14, Issue 4, December 1999, Pages 381–382.
49. Roy Porter, *London: A Social History,* Cambridge, MA: Harvard University Press, first paperback edition 1998, cited edition 2001, p. 247.
50. Hugh Thomas, "John Snow: A Pioneer in Epidemiology", in Jill Stewart (ed.), *Pioneers in Public Health: Lesson from History*, London/New York: Routledge, 2017, pp. 33–39.
51. K. Park, *Park's Book of Preventive & Social Medicine,* India: Bhanot Publishers, 23rd edition, 2015, pp. 5–6.
52. Ann F. La Berge, *Mission and Method: The Early Nineteenth-Century French Public Health Movement*, UK: Cambridge University Press, First published 1992, First paperback edition 2002, pp. 1–6.
53. Debiprasad Chattopadhyay, *Marxbad,* Kolkata: Anustup, first published 1993, 4th edition 2013, pp. 11–17.
54. Fran Collyer, "Karl Marx and Frederich Engels: Capitalism, Health and the Healthcare Industry", in Fran Collyer (ed.), *The Palgrave Handbook of Social Theory in Health, Illness and Medicine,* Basingstoke: Palgrave Macmillan, 2015, pp. 35–58.
55. Friedrich Engels, *The Condition of the Working Class in England* (it was originally written in German as *Die Lage der arbeitenden Klasse in England*, first published 1945), Moscow: Progress Publishers, 1973.
56. Howard Waitzkin, "The Social Origins of Illness: A Neglected History", *International Journal of Health Services,* Vol. 11, No. 1, 1981, pp. 77–103.
57. Adam Gaffney, *To Heal Humankind the Right to Health in History,* New York: Routledge, 2018, pp. 63–65.
58. Ibid.
59. Sujit Kumar Das, *Chikitsar Kotha: Rajniti Arthaniti O Janagan*, Kolkata: Drug Action Forum, West Bengal, 2006, pp. 13–14.
60. Henry E. Sigerist, "From Bismarck to Beveridge: Developments and Trends in Social Security Legislation", *Journal of Public Health Policy,* Vol. 20, No. 4, 1999, pp. 474–496.
61. K. Srinath Reddy, "Sabar Janya Swasthyer Lakshye Gathita Uchcha-Stariya Bisheshagga Daler Boktabya", in Punyabrata Goon (ed.), *Sbara Janya Swasthya Ekti Swapna Ja Sotyi Kara Jay*, Kolkata: Guruchandai, 2017, pp. 25–26.

62. Henry E. Sigerist, "From Bismarck to Beveridge: Developments and Trends in Social Security Legislation", op. cit.
63. Alfons Labisch, "From Traditional Individualism to Collective Professionalism: State, Patient, Compulsory Health Insurance, and the panel Doctor Question in Germany, 1883–1931", in Manfred Berg and Geoffrey Cocks (eds.), *Medicine and Modernity: Public Health and Medical Care in Nineteenth and Twentieth-Century Germany*, Cambridge: Cambridge University Press, first published 1997, first paperback edition 2002, pp. 35–54.
64. "A Brief History: Universal Health Care Efforts in the US", published in the website of Physicians for a National Health Program, a US-based organization, https://pnhp.org/a-brief-history-universal-health-care-efforts-in-the-us/, retrieved on June 19, 2021.
65. Shyamal Chakraborty, *November Biplaber Eksha Bachhar*, Kolkata: Akshar Publication, 2017, p. 18.
66. Medical Service Centre, *Samajtantre Janaswasthya – November Biplab Satabarshe*, Kolkata, 2017, p. 12.
67. Rabindranath Tagore, *Rashiyar Chithi*, Kolkata: Visva-Bharati, first published 1338 BS, cited third print 1352 BS, pp. 1–3.
68. Arthur Newsholme & John Adams Kingsbury, *Red Medicine: Socialized Health in Soviet Russia*, London: William Heinemann (Medical Books) Ltd, 1934.
69. Ibid.
70. Interview with Dr. Jnanabrata Sil, Kolkata, February 3, 2019.
71. Arthur Newsholme & John Adams Kingsbury, op. cit., pp. 205–209.
72. Ibid., p. 55.
73. Henry E. Sigerist, *Medicine and Health in Soviet Union*, Bombay: Jaico Publishing House, 1947, p. 249.
74. Arthur Newsholme & John Adams Kingsbury, op. cit., pp. 276–277.
75. Ibid., p.196.
76. Price V. Fishback et al., "Births, Deaths, and New Deal Relief during the Great Depression", *The Review of Economics and Statistics*, Vol. 89, No.1, February 2007, pp. 1–14.
77. John Maynard Keynes, *The General Theory of Employment, Interest, and Money*, Germany: Macmillan, 1936.
78. Howard Waitzkin, *Medicine and Public Health at the End of Empire*, New York: Routledge, 2011, p. 65.
79. Veeranarayana Kethineni, "Political Economy of State Intervention in Health Care", *Economic & Political Weekly*, October 19, 1991, pp. 2429–2431.

80. David Garland, *The Welfare State: A Very Short Introduction*, Oxford: Oxford University Press, p. 26.
81. Ibid., p. 27.
82. Rahul Mukherjee, "Jukta Rajyer Jatiya Swasthya Parisheba?", *Swasthyer Britte*, Vol. 2, No. 3, February–March 2013, pp. 58–59.
83. "The Socialist Medical Association and the Foundation of the NHS", Address to the 50th Anniversary Conference of The Socialist Medical Association by Dr Leslie Hilliard (1980), available at: https://www.sochealth.co.uk/national-health-service/the-sma-and-the-foundation-of-the-national-health-service-dr-leslie-hilliard-1980/, retrieved on 25.06.2023.
84. Ronan Burtenshaw, "How the NHS Was Won", *Tribune*, July 5, 2019, https://tribunemag.co.uk/2019/07/how-the-nhs-was-won, retrieved on 08.04.2023.
85. Ibid.
86. Sthabir Dasgupta, *Swasthya Niye Bad-bisangbad*, Kolkata: Ananda Publishers, 2020, pp. 250–253; John Stewart, *"The Battle for Health": A Political History of the Socialist Medical Association, 1930–51*, New York: Routledge, 2018 (First published by Ashgate Publishing in 1999).
87. Amartya Sen, *Development as Freedom*, New York: Alfred A. Knopf, 2000, pp. 50–53; Amartya Sen, "Atimari Sesh Hale Abar Dekha Habe Amader, Natun Prithibir Mukh Dekhbo?", *Anandabazar Patrika*, April 17, 2020, https://www.anandabazar.com/editorial/global-economy-social-equality-after-covid-19-pandemic-amartya-sen-on-reality-expectations-dgtl-1.1137691, retrieved on April 18, 2020.
88. Rahul Mukherjee, "National Health Service Ki?", *Swasthyer Britte*, Vol. 6, No. 6, August–September 20017, pp. 48–50.
89. Irfan Habib & Vivekananda Jha, *Mauryan India*, New Delhi: Tulika Books, 2004.
90. S. Ali Nadeem Rezavi, "Physicians as Professionals in Medieval India", in Deepak Kumar (ed.), *Disease & Medicine in India: A Historical Overview*, New Delhi: Tulika, First published 2001, Reprint 2012, p. 47.
91. Chittabrata Palit and Tinni Goswami, "Sanitation, Empire, Environment: Bengal (1980–1920)", in *Proceedings of the Indian History Congress*, Vol. 68, Part One, 2007, pp. 731–744; Debabar Banerji, "Landmarks in the Development of Health Services in India", in Imrana Qadeer et al. (eds.), *Public Health and the Poverty of Reforms: The South Asian Predicament*, New Delhi: SAGE Publications, 2001, p. 39.
92. Imrana Qadeer, "Continuities and Discontinuities in Public Health: The Indian Experience", in Amiya Kumar Bagchi & Krishna Soman (eds.), *Maladies, Preventives and Curatives: Debates in Public Health in India*, New Delhi: Tulika, 2005, pp. 79–94.

93. Mark Harrison, *Public Health in British India: Anglo-Indian Preventive Medicine 1859–1914*, Cambridge: Cambridge University Press, 1994, p. 61.
94. Kabita Roy, *History of public Health: Colonial Bengal 1921–1947*, Kolkata: K.P Bagchi, 1998, p. 6.
95. Ibid., p. 5.
96. Chittabrata Palit, "Epidemics and Empire: A Critique of Public Health policy in Colonial India", in Chittabrata Palit and Achintya Dutta (eds.), *History of Medicine in India: The Medical Encounter*, New Delhi: Kalpaz Publications, 2004, pp. 35–47.
97. Anil Kumar, *Medicine and the Raj: British Medical Policy in India, 1835–1911*, New Delhi: Altamira, 1998, pp. 88–90.
98. Geraldine Forbes, *Women in Colonial India: Essays on Politics, Medicine, and Historiography*, New Delhi: Chronicles Books, 2008, p. 86.
99. Srilata Chatterjee, *Western Medicine and Colonial Society: Hospitals of Calcutta, c.1757–1860*, Delhi: Primus Books, 2017, p. 183.
100. Moumita Chakraborti, "Tracing Medicine and Politics in Colonial Bengal, c. 1920–c.1940", *Journal of the Asiatic Society*, Vol. LX, No. 2, 2018, pp. 49–68.
101. Imrana Qadeer, "Continuities and Discontinuities in Public Health: The Indian Experience", op. cit.
102. Chittabrata Palit, "Epidemics and Empire: A Critique of Public Health policy in Colonial India", op. cit.
103. Ibid.
104. Mark Harrison, "Quarantine, Pilgrimage, and Colonial Trade: India 1866–1900", *Indian Economic and Social History Review*, Vol. 29, No. 2, 1992, pp. 117–144.
105. Alfred Crosby, *Ecological Imperialism: The Biological Expansion of Europe, 900–1900,* Cambridge: Cambridge University Press, 1993.
106. Arabinda Samanta, *Rog Rogi Rashtra: Unish Shataker Bangla*, Kolkata: Progressive Publishers, 2004, p. 39.
107. K. Sujatha Rao, *Do We Care? India's Health System*, New Delhi: Oxford University Press, 2017, p. 8.
108. David Arnold, "Touching the Body: Perspectives on the Indian Plague, 1896–1900", in Ranajit Guha (ed.), *Subaltern Studies V,* Delhi: Oxford University Press, 1987, pp. 55–90.
109. David Arnold, "The Rise of Western Medicine in India", *Lancet,* Vol. 348, October, 1996, pp. 1075–1078.
110. Mark Harrison, *Disease and Modern World: 1500 to the present day*, op. cit., p. 139.

111. Michel Foucault, *Discipline and Punish: The Birth of the Prison* (Translated from the French by Alan Sheridan), New York: Vintage Books, Second edition 1995, p. 197.
112. Anirban Mukhopadhyay, "Saratbabur Quarantine, Bankimer Marak, Bangla Sahitye Mahamari", *Anandabazar Patrika*, Kolkata, April 7, 2020.
113. Kumar Rana, "Ora Kintu Perechhe", *Anandabazar Patrika*, April 7, 2020, p. 4.
114. Arabinda Samanta, *Malarial Fever in Colonial Bengal, 1820–1939: Social History of an Epidemic*, Kolkata: Firma KLM, 2002.
115. Achintya Kumar Dutta, "Tracking Kala-Azar: The East Indian Experience and Experiments", in Biswamoy Pati and Mark Harrison (eds.), *Society, Medicine and Politics in Colonial India*, London: Routledge, 2018, 302–303.
116. Poonam Bala, *State and Indigenous Medicine in Nineteenth and Twentieth-Century Bengal: 1800–19*, Unpublished thesis, University of Edinburgh, 1987, p. 248.
117. Achintya Kumar Dutta, "Tracking kala-azar", in Biswamoy Pati and Mark Harrison (eds.), *Society, Medicine and Politics in Colonial India*, London/New York: Routledge, 2018.
118. Roger Jeffery, *The Politics of Health in India*, Berkeley: University of California Press, 1988, p. 98.
119. D Banerji, "Social and Cultural Foundations of Health Services System", *Economic and Political Weekly*, Vol. 9, No. 32/34, August 1974, p. 1334.
120. Nabaparna Ghosh, *A Hygienic City-Nation: Space, Community, and Everyday Life in Colonial Calcutta*, New Delhi: Cambridge University Press, 2020, pp. 25–67.
121. Speeches Delivered in India, 1884–1888 by the Marquis of Dufferin and Ava, London: John Murray, Albemarle Street, Calcutta: Thacker, Spink & Co. Bombay: Thacker & Co., Limited, 1890, p. 240.
122. Dhrub Kumar Singh, "'Clouds of Cholera' and Clouds around Cholera, 1817–70", in Deepak Kumar (ed.), *Disease & Medicine in India: A Historical Overview*, New Delhi: Tulika, first published 2001, reprint 2012, pp. 153, 155.
123. Sunil S. Amrith, "Health in India since Independence", BWPI Working Paper 79, Manchester: Brooks World Poverty Institute, University of Manchester, February 2009, pp. 10–11.
124. Kabita Ray, "Voluntary Associations and Public Health in Bengal 1900–1947", in Chittabrata Palit and Achintya Kumar Dutta (ed.), *History of Medicine in India: the Medical Encounter*, op. cit., pp. 327–338.
125. Projit Bihari Mukharji, *Nationalizing the Body: The Medical Market, Print and Daktari Medicine*, London: Anthem Press, 2009, p. 136.

126. Tapas Basu, *Shatabarsher Aloke Ramakrishna Mission*, Kolkata: Patraput, 1998, pp. 418–419.
127. Swami Gamvirananda, *Yuganayak Vivekananda*, Vol. 3, Kolkata: Udbodhan Karjalay, 1373 BS (1st ed.), p. 103.
128. Swami Vivekananda, *Prachya O Paschatya*, Kolkata: Udbodhan Karyalaya, 1316 BS (3rd ed.), p. 60.
129. Kabita Ray, "A ministering angel", *The Statesman*, February 2, 2017.
130. Amiya Kumar Hati, "Rabindranath O Janaswasthya", *Janaswasthya Katha*, January–June, 2012, pp. 12–15.
131. Abanindranath Tagore, *Jorasankor Dhare*, Kolkata: Visva-Bharati Granthalay, 1351 BS, pp. 125–126.
132. Nripen Bhoumik, *Rabindranath Thakur: Swasthya o Swasthya-Bhabna*, Kolkata: Ananda Publishers, 2012, pp. 99–101.
133. Rabindranath Tagore, *Sahaj Path, Part-2*, Kolkata: Visva-Bharati, first published 1337 BS (1930).
134. Biswajit Roy, "Rabindranath Bujhechhilen Byadhir Sange Larayer Mulmantra Samajik Duratwa Atikram Kara", Anandabazar Patrika, May 8, 2020, https://www.anandabazar.com/editorial/rabindranath-tagore-formed-a-voluntary-team-to-combat-against-endemic-dgtlx-1.1146688, consulted on June 11, 2020.
135. Rabindranath Tagore, "Pallisamaj Sangbidhan", in Pulin Behari Sen (ed.), *Swadeshi Samaj*, Kolkata: Visva-Bharati, 1962, pp. 65–67.
136. Amiya Kumar Hati, "Rabindranath O Janaswasthya", op. cit.
137. Nripen Bhoumik, *Rabindranath Thakur: Swasthya o Swasthya-Bhabna*, op. cit., pp. 99–104.
138. Ibid.
139. Shailen Kumar Bandyopadhyay (translator), *Mohandas Karamchand Gandhi: Palli Punargathan*, (Rebuilding of Our Villages, edited by Bharatan Kumarappa), Kolkata: Gandhi Smarak Nidhi, Second print 1962, first published 1961, pp. 17–29.
140. Debabar Banerji, "Retrieval of the Approach of Primary Health Care (PHC) in Public Health", C Ramachandran Memorial Lecture 2006, https://pdfs.semanticscholar.org/d6b8/07ab3208abd60e084c51a69521d15424d80c.pdf, retrieved on June 11, 2020.
141. David Arnold, "Death and the Modern Empire: The 1918–19 Influenza Epidemic in India", *Transactions of the Royal Historical Society*, Vol. 29, 2019, pp. 196–197.
142. F. Norman White, A Preliminary Report on the Influenza Pandemic of 1918 in India, Simla, 1919, p. 12.
143. Isaiah Azariah, "Dr. Ida Scudder and The Revolution in Indian Medical Education", *Journal of Third World Studies* (University Press of Florida),

Vol. 7, No. 1, Historical and Contemporary Third World Problems and Issues, Spring 1990, pp. 133–143

144. Partha Dutta, "Health and Healing in Colonial Bengal: The Christian Missionaries and the Imperial Impact", *Vidyasagar University Journal of History*, Vol. VI, 2017–2018, pp. 87–95.
145. Ibid.
146. Sujata Mukherjee, *Gender, Medicine, and Society in Colonial India: Women's Health Care in Nineteenth and Early Twentieth-Century Bengal*, New Delhi: Oxford University Press, 2017, p. xi.
147. Akshaykumar Dutta, *Bahya Bastur Sahit Manab Prakritir Sambandha Bichar*, Vol. 1, Kolkata: Sanskrit Press, 1851.
148. Akshaykumar Dutta, *Dharmaneeti*, Part I, Kolkata: Sanskrit Press, 1863 (4th ed.).
149. Asitkumar Bhaṭṭacharya, *Akshaykumar Dutta*, India: Sahitya Akademi, 1996, pp. 28–44.
150. Dharmadas Basu, *Swasthya-Raksha O Sadharan Swasthya-Tattwa*, Vol. 1, Calcutta: H. M. Mookerjea & Co, 1885.
151. Ibid., p. 2.
152. Jadunath Mukhopadhyay, *Dhatrishiksha Ebang Prasutishiksha,* Chinsura: Chikitsabodhak Press, 1875.
153. Pashupati Bhattacharya, *Ahar O Aharya*, Kolkata: Visva-Bharati, 1347 BS (1940).
154. Chunilal Bose, *Palli Swasthya*, Published by Jyotiprakash Bose, Kolkata, 1916.
155. Ibid.
156. Ibid.
157. Chunilal Bose, *Sharir Swasthya-Bidhan*, Kolkata: Kantik Press, 1913.
158. Subodh Chandra Sengupta & Anjali Basu (eds.) *Sansad Bangali Charitabidhan*, Kolkata: Sahitya Sangsad, first published 1976, pp. 75–76.
159. Ranatosh Chakraborty, *Bismritapray Bengali Bijnani*, Vol. 2, Kolkata: Jnan Bichitra, 2013, 52–55.
160. *Swasthya Samachar*, Vol. 1, No. 1, Baishakh, BS 1319 (1912 AD).
161. *Swasthya*, Vol. 1, No. 1, Chaitra BS 1329.
162. *Swasthya*, Vol. 2, No. 7, Bhadra BS 1331.
163. Shyamal Chakraborty, "Unish-Bish Shataker Bangla Bijnan Patrika", in Muntasir Mamun (ed.), *Dui Shataker Bangla Sambad Samaikpatra*, Kolkata: Pustak Bipani, 2000, p. 313.
164. Projit Bihari Mukharji, *Nationalizing the Body: The Medical Market, Print and Daktari Medicine*, op. cit., p. 160.
165. *Anubikshan*, Vol. 1, No. 1, Shraban, BS 1282 (1875).

166. Pradip Kumar Bose (ed.), *Health and Society in Bengal: A Selection from Late 19th-Century Bengali Periodicals*, New Delhi: SAGE Publications India, 2006, p. 277.

 Chikitsa Sammilani was published as a monthly magazine from 1884 onwards (BS 1291) and was edited at different times by Annadacharan Khastagir, Abinash Chandra Kabiratna, Pulinchandra Sanyal and Sitalchandra Kabirama. In its first two years, it was published from 132 Maniktala Street, Calcutta and then from 227 Cornwallis Street. This periodical had three separate sections. for allopathy, homeopathy and ayurveda, respectively.
167. *Chikitsak O Samalochak*, Vol. 1, No. 2, Falgun BS 1301 (1895) (name of the editor is not mentioned).
168. Krishanu Bhattacharyya, *Bijnanee Dr Gopalchandra Chattopadhyay: Malaria O Sankramak Rog Nibaraner Udyog*, Sodepur: Hemprabha, 2004, pp. 32–33.
169. Ibid., p. 34.
170. Kishorimohan Bandyopadhyay, "Malaria Nibarani Samitir Janma Karma Katha", *Swasthya*, Vol. 2, No. 9, Kartik, BS 1331, pp. 279–287.
171. Ibid.
172. Gopalchandra Chattopadhyay, "Malaria Nibarani Samabay Samiti", *Swasthya*, Vol. 2, No. 7, Bhadra, BS 1331, pp. 195–197.
173. Ranatosh Chakraborty, *Bismritapray Bangali Bigyani*, Kolkata: Jnan Bichitra, 2010, pp. 70–73.
174. Rabindranatha Tagore, "Samabaye Malaria Nibaran", *Rabindrarachanabali*, Vol. 13, Kolkata: West Bengal Government, 1990, pp. 795–798; Rabindranatha Tagore, "Malaria", Rabindrarachanabali, Vol. 13, op. cit., pp. 798–803.
175. *The Lancet*, Vol. 205, No. 5304, April 25, 1925, p. 891.
176. Surendranath Banerjea, *A Nation In Making*, Bombay/Calcutta/ Madras: Oxford University Press, Second Impression, 1925, pp. 355–256.
177. Kabita Ray, *History of Public Health: Colonial Bengal 1921–1947*, Kolkata: K.P Bagchi & Company, 1998, pp. 65, 71–72.
178. "Malaria Control at Birnagar", *The Modern Review*, Vol. XLI, No. 3 (Whole No. 243), March 1927, p. 339.
179. Soroj Nalini Dutta Memorial Association, http://www.sarojnalinidutt-memorialassociation.com/ retrieved on February 20, 2021.
180. Government of India, *Annual Report of the Public Health Commissioner with the Govt. of India*, Delhi: Office of the Superintendent of Government Printing, India, 1933, p. 276.
181. Edward Blunt (ed.), *Social Service in India*, London: His Majesty's Stationery Office, reprinted 1946 (1st ed. 1939), pp. 383–384.

182. Achintya Kumar Dutta, *Trauma in Public Health: Tuberculosis in Twentieth-Century India*, Kolkata: K.P. Bagchi & Company, 2018; Suvankar Dey, "Fighting the invisible enemy: In search of the history of tuberculosis in Colonial Bengal", in *Journal of People's History and Culture*, Vol. 6, No. 1, January 2020, pp. 40–46.
183. D. Mark Anderson, "Was the First Public Health Campaign Successful? The Tuberculosis Movement and its Effect on Mortality", Discussion Paper, IZA–Institute of Labor Economics, Germany, February 2017, pp. 6–8.
184. Amiyajiban Mukhopadhyay, *Rogta Jakhon TB*, Kolkata: Bengal Tuberculosis Association, first published 1941, pp. 200–211.
185. Pamphlet of Bengal Tuberculosis Association, date not mentioned.
186. Amiyajiban Mukhopadhyay, *Rogta Jakhon TB*, op. cit., 211–213.
187. Pamphlet of Bengal Tuberculosis Association, date not mentioned.
188. Ibid.
189. Md Abdullah Rasul, "PRC-er Gourabmay Oitjya", in *People's Relief Committee-er Dyutimay Itibritta*, a publication on the occasion of Diamond Jubilee Year of PRC, Kolkata, 2003, pp. 7–8.
190. Subal Bera, "People's Relief Committee-er Gorar Kotha", in *People's Relief Committee-er Dyutimay Itibritta*, op. cit., pp. 30–31.
191. Ibid.
192. Naresh Banerjee, "People's Relief Committee-er Sankhipta Itihas", in *People's Relief Committee-er Dyutimay Itibritta*, op. cit., pp. 42–80.
193. Saroj Mukhopadhyay, *Bharater Communist Party O Amra*, Dwitiya Khando (1942–1947), Kolkata: National Book Agency, 1986, p. 170.
194. Henry E. Sigerist, *Socialised Medicine in the Soviet Union*, London: Victor Gollancz, Ltd., 1937.
195. Pashupatinath Chattopadhyay, "Arundake Jeman Dekhechhi", in *Smaranika: Dr Arun Sener Uddeshe Shraddhanjali*, Kolkata: Arun Sen Memorial Committee, 1996, pp. 42–51.
196. Nataraj Malakar, "Janasebar Itihas" (Letter), *Anandabazar Patrika*, Kolkata, May 29, 2021, p. 4.
197. Pashupatinath Chattopadhyay, *Students Health Home*, Kolkata: Arun Sen Memorial Committee, 2001, pp. 3–9.
198. Ibid.
199. Ibid.
200. Official Records of the World Health Organization, No. 2, Report of the International Health Conference (United Nations document E/772), New York, June 1948, pp. 5–6.
201. K. Evang, "Political, National and Traditional Limitations to Health Control", in Gordon Wolstenholme and Maeve O'Connor (eds.), *Health of Mankind*, London: J. & A. Churchill Ltd, 1967, pp. 196–211.

202. Ibid.
203. Ibid., p. 100.
204. Ibid., p. 100.
205. https://www.who.int/about/who-we-are/frequently-asked-questions, retrieved on December 9, 2019.
206. https://digitallibrary.un.org/record/670964?ln=en&p=Resolution+217%28III%29+A, retrieved on December 9, 2019.
207. Universal Declaration of Human Rights (UDHR), https://www.un.org/en/udhrbook/pdf/udhr_booklet_en_web.pdf, retrieved on December 10, 2019.
208. Edward Shorter, "The History of the Doctor–Patient Relationship", in W.F Bynun and Roy Porter (eds.), *Companion Encylopedia of the History of Medicine*, volume 1 & 2, London & New York: Routledge, first published 1993, reprinted 1994, pp. 783–800.
209. Amor Benyoussef & Barbara Christian, "Health Care in Developing Countries", *Social Science and Medicine,* Vol. 11, No. 6–7, 1977, pp. 399–408.
210. Raghunandan and Amit Sengupta, "Primary Health Care in Rural India: Towards Alternative Strategies", in S Bhattacharya (ed.), *Interaction of Health & Social Sciences* (Selected papers of Seminar Sponsored by the Calcutta University and UNICEF, Calcutta, December 1 & 2, 1990), Health and Social Sciences Seminar Committee, University College of Medicine, Calcutta University, 1991, pp. 73–100.
211. Ruth Sidel & Victor W Sidel, *The Health of China*, Boston: Beacon Press, 1982, pp. 19–34.
212. David M. Lampton, "Public Health and Politics in China's Past Two Decades", *Health Services Reports*, Vol. 87, No. 10, December, 1972, published by Association of Schools of Public Health, pp. 895–904.
213. Ruth Sidel & Victor W Sidel, *The Health of China*, op. cit., pp. 19–34.
214. "Directive on Public Health" (June 26, 1965) from Long Live Mao Tse-tung Thought, a Red Guard Publication, in *Selected Works of Mao Tse-tung*, available from https://www.marxists.org/reference/archive/mao/selected-works/volume-9/mswv9_41.htm#n1, retrieved on 27.11.2020.
215. "Chaina's Village Doctors take great strides", available from (http://www.who.int/bulletin/volumes/86/12/08-021208/en/) retrieved on March 4, 2018.
216. Ruth Sidel & Victor W Sidel, *The health of China*, op. cit., i–iv.
217. https://www.marxists.org/archive/guevara/1960/08/19.htm, retrieved on August 6, 2019.

218. Tarun Mondal, "Cuba-er Swasthya Byabastha", *Swasthya Bikshan*, Kolkata: Medical Service Centre, Vol. 7, No. 2–3, April-June; July–September 2001, pp. 23–34.
219. Carmelo Mesa-Lago, "Economic and Social Balance of 50 Years of Cuban Revolution", 2009, https://pdfs.semanticscholar.org/e79e/8d3ce5009b1db6807707c0ff3f27e609d99a.pdf, retrieved on August 6, 2019.
220. Edward W. Campion and Stephen Morrissey, "A Different Model—Medical Care in Cuba", *New England Journal of Medicine*, Vol. 368, No. 4, January, 2013, pp. 297–299.
221. Imrana Qadeer, *Public Health in India: Critical Reflection*, Delhi: Danish Book, 2011, p. 66.
222. Lorraine S. Wallace, "A View of Health Care around the World", *Annals of Family Medicine*, Vol. 11, No. 1, January/February 2013, p. 84.
223. "The Fight for Medicare", https://www.cbc.ca/history/EPISCONTENTSE1EP15CH2PA4LE.html, retrieved on October 22, 2021.
224. *World Nutrition* (Journal of the World Public Health Nutrition Association), Volume 5, Number 4, April 2014.
225. Harsh Sethi, "Alternative Development Strategies: A Look at Some Micro Experiments", *Economic and Political Weekly*, Vol. 13, No. 31/33, Special Number, August 1978, pp. 1307–1316.
226. Jayanta Kumar Ray, "Organising Villagers for Self-reliance: A Study of *Gonoshasthya Kendra* in Bangladesh", *The Calcutta Historical Journal* (edited by Amalesh Tripathi, Department of History, University of Calcutta,), Vol. V, No. 1, July–December, 1980.
227. David Werner, *Where There is No Doctor*, USA: Hesperian, first English edition 1977; 11th printing 2010.
228. David Werner, "Rising up in Latin America", *World Nutrition*, Volume 5, Number 4, April 2014, pp. 344–345.
229. *Jekhane Daktar Nei*, Bangladesh: Gonoshasthaya Kendra, 1390 BS.
230. *Prayojaniya Osudher Byabahar*, Dhaka: Ganaprakashani, 1992.
231. Jayanta Bhattacharya, "Sakaler Janya Swasthya Theke Swasthya Parishebar Mukta Bazar", *Ekak Matra*, Kolkata, Vol. 17, No. 1, July 2016, pp. 8–11.
232. Primary Health Care: Report of the International Conference on Primary Health Care Alma-Ata, USSR, 6–12 September 1978—jointly sponsored by the World Health Organization and the United Nations Children's Fund, World Health Organization, Geneva, 1978, pp. 11–13.
233. Ibid., pp. 2–32.
234. Ibid., pp. 3–5.
235. Ibid.
236. World Health Organization, *From Alma-Ata to the Year 2000: Reflections at the Midpoint,* Geneva: WHO, 1988, p.3.

237. Halfdan Mahler, “The Meaning of Health For All by the Year 2000”, in *World Health Forum*, Vol. 2, No. 1, WHO, 1981, pp. 5–22.
238. Susan B. Riffkin, and Gill Walt, “Why Health Improves: Defining the Issues Concerning Comprehensive Primary Health Care and Selective Primary Health Care”, *Social Science and Medicine*, Vol. 23, No. 6, 1986, pp. 559–566.
239. Jan Swasthya Abhiyan, *Whatever Happened to Health For All by 2000 AD!,* Chennai: National Coordination Committee, 2000, pp. 6–10.
240. Irfan Habib, *Man and Environment: The Ecological History of India*, Delhi: Tulika Books, 2010.
241. K. Srinath Reddy, *Make Health in India: Reaching a Billion plus*, Hyderabad: Orient BlackSwan, 2019, pp. 1–8.
242. The Preston curve is an empirical cross-sectional relationship between life expectancy and real per capita income. It is named after Samuel H. Preston who first described it in 1975.
243. K. Srinath Reddy, op. cit., p. 5.
244. Ibid., pp. 5–8.
245. Kasturi Sen, “Introduction: Restructuring Health Services—Public Subsidy of Private Provision”, in Kasturi Sen (ed.), *Restructuring Health Services: Changing Contexts and Comparative Perspectives*, United Kingdom: Zed Books Ltd, 2003, pp. 1–2.
246. Sumanta Roy, “Marxists vs Paternalists vs Liberals: Where Healthcare Stands in India”, *Down to Earth*, 29 June 2020, https://www.downtoearth.org.in/blog/health/marxists-vs-paternalists-vs-liberals-where-healthcare-stands-in-india-72022, retrieved on November 20, 2020.
247. Susanne MacGregor, “Welfare, Neo-Liberalism and New Paternalism: Three Ways for Social Policy in Late Capitalist Societies”, *Capital & Class*, Vol. 23 No. 1, Spring 1999, pp. 91–118.
248. David Sanders, “Twenty Five Years of Primary Health Care: Lessons Learned and Proposals for Revitalisation”, in Ravi Narayan and Unnikrishnan P V (eds.), *Health for All now: Revive Alma Ata*, People’s Health Movement, Bangalore, India, 2003, pp. 1–10.
249. David Werner, “The Alma Ata Declaration And The Goal Of ‘Health For All’ 25 Years Later Keeping The Dream Alive”, in Ravi Narayan and Unnikrishnan P V (eds.), *Health for All Now: Revive Alma Ata*, op. cit., pp. 15–18.
250. Ibid.
251. Jan Swasthya Abhiyan, *Whatever Happened to Health For All by 2000 AD!*, op. cit.; Gavin Mooney, “Neoliberalism is Bad for Our Health”, in *International Journal of Health Services*, Volume 42, No. 3, 2012, pp. 383–401.

252. Adam Gaffney, *To Heal Humankind the Right to Health in History*, op. cit., pp. 3–4.
253. Margaret Whitehead et al., "Equity and health sector reforms: can low-income countries escape the medical poverty trap?" in *The Lancet*, Vol. 358, September 8, 2001, pp. 833–836.
254. World Health Organization, Fifty-Eighth World Health Assembly, *Sustainable Health Financing, Universal Coverage and Social Health Insurance*, WHA 58.33, Geneva, 2005, pp. 126–129.
255. Universal Health Coverage, WHO, https://www.who.int/healthsystems/universal_health_coverage/en/#:~:text=Universal%20health%20coverage%20is%20defined,the%20user%20the%20financial%20hardship., retrieved on December 2, 2020.
256. Indranil Mukhopadhyay, "National Health Policy 2017: Securing Interests of Profits", in Imrana Qadeer, K. B. Saxena and P. M. Arathi (eds.), *Universalising Healthcare in India: From Care to Coverage*, Delhi: Aakar Books, 2021, p. 40.
257. United Nations, Department of Economic and Social Affairs Sustainable Development, https://sdgs.un.org/goals, retrieved on October 22, 2021.
258. "News", *Health Education Research*, Vol. 8, No. 2, June 1993, pp. 297–304. María Hamlin Zúniga, "The International People's Health Council", *Development in Practice*, Vol. 3, No. 1, February, 1993, pp. 59–61.
259. María Hamlin Zúniga, "The International People's Health Council", op. cit.
260. The People's Charter for Health—People's Health Movement, People's Health Assembly held at Dhaka, Bangladesh in December 2000.
261. Ibid.
262. The People's Health Movement (PHM) has national-level groups or branches, called "country circles," in many countries around the world. In India, the Jan Swasthya Abhiyan serves as the PHM country circle.
263. Ibid.
264. Ravi Narayan et al., "The People's Health Movement", May 29, 2020, Available at: https://oxfordre.com/publichealth/view/10.1093/acrefore/9780190632366.001.0001/acrefore-9780190632366-e-54#acrefore-9780190632366-e-54-bibItem-0057, retrieved on December 12, 2020.
265. People's Health Movement et al., *Global Health Watch 2: An Alternative World Health Report*, London: Zed Books, 2008, pp. 361–363.
266. Ranja Sengupta, "Privatisation, Healthcare and Social Movement in El Salvador: Solidarity brings Victory", in *International Development Economics Associates*, August 13, 2003. Available at: http://www.networkideas.org/news/aug2003/news13_El_Salvador.htm, retrieved December 5, 2020.

267. Howard Waitzkin, *Medicine and Public Health at the End of Empire*, New York: Routledge, 2011, p. 172.
268. People's Health Movement et al., *Global Health Watch 5: An Alternative World Health Report,* London: Zed Books, 2017, pp. 369–379.
269. People's Health Movement et al., *Global Health Watch 4: An Alternative World Health Report,* London: Zed Books, 2014, pp. 368–376.
270. Ibid.
271. World Health Organization, Declaration of Astana. Geneva: World Health Organization, WHO/HIS/SDS/2018.61. Available from: https://www.who.int/primary-health/conference-phc/declaration, retrieved on 19.01.2022.
272. People's Health Movement, Declaration of the Fourth People's Health Assembly—PHA4, Savar, Bangladesh, November 15–19, 2018. Available from: https://phmovement.org/declaration-pha4/, retrieved on January 19, 2022.

CHAPTER 3

Diagnosing the Maladies of Health System: A Critical Analysis

At the 1978 Alma-Ata Conference, the first international conference on universal health care, it was declared that the state should be responsible for providing health services to the people to achieve "Health for All by 2000." If the state does indeed have to carry out this responsibility, it is necessary for it to formulate an explicit health policy "that refers to decisions, plans, and actions that are undertaken to achieve specific health care goals within a society."[1] Michael Gideon Marmot, a professor of public health, once commented that "health is political"[2] and that one should "put health equity at the heart of all policy-making."[3] Health policy, in particular, is influenced by socio-economic, cultural, and educational factors and policies. Furthermore, political ideologies play a major role in formulating health policies.[4] But health policymaking and health planning are not simply a post-Alma Ata phenomenon. They also have a strong historical basis. In India, organized health policy was introduced during the colonial period. However, the imperialist government's health policy was 'minimalist,' which was a method of sustaining colonial rule in India.[5] Most of the scholars who have worked on health and medicine under the Raj, such as Kabita Ray,[6] Anil Kumar,[7] J.C. Hume,[8] and V.R Muralledharan,[9] pointed out that colonial medical policy emphasized the needs of the British military and civilians. This chapter offers a critical study of the history of the health system and health policies in India. This discussion is

© The Author(s), under exclusive license to Springer Nature Switzerland AG 2025

N. Malakar, *Historicising the People's Health Movement in West Bengal, India*, https://doi.org/10.1007/978-3-032-02696-5_3

divided into two broad sections—the first traces the evolution of the health system in India in general; the second explores its trajectory within the specific context of West Bengal.

Health Policy of India

1938–1947

The colonial government was compelled to give the Indian people some opportunity to access health services for economic reasons.[10] In colonial India, the main taxpayers had been native peasants whose death in ill-health would result in a loss of revenue. In addition, there was growing pressure from the political movement on the Raj. This pressure also came from the international business community who saw an India full of epidemics as an impediment to free trade.[11]

During the freedom movement, nationalist leaders were concerned about the health of the people. On the eve of independence, several eminent Indian medical professionals—including Dr. B.C. Roy, Dr. A.R. Ansari, Dr. Khan Saheb, Hakim Ajmal Khan, Dr. Jeevraj Mehta, and Dr. N.M. Jaisoorya—held leading roles in the national freedom movement. Influenced by the welfare state model in the United Kingdom and the socialized health services of the Soviet Union, they advocated for the establishment of a more equitable and accessible health system. This demand was to become a key component of the broader anti-colonial struggle.[12] In his presidential address given at the Haripura Congress (1938), Subhas Chandra Bose talked about the problem of the disease of countrymen. He felt the need to form a commission to draw up a comprehensive plan of reconstruction.[13] In the same year, the National Planning Commission of the Indian National Congress was established. This committee went on to establish a sub-committee on National Health under the chairmanship of Colonel Santok Singh Sokhey of the Indian Medical Service. The sub-committee submitted an interim report in 1940.[14] The sub-committee advised that:[15]

- India should adopt a form of health organization, in which both curative and preventive functions are suitably integrated and administered through one agency.
- Such an integrated system of health organization can be worked only under State control. It is, therefore, recommended; that the

preservation and maintenance of the health of the people should be the responsibility of the State.

Health planning in India was also related to post-war reconstruction in various other areas of policy, such as industry, agriculture, and social security. "The plans for India's health service also coincided with the publication of the so-called Bombay Plan…an economic plan which used socialist language…"[16] In 1943, in the last phase of colonial rule in India, the government appointed a committee named the *Health Survey and Development Committee*, under the chairmanship of Joseph Bhore, to make a survey then existing health conditions and devise a plan for the future development of health services. In 1946, the committee (popularly known as the *Bhore Committee*) submitted its historic report in four volumes.[17] In its first volume, the committee drew a picture of public health in British India. It revealed that, in addition to the general death rate, both infant mortality and maternal mortality rates were very high in comparison with other countries such as Canada, England and Wales, Italy, Java, Japan etc.; most of these fatalities were from communicable diseases such as cholera, plague, smallpox, and diarrhoea. The causes of high mortality and morbidity were illiteracy, poor public hygiene, sufficient nutrition, and adequate preventive and curative health services.[18] The committee recommended both long-term and short-term programs to develop the health condition of the country. It emphasized preventive service and an infrastructural network, and the training up of so-called 'social physicians.' It also recommended that:[19]

- No individual should lack access to medical care because of inability to pay for it.
- The services should make adequate provision for the medical care of the individual in the curative and preventive fields and for the active promotion of positive health.
- These services should be placed as close to the people as possible, in order to ensure their maximum use by the community, which they are, meant to serve.

It is pertinent to note that in their reports both the sub-committee of the NPC and the Bhore Committee mentioned that an independent India should take responsibility for the health of its people. According to Roger Jeffery, "both reports looked toward a socialized system of health services in which public health provisions dominate and eventually replace private medical practice. Both supported insurance-based services for industrial workers, but accepted that this was impractical for the mass of the Indian population in the foreseeable future."[20]

1947–1983

The report of the Bhore Committee provided the 'blueprint' for health policy in independent India, perceived by the *First Health Ministers Conference* in 1948.[21] The committee recommended a three-tier plan for health organizations: primary units, secondary units, and district hospitals. In accordance with the recommendations, primary health centers (PHCs) began to be formed in the early 1950s by the union government.[22] The first two Five-Year Plans followed the recommendations of the Bhore Committee. In 1959, the government set up the *Health Survey and Planning Committee*, chaired by Dr. A.L. Mudaliar, to survey the progress of health since 1946. It found that the quality of health services provided by primary health care was inadequate and thus it proposed an improvement in health services networking.[23]

In the 1950s and 1960s, the health sector in India focused on the control of epidemics. Mass campaigns were launched to eradicate different diseases such as malaria and tuberculosis (TB). In that period India succeeded in fighting against communicable diseases and was able to reduce the death rate from these causes.[24] However, the emphasis of those separate countrywide campaigns was on technology-centric approaches (so-called vertical programmes) to prevent malaria, smallpox, leprosy, filarial, cholera, tuberculosis, and so on.[25] In the early years following independence, health policy in India reflected an 'uneasy coexistence' between two contrasting models. The Gandhian, community-based approach emphasized rural development through environmental sanitation, nutrition, health education, and training local women and paraprofessionals, aiming for holistic improvement in public health. In contrast, Nehru's model prioritized rapid industrialization and modernization through a centralized, technology-driven, top-down strategy. It was assumed that economic growth would eventually improve health outcomes. By the late 1950s, the slow pace of the Gandhian model led to its increasing marginalization. The Nehruvian approach became dominant, focusing on curative services and single-disease control programs supported by international aid.[26] For instance in 1953, the *National Malaria Eradication Programme*

(NMEP) was launched in collaboration with the *Technical Cooperation Mission* of the United States of America and technical advice of the World Health Organization (WHO). At that time, *Dichloro Diphenyl Trichloroethane* (DDT) spraying was an aspect of the malaria prevention program. Instead of improving the socio-economic condition, there was an effort to prevent tuberculosis through vaccination with *Bacille Calmette-Guerin* (BCG). All of these programs depended on international organizations like the *United Nations International Children's Emergency Fund* (UNICEF), the WHO and the *Rockefeller Foundation* for essential chemicals and vaccines.[27]

Vertical programs are often favored by decision-makers because they are supported by powerful funders, are easier to evaluate, and offer clear, measurable outcomes. When targets are well-defined—such as reducing cases of a specific disease—it is simpler to demonstrate success. In contrast, broader health system approaches may result in modest improvements across multiple areas, which are harder to quantify and attribute directly.[28] This ease of evaluation makes vertical programs attractive to policymakers seeking visible, reportable achievements. The colonial government emphasized specific diseases such as plague and cholera, which posed immediate threats to British officials, soldiers, and urban centers. The primary aim was not to improve general public health, but to contain epidemics that disrupted trade, endangered European lives, and threatened colonial control. Continuing the colonial policy, the post-colonial government in India also focused on vertical health policies. In both colonial and post-colonial contexts, rulers have often used vertical programs to gain political advantage by showcasing quick, tangible results that serve administrative or electoral goals.

Imrana Qadeer argues that, following Independence, India's public health system experienced a major shift as the experienced officers of the Indian Medical Service (IMS) left and the service itself was abolished. This vacuum was filled by personnel with military backgrounds, who applied rigid, top-down strategies to health programs—such as the use of 'beats' and 'hire and fire' approaches seen in the National Malaria Eradication Programme. Medical education and research followed British and later American models, which were hospital-centric and technocratic, largely ignoring the social and environmental determinants of health. Even departments of Preventive and Social Medicine paid little attention to structural issues, focusing instead on individual behavior. Planning documents like the Bombay Plan and Bhore Committee Report emphasized medical institutions, vertical disease control programs, and external expertise, rather than developing integrated, community-based systems.[29]

During the two decades following independence, the development of public health and health services was on the rise. This period may be termed "the Golden Two Decades of Public Health in India."[30] But the degradation of health services had become apparent in early 1967. The government thought that "the fruits of development are being eaten away by the exponential growth of population." Thus, it was felt that family planning policy had to be undertaken.[31] In 1952, India became the first country in the world to adopt a family planning program. In 1967, on the basis of recommendations of the Planning Commission-led assessment, the *Ministry of Health* was renamed the *Ministry of Health and Family Planning*.[32] From the fourth Five-Year Plan (1969–1974) onward, a large proportion of the health budget was allocated to family planning,[33] at a time when the expenditure on health services was shrinking.[34] In the words of Debabar Banerji: "The year 1967 marked the beginning of a steep decline in the health services, culminating in the present state of its serious 'sickness'. An all-out effort to push forward the Family Planning Program at all costs had a devastating impact on the wider provision of health services."[35]

As India settled down in the 1960s and 1970s, both population and per capita income were increasing gradually. As a result, patients who had a little bit of money and were dissatisfied with the levels of rural health care could travel to urban areas to obtain health services in city hospitals.[36] The government made no attempt to improve the quality of health care. K Sujatha Rao wrote, "instead of addressing this growing demand, public policy shifted its attention to population control through expanding access to contraceptives."[37] Around that time, issues relating to nutrition, water, and sanitation were separated from the Department of Health. While matters of water and sanitation were assumed by the Department of Rural Development, and nutrition became the responsibility of the Department of Women and Child Development. The inadequate attention paid to the improvements in public health care caused the growth of private diagnostic clinics and nursing homes, in both urban and semi-urban areas.[38] Rama V. Baru wrote in her thesis that in India, "although the presence of private institutions was small during the fifties and sixties, from the seventies onwards there was a steady growth in this sector."[39]

From the late 1960s, India's priority was on family planning rather than the launching of public health campaigns and expanding public investment to assure universal access to nutritious food, pure drinking water, education, and environmental sanitation.[40] Neglecting rural health, the administrators prioritized curative services, which were 'expensive' and 'urban-based.' Public funds were used to make hospitals for the elites, many of which had modern medical technology.[41] Several scholars have argued that the development process in India was primarily elite-centric. As a result, people-centric or alternative development approaches were largely overlooked, leading to the emergence of several protest movements across the country.[42]

It is important to highlight that the prioritization of urban over rural health characterized both the colonial and post-colonial periods in India. In this respect, the case of colonial Bengal offers valuable insights. The inadequacy of hospitals and dispensaries—especially in rural areas—was repeatedly raised by members of the Bengal Legislative Assembly. In 1937, several legislators voiced their concerns about the lack of adequate medical relief in the area. Syed Nausher Ali, then minister-in-charge of the Medical and Public Health Department, also acknowledged that, in the mofussil areas, there were, practically speaking, very few hospitals or dispensaries maintained by the government.[43] The population served by each medical institution was significantly higher in rural areas than it was in urban centers. In 1940, for instance, rural areas (including all municipalities, with the exception of Calcutta) had only one dispensary for every 30,000 people across approximately 40 square miles. In 1941–1942, the average urban population served by a single medical institution was 19,730, whereas in rural areas it was as high as 37,996. Given that nearly 90 per cent of the population lived in rural regions, the inaccessibility of medical relief effectively amounted to a denial of care. During one session of the Bengal Legislative Assembly, one speaker even said that it seemed like a 'criminal conspiracy'—as if poor patients in the mofussil were left to die so that they would not make embarrassing demands for comfort and well-being.[44]

However, one important point, as Madhvi Gupta and Pushkar have argued, is that although India's urban infrastructure has undoubtedly improved over time, serious deficiencies still persist in the provision of public services in this area. While urban areas generally offer better amenities than rural regions, access to clean water, sanitation, affordable health care, and other essential services remains inadequate—particularly for low-income and marginalized populations. These gaps have a direct impact on health outcomes. Contrary to common perception, the health status of the urban poor is not significantly better than that of their rural counterparts; in fact, on several key health indicators, the urban poor fare worse.[45]

The colonial legacy in health services—especially the poor condition of government-run healthcare—will be explored in greater detail in the second half of this chapter, with particular attention to the health system in West Bengal.

In 1981, a study group set up jointly by Indian Council of Social Science Research (ICSSR) and the Indian Council of Medical Research (ICMR) stated in its report:

> We do believe that several of the assumptions on which the present system is based are wrong. For instance, there is no distinction between planning for "health" and that for "health services" so that little or no attention has been paid to the social, economic, political and cultural dimensions of health…The imported and inappropriate model of health services is top-heavy, over-centralized, heavily curative in its approach, urban and elite oriented, costly and dependency-creating.[46]

Actually, in shaping its health policy, post-independence India largely followed the path laid down by its colonial rulers. The dominant approach focused on curative measures—treating diseases by removing germs from the body—while largely neglecting preventive measures. Consequently, during the first phase of India's health policy (1947–1983), the government initiative in the health sector failed to achieve significant success. Until 1983, India did not have a formal national health policy; instead, actions in the health sector were guided by the recommendations of various committees and commissions formed at different times.[47] After the Alma-Ata Declaration, India accepted the goal of 'Health for All by 2000 AD.' The Planning Commission formed a *Working Group on Health* to determine the program to achieve this goal. The specific program for the sixth *Five-Year Plan* (1980–1985) was drawn up with that perspective in mind.[48] In 1981, Prime Minister Indira Gandhi participated in the 34th World Health Assembly in Geneva. Speaking there, she remarked that "…we must stress the need for a health revolution in developing countries, not only to wipe out diseases and to make available specialized treatment, but what is equally essential, to provide basic health care and to take preventive measures."[49]

1983 and After

In 1983, the government of India framed the first *National Health Policy* (NHP), influenced by the Alma-Ata Declaration (1978) and the recommendations of the ICSSR and ICMR's joint panel (1981).

The NHP report (1983) revealed the following: that infant mortality and maternal mortality rates were very high; that about one-third of total deaths occurred among children below 5 years of age; that infant mortality was around 129 per 1000 live births; that only 31 per cent of the rural population could access drinking water and just 5 per cent enjoyed basic sanitation; and that the major and important causes of disease and mortality were socio-economic oriented, such as poverty, lack of safe drinking water, poor environmental sanitation, and so on. Additionally, although the government spent huge amounts of money on family planning, the pace of population growth continued.[50] In the NHP report (1983), it was stated that:

> The existing situation has been largely engendered by the almost wholesale adoption of health manpower development policies and the establishment of curative centres based on the Western models, which are inappropriate and irrelevant to the rural needs of our people and the socio-economic conditions obtaining in the country. The hospital-based, disease and cure-oriented approach towards the establishment of medical services has provided benefits to the upper crusts of society, especially those residing in the urban areas...Furthermore, the continued high emphasis on the curative approach has led to the neglect of the preventive, promotive, public health and rehabilitative aspects of health care.[51]

However, the objective of NHP was to attain the goal of 'Health for All by 2000 AD' by providing "universal comprehensive primary health care services," something which was recommended by the Alma-Ata Declaration. In fact, NHP highlighted all elements of primary health care mentioned in the declaration.[52] In the 1980s, rural health care received particular special attention. The Sixth and Seventh Five-Year Plans (1980–1985 & 1985–1990) emphasized the need to build infrastructure to provide primary health care services. The target was to set up one PHC for every 30,000 people and one sub-centre (SC) per 5000 people in plain areas. This target was more or less achieved in most states. In accordance with rural health statistics in India, in December 1995, 7873 SCs and 1556 PHCs were established in West Bengal.[53] The Report of the

Independent Commission on Health in India published by the Voluntary Health Association of India (VHAI) stated that "Though the infrastructure exists in most areas, it is grossly underutilised because of poor facilities, inadequate supplies, insufficient effective person-hours, poor managerial skills among doctors, and lack of proper monitoring and evaluating mechanisms."[54] The government also emphasized the quantity, rather than the quality, of the PHCs and SCs. NHP was opposed to 'vertical' programs which were imposed from above on the people. Along with the old programs, many new 'vertical' programs, such as AIDS control and the *Revised Tuberculosis Control Programme* (RTCP) were launched in the early 1990s. Funding agencies such as the *World Bank* also focused on 'vertical' programs. It gave priority to AIDS rather than diseases such as tuberculosis, diarrhoea, and malaria.[55] Thus, by neglecting public health, India focused on controlling specific diseases repeatedly and launched a large number of programs.

The government's commitment to the health policy was not reflected in its implementation; there was a large gap between the commitment and the reality. The government did not meet the basic needs of the people, and expenditure in the health sector began to decline gradually. In the 1970s, the Keynesian economy and welfare state theory lost its popularity in capitalist countries such as the USA and the countries of Western Europe. Ronald Wilson Reagan, the president (1981–1989) of the USA and Margaret Hilda Thatcher, the UK prime minister (1979–1990), blamed the welfare state for the economic problems of capitalist countries. They popularized the idea of neo-liberal statesmanship in the 1980s. The two pillars of that policy were 'individuals' and 'markets' and the keynote was to narrow the power and scope of the state.[56]

Neo-liberal economic policy began headway in India during the 1990s. The effects of Liberalization–Privatization–Globalization (LPG) were felt in the area of public health. The *World Bank* (WB) and the *International Monetary Fund* (IMF) launched the *Structural Adjustment Programme* (SAP) globally in 1981, which were imposed on indebted Third World countries, to secure their loan repayments. In India, the structural adjustment package was introduced in July 1991, just one month after the formation of a new government with Narasimha Rao as prime minister and Dr. Manmohan Singh as finance minister. The government found that it had very low levels of foreign exchange reserves. The government soon applied for a loan of \$2.3 billion from the IMF and began fulfilling the 'anticipatory conditionalities,' including two successive devaluations and the withdrawal of export subsidies, to smooth the passage of the application. The annual budget of July 1991 fully reflected the structural adjustment package, which came to be known as the New Economic Policy (NEP). The package introduced in 1991 was sarcastically described as 'the LPG model' because of its incorporation of liberalization, privatization, and globalization as its essential components.[57] The conditions of loan under SAP were very strict. In accordance with them, it was forced to reduce expenditure in health care, to introduce service charges in public hospitals, and to hand over the responsibility for government institutions, even hospitals, to the private sector. India was also opened up to foreign multinational companies. As a result, agencies such as the WB and the IMF began to play a major role in directing policy in India, as it did in other developing countries.[58] The union health budget was slashed by a massive 20 per cent in 1992–1993 (without even accounting for inflation), from Rs. 302 crores in 1991–1992 to Rs. 244 crores in 1992–1993.[59]

The World Bank began to actively promote health sector reform (HSR).[60] This started with an influential document titled *Financing Health Services in Developing Countries: An Agenda for Reform*[61] in 1987, which was followed up by a 1993 report titled *Investing in Health*,[62] the bank promoted this policy, which curtailed the role played by the state in the delivery of health care services. *Financing Health Services in Developing Countries* criticized the 'inefficiency' of publicly provided primary health care in developing countries and advocated private sector involvement as the remedy. Though the World Bank acknowledged the role of government efforts in *Financing Health Services*, it advocated for a 'different approach' that would include four policies: charging the users of government health facilities; providing insurance or other risk coverage; using non-government resources effectively; and decentralizing government health services.[63] Similarly, *Investing in Health* focused on market-oriented reforms such as recovering expenses by charging fees for services.[64]

In the 1980s and 1990s, the agenda of the *World Bank* and the IMF encouraged privatization in the health sector. The government of India started to give concessions to multinational companies and subsidies on the import of medical equipment. During that time, many multinational companies entered the Indian market. International health insurance companies were allowed by government policy in India.[65] Although the government had cut back the outlay of public health and health care since the 1980s, in the 1990s health expenditure fell dramatically. The Bhore Committee recommended that the government should spend 12 per cent of its total expenditure on health services; after the first Five Year Plan, however, it never rose above 3 per cent. Government failed to provide health care services to the common people.[66] The target of 'Health for All by 2000' had been forgotten. Since the 1990s, the incidence of huge private hospitals had begun to grow rapidly. We know that the privatization of health services means the development of profit-based sophisticated curative health care. Government had no control over the private health care system.[67] Imrana Qadeer and Indira Chakravarthi remark that "India chose massive privatization of its medical care services. Today, it is amongst the most privatized health care systems along with Laos, Burundi, Pakistan, Myanmar etc....privatization does not help the marginalized, it only furthers their marginalisation."[68]

The effect of privatization on the health system can be observed in various fields such as drugs, medical equipment, health care, and medical education. However, the development of private health services was not a new phenomenon. In the pre-liberalization period, private health care meant small nursing homes (5–10 beds), doctors' clinics, and dispensaries, which were characterized by a domestic environment. At that time, there was a less commercial relationship between the physician and the patient. People used to receive services from nursing homes for the treatment of small diseases or surgery. Generally, they depended on government hospitals only for the treatment of critical diseases.[69] As a result, the private medical care system did not grow in any true sense at that stage. In the era of liberalization, however, medical care had become a commodity. Advances in medical technology facilitated the commercialization of medical care, resulting in an increase in the number of corporate hospitals. In India, private hospitals accounted for 14 per cent of the total hospitals in 1974; by 1993, the number had increased to 58 per cent. Most hospitals, whether public or private, were located in the urban areas. According to the statistics of 1997, 84 per cent of the total hospital beds were in the urban areas, despite 75 per cent of the country's total population living in the villages.[70]

Until the 1980s, the private sector could be described as being a cottage industry. It was the opening of the Apollo Hospital in Chennai in 1983 that marked the inauguration of the corporatization of health care in India. In the late 1970s and 1980s, some non-resident Indian doctors returned to India, creating pressure on the government to provide concessions and subsidies for the establishment of corporate hospitals. Prathap Reddy, a cardiologist who had long practised in the USA, returned to India in the late 1970s and lobbied with the Indian political class and bureaucracy to create favorable business conditions for corporate hospitals. He modelled the Apollo Hospital on the multi-specialty hospitals he had located in the USA.[71] This drive was joined by many corporate groups and non-resident Indians, such as the Escorts Groups, the Standard Organic Group, the Surlux Diagnostics Centres, the United Breweries Group, and the Hindujas, Goenkas, Birlas, and Modis.[72] Apollo Hospitals expanded to Hyderabad by 1988 and to New Delhi in 1996. By 1993, Apollo Hospitals began to place large advertisements in the national press congratulating themselves on their service to the nation. Apollo has continued to expand in India and beyond. Prior to the 1980s, India had different private hospitals based on specialization. The Apollo Hospital changed that concept. They had the byline "All departments under one roof."[73] This is the way in which, after liberalization, corporate hospitals and multinationals entered Indian health care. India witnessed an 'explosive growth' and the medical tourism industry in India expanded with the establishment of major corporate hospitals and large private investments. For instance, sophisticated medical facilities provided by the corporate health care industry in Kolkata attracted a large influx of both domestic and foreign patients from neighboring countries such as Bangladesh, Myanmar, Bhutan, and Nepal.[74]

The common people were deprived of public health services. The dilapidated state of the public health system was described in the National Health Policy (NHP) 2002. This expressed the view that the inadequate outdoor and indoor medical facilities caused overcrowding in hospitals. It also outlined the process of exploitation of people by the private medical system.[75] Being concerned about the pathetic condition of the health system in India, the government planned, in NHP-2002, that public expenditure on health should rise to 2 per cent of GDP by 2010.[76] However, NHP-2002 welcomed the participation of the private sector in health services in the same way as the NHP-1983 had invited non-governmental organizations.[77]

In 2005, the government's report[78] again revealed a picture of the country's abysmal health scenario. The report showed that India's public health indicators were lower than those in many other countries. Even neighboring countries such as Bangladesh, Nepal, Sri Lanka, which were once under colonial rule like India, were ahead in the health index. According to the report, in India, the infant mortality rate at (IMR) at the time was 68 per 1000 live births, compared with 66 in Bangladesh, 64 in Nepal, and 8 in Sri Lanka. Pakistan had eradicated smallpox, polio, and guinea worm disease before India. The report stated that "although we account for 16.5% of the global population, we contribute to a fifth of the world's share of diseases; a third of the diarrhoeal diseases, TB, respiratory, and other infections and parasitic infestations, perinatal conditions, a quarter of maternal conditions, a fifth of nutritional deficiencies, diabetes, CVDs, and second largest number of HIV/AIDS cases after South Africa."[79] The following table is an indicator of the comparative study between India and other countries.

India in comparison with other countries

Indicator	*India*	*China*	*USA*	*Sri Lanka*	*Thailand*
IMR/1000 live-births	68	<30	2	8	15
Under-5 mortality /1000 live-births	87	37	8	15	26
Fully Immunized (%)	67	84	93	99	94
Births by skilled attendants	43	97	99	97	99
Health expenditure as % of GDP	4.8	5.8	14.6	3.7	4.4
Government share of total expenditure (%)	21.3	33.7	44.9	48.7	69.7
Government health spending to total government spending (%)	4.4	10	23.1	6	17.1
Per capita spending in international dollars	96	261	5274	131	321

Government of India, *Report of the National Commission on Macroeconomics and Health*, New Delhi: Ministry of Health & Family Welfare, 2005, p. 16

It is clear that low levels of expenditure in the health sector were responsible for the deterioration of public health in India. In the period between 1990 and 2001, only 0.5 per cent of the public health expenditure was spent on preventive and promotive health services. Public spending on National Health Programmes (NHP) should have been minimum Rs. 11,210 crores, but the combined expenditure of the states and the union government was an estimated Rs 5563 crores in 2001–2002.[80] As a result, more people had become ill. Because of shortages in the government medical system people were obliged to attend private hospitals. They had to spend well beyond their capacity, often having to take out loans or sell their possessions to get money for treatment.

According to a survey conducted in eight districts across the country, private hospitals in India treated 75 per cent of non-communicable diseases (mental health, dental health, cancer, orthopedics, vascular) and 40 per cent of communicable diseases.[81] As stated above, more than 40 per cent of total hospitalized people in India had to borrow heavily or sell property to pay for treatment; on average, 58 per cent of their total annual family expenses were spent on medical treatment; and 25 per cent of hospitalized people fell below the poverty line through the payment of hospital bills.[82] It is clear, therefore, that the failure of state-provided health services strengthened the profit-oriented private health sector.

It was also observed that there was a huge difference between the rural and urban areas in terms of the provision of health services. The *National Rural Health Mission* (NRHM) was launched in 2005 by Prime Minister Manmohan Singh throughout the country with a special focus on 18 states where public health indicators and infrastructure were particularly weak. The Mission aimed to offer accessible, affordable, and quality health care to rural people, especially vulnerable sections in the country. Within its seven-year time frame (2005–2012), the mission sought to reduce the infant mortality rate (IMR), the maternal mortality rate (MMR), and the total fertility rate (TFR). To that effect, the Mission included many strategies, such as increasing budgetary outlays for health, decentralization, community participation, community monitoring system, strengthening the health service delivery infrastructure etc. The NRHM introduced *Janani Suraksha Yojana* (JSY) to reduce IMR and MMR and engaged trained voluntary health workers (Accredited Social Health Activists [ASHA]) to facilitate access to health services. The NRHM may be regarded as a major milestone in India.[83]

The 'right to health' was also recognized by the government. Prime Minister Manmohan Singh stated that "we recognize health as an inalienable human right that every individual can justly claim."[84] In the Indian Constitution, however, health has not been recognized as a fundamental right. Rather, it was included in the directive principles. In his remarks, Singh also observed that "so long as wide health inequalities exist in our country and access to essential health care is not universally assured, we would fall short in both economic planning and in our moral obligation to all citizens."[85]

The *National Rural Health Mission* was the first step towards the establishment of *Universal Health Coverage*. It was, however, only a partial success. Indeed, it turned from 'comprehensive primary healthcare' to the idea of a 'selective primary health care' program. It focused on communicable diseases and infant and child health, but did not cover non-communicable diseases (snakebites, mental health, eye care, oral health, and so on). Therefore, NRHM did not achieve the aims of the *Millennium Developments Goals* by 2015, in line with the plans laid out at the United Nations in 2000.[86]

In 2010, the Planning Commission formed a *High Level Expert Group* (HLEG), chaired by Dr. K. Srinath Reddy, to formulate recommendations for *Universal Health Coverage* (UHC). The HLEG on UHC submitted its report to the Planning Commission of India in 2011.[87] The report was particularly crucial for policymaking in India. It highlighted the government's responsibility in providing health services to the country's people. HLEG pointed out that "Ensuring equitable access for all Indian citizens resident in any part of the country, regardless of income level, social status, gender, caste or religion, to affordable, accountable and appropriate, assured quality health services (promotive, preventive, curative and rehabilitative)…"[88]

To fulfil the goal of UHC, the HLEG proposed many recommendations. These were similar to those outlined by the Bhore Committee (1946). They included the following:

- Government (union and states government combined) should increase public expenditure on health from the current level of 1.2 per cent of GDP to at least 2.5 per cent by the end of the 12th plan, and to at least 3 per cent of GDP by 2022.
- Ensure availability of free essential medicines by increasing public spending on drug procurement.
- Do not levy any kind of fees for use of health care services under the UHC.
- Do not use insurance companies or any other independent agents to purchase health care services on behalf of the government.
- Purchases of all health care services under the UHC system should be undertaken either directly by the union and state governments through their departments of health or by quasi-governmental autonomous agencies established for the purpose.[89]

Some impacts of the recommendations of HLEG were seen in the 12th Five-Year Plan (2012–2017). But public spending on health in the *plan* was not increased in accordance with the recommendations of HLEG. HLEG argued that if the government increased expenditure on health, out-of-pocket (OOP) expenditure would be reduced. The 12th Plan recommended an increase in spending on health, from 1.04 per cent in 2011–2012 to 1.87 per cent of the GDP by the end of that plan (2017). The government proposed the development of the *Public –Private Partnership* (PPP) model. It proposed that the private sector could "claim up to 20 per cent of the project cost as grant from the Government" to construct medical hospitals and colleges.[90] Through this PPP model, the government assisted in the growth of the private sector in health care. This privatization of health care is a major challenge to universal access. Unfortunately, there was no wide-ranging discussion of regulating the private sector in the report of the HLEG. Rama V Baru wrote "though the challenge of regulating the private sector in Indian healthcare has emerged as a major public policy concern, HLEG report is largely silent on this aspect."[91]

In 2014, India witnessed a political change. Under the leadership of Narendra Modi, the BJP (Bharatiya Janata Party) came to power. This new government formed the National Institute for Transforming India (NITI) Aayog replacing the age-old Planning Commission. In its first budget, the Modi government reduced health care expenditure by 20 per cent,[92] endangering many disease control programs. A draft National Health Policy-2015 (DNHP-2015) was also published by the government. After much debate, two years later, the government issued the National Health Policy-2017 (NHP-2017).[93] This document proposed that government spending on health should be increased to 2.5 per cent of GDP by 2025. Though it supported the public financing of health, it invited the private sector to become involved in advanced health care. It stated that "purchasing care after due diligence from non-government hospitals as a short-term strategy till public systems are strengthened." Yet there was no details of how the public health system would be strengthened. NHP-2017 also recommended the use of health insurance schemes to cover secondary and tertiary health care services.[94] At the very outset, it would be better to have a clear understanding regarding the government expenditure on health. For that purpose, we can go through a table to have an idea of a somewhat gradual curtailment of allocation of funds on health as compared to GDP.

Trend in public expenditure on health

Year	*Public expenditure on health as percentage of GDP*
2009–2010	1.12
2010–2011	1.07
2011–2012	1.10
2012–2013	1.09
2013–2014	1.00
2014–2015	0.98
2015–2016	1.02
2016–2017	1.17
2017–2018	1.28

Government of India, *National Health Profile 2018*, Chapter Four: Health Finance Indicators, Central Bureau of Health Intelligence, Ministry of Family Welfare, p. 172

The above table shows that public financing for health ranged from around 0.9 to 1.2 over the past one decade.

The emergence of an insurance-centric health care model proved disastrous as far as public health is concerned. In India, the health insurance market has grown significantly from the mid-2000s. T, Sundararaman wrote "a number of studies and National Sample Surveys show that existing government health insurance schemes, which already claim to cover close to 40 crore people, are failing to provide financial protection."[95] In 1963, the prominent economist Kenneth J. Arrow showed the limitations of health insurance, focusing principally with 'moral hazard.' He argued that health care in the public domain is different from that in the competitive market.[96] Nevertheless, in 2018 Prime Minister Narendra Modi launched Pradhan Mantri Jan Aarogya Yojana (PMJAY) (it was called *Modicare*, being comparable with *Obamacare* in the USA). It was the largest insurance scheme in the world, which would cover 10 crore families for secondary and tertiary care as claimed by the government.[97] Indeed, the implementation of PMJAY was a political strategy of the BJP to win the 2019 national elections. However, PMJAY is not the first government-run health insurance program in India. In 2008, the National Congress party-led UPA (United Progressive Alliance) government launched *Rashtriya Swasthya Bhima Yojana* (RSBY), which enrolled the Below Poverty Level (BPL) families. Their insurance premiums were paid by the government. Beneficiary families under the scheme could avail the health care up to a maximum of Rs 30,000 per annum according to their choice from listed hospitals.[98] But Soumitra Ghosh and Nabanita Datta Gupta in a paper opined that the RSBY failed to put any impact on financial protection.[99]

The benefit of health insurance is fully related to curative care. In addition, these schemes do not include out-patient department (OPD) treatment, on which a large number of patients depend. No one would receive an insurance payment without admission to hospital; most of the time, however, people have to spend money for treatment without receiving hospitalization. This insurance-centric health care system favored private hospitals and insurance companies. Taxpayers' money goes into the pockets of private insurance companies. With regard to RSBY, it was stated that "the plan presents a way for insurance companies to market themselves and develop brand awareness."[100] In discussing PMJAY, K. Sujatha Rao, a former Union secretary of the Ministry of Health and Family Welfare, wrote that "the poor dislike hospitalisation due to the indirect income losses they face. Therefore, effective primary care and insurance against out-patient care would be more valuable for them…"[101] According to her, in the PMJAY this aspect was overlooked by the government.[102] We may also consider another insurance scheme known as *Pradhanmantri Fasal Bima Yojana* (PMFBY) when trying to understand the anti-people aspect of the insurance policy. Drawing on the example of Maharashtra, renowned journalist P. Sainath observed that:

> Some 2.80 lakh farmers sowed soya in their farms. In a district, the farmers paid a premium of Rs. 19.2 crore, the state government and the central governments paid Rs. 77 crore each, amounting to a total of Rs. 173 crore, which was paid to Reliance insurance…The entire crop failed and the insurance company paid out the claims. Reliance paid Rs. 30 crore in one district, giving it a total net profit of Rs. 143 crore without investing a single rupee.[103]

Private health insurance originated in the USA. This was a country which lagged behind many European countries in health indicators, despite having an excellent quality of health care. America's healthcare system is the most costly in the industrialized world. The main problem in America was that of inequality; around 20 per cent of people were deprived of health insurance. It was difficult to reform the health system of America because of the dominance of the health insurance business and deep political resistance against the very idea of a 'socialized' health care system. In contrast, Canada achieved more health outcomes at a lower cost than America through state-provided health care.[104] Hence, in the United States, health activists demanded direct free health care delivery for all.

The 'Healthcare Access Quality' (HAQ) Index of 'Global Disease Burden Study 2015' (GBD) was published in the *Lancet* Journal. The study compared the accessibility and quality of health care services of 195 countries between 1990 and 2015. It was based on death rates caused by 32 diseases that could be eliminated through proper treatment. Andorra (score of 95) stood at the top of the table in the HAQ index. It was followed by Iceland, Switzerland, Sweden, Norway, Australia, Finland, Spain, the Netherlands, Luxembourg, Japan, and Italy successively. With a score of 44.8, India ranked 154th out of 195 countries. On the subcontinent, India scored lower than Sri Lanka (72.8), Bhutan (52.7), Bangladesh (51.7), and Nepal (50.8). India's situation was just slightly better than either Pakistan (43.1) or Afghanistan (32.5).[105] In terms of neonatal death rates, India scored just 14 out of 100, which was lower than even Somalia (21/100) and Afghanistan (19/100). In the case of tuberculosis disease, India's score (26) was lower than both Congo (30) and Pakistan (29).[106]

The immunization rates of India are also disappointing, with India's rates being among the lowest in the globe. UNICEF's *State of the World's Children* report, released in 2012, found that India lagged behind the 'least developed countries' in Sub-Saharan Africa in terms of general immunization such as DPT, polio, measles, hepatitis B. The only exception was the BCG vaccine. Other South Asian countries, including Nepal and Pakistan, were ahead of India in terms of immunization rates. Jean Drèze and Amartya Sen observed that "Bangladesh has achieved immunization rates of around 95 per cent for each vaccine…Child immunization rates in India increased very slowly in the 1990s and early 2000s, while Bangladesh closed most of the immunization gap over the same period."[107]

Some capitalist countries, such as Sweden, had very advanced health systems, but with no private hospitals. The local government ran the hospitals, which were larger than the corporate hospitals to be found in India. Local governments catered for the health facilities for all of the country's citizens. Nurses played a significant role in Sweden's health system.[108] We have seen that in India poor environmental conditions are one of the most significant causes of ill-health. The nation's government largely neglected environmental issues. In contrast, developed countries like the USA and the UK assured a healthy environment. Even India's neighbor, Sri Lanka, placed a focus on public health. In spite of its low GDP growth rates, Sri Lanka spent money on developing its public health system, spending 0.02 per cent of GDP on public health. A system of public health inspectors played an important role in controlling the spread of communicable diseases in the country.[109]

According to Amartya Sen, the development of health is dependent on the provision of a sufficient level of primary health care. In this context, he has focused on general failures in the system in India. He pointed out that, first, India neglected primary health care; second, India depended on private health care; and third, there was a lack of general public discussion around the issue of health care in the country (a public discussion on healthcare could help develop effective health policymaking).[110] India's major problem of inequality is another obstacle to universalizing health care. This has been increasing rapidly with the introduction of LPG in

India since the 1990s; the rich have become richer whereas the poor have to struggle hard even to secure food and primary health care.[111] But the government did not take steps to improve the conditions of the poor. Indeed, in 2019, the government further reduced taxes on the corporate sector.[112]

To overcome India's health crisis, Drèze and Sen proposed two approaches: one is to make the state-provided health service more effective than the private health service; and the second is to place a greater emphasis on primary health care and preventive medicine.[113]

But the government of India did not meet the primary health care needs of the people. No political party kept its promises once it came to power. Dr. Halfdan Mahler, the former WHO director general, once noted that "health is politics and politics is health on a large scale. If you really want to move healthy public policies forward in a big manner then you have to have the political dynamite that is necessary."[114] But in our country 'political will' has not been seen to assure universal access to health care.

Health Policy of West Bengal

In accordance with the Indian constitution, the responsibility for public health lies primarily with the state governments and union territories,[115] including the implementation of health programs of the union government. Therefore, any meaningful analysis of health policy in India must consider not only national-level developments but also state-specific experiences. As this study focuses on West Bengal, it becomes essential to examine how the state's health policy evolved—both in alignment with, and in divergence from, national trends. While the previous sections provided an overview of India's national health policy, this section traces the development of West Bengal's health system since independence. Particular attention is given to how Bengal navigated broader processes, such as the privatization of health care,[116] and whether its approach produced distinctive outcomes. This section is structured chronologically to present a clear evolution—from the early years after independence to the policies adopted during and after liberalization—highlighting continuities, changes, and policy outcomes within the state's unique political and administrative context.

1947–1977

From the very beginning, the state of Bengal had a separate department of health to cater state-sponsored health services to people in West Bengal. In 1948, Chief Minister (1948–1962) Dr. Bidhan Chandra Roy (1882–1962) himself was the minister in charge of the Department of Health.[117]

In the wake of the 1943 famine, almost 20 million people in the Bengal province suffered from cholera, smallpox, or malaria in 1943–1944. Even after independence, Calcutta experienced outbreaks of cholera and smallpox epidemics with high mortality rates. Between 3 January and 8 May 1948, some 1326 people died of cholera and 4861 died of smallpox in Calcutta.[118] A government report for 1950 showed that the influx of refugees from East Bengal was an outrageous threat to the public health of newly born West Bengal. There were pervasive outbreaks of cholera and smallpox in refugee colonies and camps due to the overcrowding. The West Bengal government appointed mobile medical and public health staff to take measures against the epidemic.[119] This resulted in a degree of improvement in different aspects of public health. The infant mortality rate was very high at this time; however, there was a declining mark compared to the previous year. Although the plague disease reached its peak in 1949, the rate of transmission began to decline in 1950.[120] That report stated that one of the formidable diseases was tuberculosis, which was causing gigantic losses to the country. To address the problem, the West Bengal government added more beds to existing hospitals and sanatoria. In addition, as a preventive measure, the BCG campaign was launched in April 1949. To provide medical and public health services to the rural population, *union* and *thana* health centers were also established.[121]

Following independence, West Bengal established a well-thought-out framework for its health infrastructure well. To reduce the pressure on the Infectious Diseases Department of Nil Ratan Sircar Hospital (NRS), in 1951, the state government assumed the initiative, establishing a 150-bed hospital in Beliaghata, Kolkata to address the issue of infectious diseases.[122] Bidhan Chandra Roy gave the top priority to community development. He made effective changes in the arena of health care through the creation of primary health centers. As a result, significant success was achieved in respect of the prevention of diseases such as malaria, cholera, and smallpox.[123] Since Roy himself was a doctor, he could easily comprehend the problems prevalent in the health system. Therefore, in the First and

Second Five-Year Plans, West Bengal spent 42.7 per cent and 37.64 per cent, respectively, on social services such as education, public health, and health service of its total allocation.[124] Dr. Roy understood that "the standard of living of most of our people is so low that better nutrition, better health, and better education are necessary preliminaries for efficient production of wealth..."[125]

In 1959, the Government of West Bengal attempted to improve its health care infrastructure based on the recommendations of the Bhore Committee (1946). The then Health Secretary and Director of Health Services in West Bengal Dr. (Lt. Gen.) D. N. Chakraborty played a pivotal role in that process. *Primary Health Centers* (PHCs) were set up at the community development block (C D Block) level and *Subsidiary Health Centers* (SHCs) were placed below PHCs. With the exception of Punjab, there were no state-run SHCs below the block level at that time. Previously West Bengal had district hospitals and sub-divisional hospitals. After the reform, however, PHCs and SHCs were developed.[126] In 1958, the government also tried to make *West Bengal Health Service* (WBHS) organized and uniform.[127] In this regard, *The Health Service (Cadre, Pay and Allowance) Rule 1958* was introduced. The rule stated "All post in the unified cadre of the West Bengal Health Service shall be made non-practicing with effect from the 1st January 1958."[128]

The Cadre of the WBHS was reorganized in April 1965.[129] Gouripada Dutta, a doctor by profession as well as a Left politician, acknowledged the laudable efforts of Dr. D.N. Chakraborty. Indeed, a number of states had gradually remodelled their structure of health service on the lines of West Bengal and the creation of *Central Health Services* (CHS) was essentially a reflection of the WBHS. It was also realized that the WBHS would serve as the nucleus of a future nationalized health service.[130]

In the 1960s, the health care service of medical colleges and adjoining hospitals in Kolkata was of relatively good quality.[131] However, outside the city, in the district towns or villages, the picture was completely different. Although there were a small number of MB (Bachelor in Medicine) and LMP (Licentiate Medical Practitioner) doctors in rural West Bengal, patients had to rely on 'quack' doctors or practitioners of other methods of medicine for treatment.[132]

The state of rural health in immediate post-colonial West Bengal closely resembled the conditions prevalent during the colonial period. As Kabita Ray writes, colonial Bengal was confronted with a peculiar phenomenon: a concentration of medical practitioners in urban areas, resulting in a stark shortage of qualified doctors in rural districts. The doctor-to-population ratio in urban regions was approximately three and a half times higher than in rural areas. Consequently, the rural population had significantly less access to modern, scientific medical care compared to their urban counterparts. Letters to the editors of various newspapers frequently highlighted the acute scarcity of doctors in Bengal's villages. Some reports noted that there were places where not even quack doctors or licensed compounders were available—let alone qualified physicians.[133]

In pre-independence India, there were two types of medical practitioners in modern medicine: university graduates, who had completed a five-and-a-half-year degree course at medical colleges; and licentiates, who had completed a shorter three-to-four-year course at medical schools, graduating with a Licence of Medical Practice (LMP). The Bhore Committee advocated for the establishment of a 'basic' doctor of modern medicine, emphasizing the importance of five-and-a-half years of university education as the foundation of the health system, while recommending the discontinuation of short-term licentiate medical courses. However, six members of the committee expressed their dissent from this recommendation, stating that "the basic doctor would not willingly fit in the rural scheme." During the 1960s, when the rural health scheme envisaged by the Bhore Committee was expected to cater to at least half of the Indian population and to employ approximately 29,000 graduate doctors, a significant number of Indian physicians migrated to the UK. This was as a result of the UK Health Minister Enoch Powell's appeal to address a staffing crisis within the rapidly expanding NHS.[134]

In 1956, it was written in the *Amrita Bazar Patrika* that "today a large section of people are keeping their faith in indigenous systems of treatment. This is due to not merely economic reasons but also to non-availability of modern medical facilities to large masses of people, particularly in remote rural areas."[135] It was also stated that "only a few years ago even the educated and enlightened families in big cities were reluctant to send patients for admission into a hospital. But now the shyness is fading away. The people have started to think differently and admission into hospitals for treatment is no longer a fearsome proposition."[136] However, there was an inadequacy of medical facilities in the district towns. On 4 August 1962, a patient named Saralabala Goswami was admitted to the paying ward of Purulia Sadar Hospital. But due to a lack of proper treatment and the negligence of doctors, the patient died after 36 hours.[137]

In 1967, the United Front, a coalition of 14 political parties, came to power, surviving in office for nearly nine months. Before assuming power, it committed to an 18-point program. The new government set itself the task of meeting "the primary needs of the people in respect of food, clothing, housing, health services and employment opportunities."[138] Within a month of its formation, the United Front government sanctioned an expenditure of 68 lakh rupees for the expansion of medical facilities.[139] In April 1967, Health Minister Nani Bhattacharya announced that a health council would be formed in each hospital to address various problems, with local MPs, MLAs, workers of different political parties, and doctors from various medical associations.[140]

The 1970s was a significant time in the history of West Bengal owing to the shift of political power. In 1972, the *Indian National Congress*, under the leadership of Siddhartha Shankar Roy, formed the government in West Bengal. Ajit Panja, the health minister, proposed that specialist doctors be sent to rural Bengal on a regular basis to provide quality medical care. However, since medicine, oxygen cylinders, and ambulances were all unavailable in rural Bengal, the government's decision had little effect on the rural population. Thus, the suffering for the healthcare of the villagers could not be alleviated. For instance, between September 15 and December 31, 1973, some 17,392 people were infected with smallpox, and 4295 of them died.[141] According to the Bureau of Intelligence, Western States, 25 per cent of boys in West Bengal were malnourished; most of the boys were infected with tuberculosis.[142] Rural people were often deprived of the medicines provided by the health centers. Average distances between health centers were 12 to 14 miles (19.3 to 22.5 km). People were unable to reach the health centers during their operating hours, which were scheduled from 8 a.m. to 11 a.m., because of the long distances involved. The health minister proposed that supplying medicines in the afternoon would solve this issue. However, the opening of evening medicine dispensaries was not able to resolve the issue. Since patients did travel a long way, it was difficult for them to return home after receiving the medicine, even in the evening. Their problems were compounded by the underdeveloped transport system. What was really needed was more health centers. In a vehement attack, on March 16, 1974, Satya Ghosal, a CPI MLA, presented an unflattering image of government hospitals to the Assembly House.[143] Even in West Bengal's approach paper to the Fifth Five-Year Plan (1974–1979), it was stated that "Emphasis should be diverted from the urban to the rural centre as far as possible. In West

Bengal this is especially important as the Calcutta metropolitan area takes a major part of the funds available for hospital, medical education and public health services."[144]

The quality of medical services in the government hospitals of Kolkata began to deteriorate in the 1970s because of the growing demand for medical care through the public institutions. In January 1974, *Jugantar* (Bangla Daily) reported on the poor condition of the R.G. Kar Hospital in Kolkata. It was found that the hospital was overcrowded in all departments, both indoor and outdoor. The government had been made aware of the shortage of beds and the lack of medical facilities in the hospital through the report of the Basu Committee, which had been formed in 1971 to assess the state of medical education and medical services in West Bengal. In 1973, Dr A.K. Basu, after whom the committee was named, had also written a letter to the chief minister about the condition of the R.G. Kar Hospital. However, the government appeared to show no concern about this matter.[145]

1977–2011

In 1977, the Left Front (LF) assumed power; it retained office in West Bengal for the next 34 years. The new government focused on matters such as rural development, including land reform or *Operation Barga* and *Panchayat* (self-government in the rural areas). The LF claimed that those two initiatives had resulted in progress in rural Bengal.[146] But Rajesh Bhattacharya remarked that "experiment was not the Marxian 'alternative'. It was the capitalist strategy."[147] But now the question is: Did the Left Front government bring about any remarkable change in the health system? That is to be probed.

Government Medical Care

Up to 1977, there was a hierarchy in the health system in West Bengal. There were, however, some changes in nomenclature in 1977. The *National Family Planning Programme* was renamed the *National Family Welfare Programme* by the Indian government. Similarly, the name of the *Ministry of Health and Family Planning* was changed to *Ministry of Health and Family Welfare*.[148] Following that, the West Bengal State Government also changed the name of the *Ministry of Health and Family Planning* to the *Ministry of Health and Family Welfare* in October of the same year.[149] In the regime of the first Left Front government, the health portfolio went to the *Revolutionary Socialist Party* (RSP), With Nani Bhattacharya being the health minister in the new cabinet.[150] At the time of United Front governments (1967, 1969–1970), he earned a great deal of respect as the health minister, because the sector achieved some improvements. The government assumed control of the management of the National Medical College and began to run evening clinics.[151] In November 1977, Nani Bhattacharya gave a positive picture in relation to public expenditure on health. He said:

> Top on the list is water supply in villages and other areas where it is scarce or 'hopelessly inadequate'. Rs 50 million has been earmarked for this to be spent by March 31, 1978. Over Rs 10 million has already been spent...The Public Health Engineering Department is strengthened. Measures to prevent diseases such as malaria and cholera and resurgence of small-pox will be taken. Out-patient departments will be improved and eight such departments are to be opened at Dum Dum, Jadavpur and Tangra. They will function like large dispensaries and be attached to big hospitals. 800 new doctors are to be recruited and 400 have already been selected. Rs 110 million have been allocated to improve the standard of treatment in hospitals. To provide better food to patients, the cost for each bed had been raised from Rs 2.50 to Rs 3.50 for tuberculosis patients. All this will cost extra Rs 7 million.[152]

Despite the increasing funds for the health sector, however, people's aspirations were not met.

On February 28, 1979, Congress MLA Satyaranjan Bapuli raised questions about the health system of the LF government in the legislative assembly. He said that the government had focused more on the party than on the infrastructural development of hospitals and other sectors; indictments had been received from doctors that there was a lack of minimal infrastructure, medicines, doctors, and medical personnel in government hospitals. Yet it had been found that Rs. 2 crores unspent money had been returned from the health department. Therefore, he argued that the shameful condition of the hospitals was not caused by the lack of money; rather, it was the result of government negligence.[153]A.K.M. Hasanuzzam an, another MLA, also brought the attention of assembly members to the poor condition of hospitals. According to him, there was no difference between the Left Front government and the previous government with regard to health administration. The government had been unable to improve the management of the hospital. Referring to his mother's treatment at ID Hospital, he observed that "people go to the hospital to save their lives, but now I see people go to the hospital to lose their lives."[154] A speech by Debaprasad Sarkar, a SUCI legislator, detailed how some low-quality drugs which had been cancelled by the health department were provided to patients. He posed the question: "does any member of assembly have anything to do with this corruption?" He also said that while the health minister had announced 'prevention is better than cure,' government spending on public health had been cut back.[155]

Responding to the deliberation, Nani Bhattacharya stated that the Ministry of Health had been fully aware that the medical system could not be expanded in line with the demand. He argued that, as a result of the growing population, hospitals became overcrowded. Public outrage over the inadequacies of the health system fell sharply on hospital staff. He added that improved hospital services could be expected by the people. But it would not be possible to change that situation suddenly because the state government did not have the money to satisfy everyone. He stated that, in response to the proposed spending of Rs. 160 crores by the state government during the Sixth Five-Year Plan (1980–1985), the Planning Commission had allocated only Rs. 60 crores. He also stated that many doctors and health workers did not perform satisfactory duties; therefore, patients were deprived of health services.[156] So he urged that "if the people cooperate with the government and be patient, I would be able to present a better picture of health next year."[157]

Shaibal Gupta wrote that the only reason for the collapse of the medical system in West Bengal was its politicization.[158] In similar remarks, MLA Debaprasad Sarkar exposed corruption in the health sector. It was alleged that teachers in the medical colleges and other medical officers were illegally recruited and that appointments were completed without the convening of any panel. These recruitments had been mainly done on the basis of 'nepotism.'[159] The 'nepotism' of the Left Front with regard to the health sector was also revealed by *The Telegraph*.[160] Partha Sarathi Banerjee, a researcher, wrote "…political control over the masses is popularly known as *'paiye deowar rajniti'* (politics of dole-giving), which is practised by all the parties vying for power. But the CPI (M) has gained mastery of this particular kind of politics by virtue of its superior and skilful party network."[161]

The second LF government, formed in 1982, had two health ministers: Dr. Ambarish Mukhopadhyay, who served as the minister-of-state-in-charge of Medical Education, Equipment and Supplies in the Department of Health and Family Welfare; and Shri Ram Naryan Goswami, who worked as the minister-of-state-in-charge of the Public Health Programme in the Department of Health and Family Welfare.[162] Both of them belong to CPI (M). Thus, the health portfolio was transferred from RSP to the hands of CPI (M). However, the scenario of the health system was unchanged.

Indeed, the West Bengal government had no specific health policy. It had no estimate of how many people would be given health care or what kind of health care would be provided. The *Health Services Association*, an association of government doctors in West Bengal, found that large numbers of the affluent population in West Bengal had received free medical care from government hospitals. There was no obstacle to stop the rich from accessing the medical services intended for the poor. In addition to residents of West Bengal, people from neighboring Bihar, Uttar Pradesh, Sikkim, Orissa, and even from Bangladesh and Bhutan, used to travel to WB to receive health care.[163] The *Health Service Association* brought this matter to the attention of the *Administrative Reform Committee*, headed by Dr. Ashok Mitra.[164] The committee report was published in 1983. Having described te plight of the hospitals, the committee made a number of recommendations: that the hospital administration should be better organized; the eligibility to receive free treatment should be specified; and that beneficiaries of government health schemes should be precluded from accessing health services in state government hospitals.[165]

The government did not follow the commission's recommendations, meaning that no positive changes were introduced into the health system. In 1983, the *NRS Medical College Hospital* collapsed as a result of the shortage of life-saving drugs. Companies stopped supplying drugs to the NRS when the West Bengal government failed to settle the due bill of Rs 86 lakh. At that time the price of medicines had risen, but the state government reduced the allocation for medicines by Rs. 8 lakh. In one incident, a boy from Midnapore who was suffering from the symptoms of a snake bite died at a hospital in Kolkata. It was alleged that the boy died without treatment due to a lack of anti-venom serum (AVS) in the hospital.[166] The government used to make the claim that no one would die of starvation in West Bengal. But when one person died due to a lack of treatment at the NRS hospital, the government argued the man was a beggar; he had died of starvation.[167] As a result, members of opposition parties became vocal in the Assembly House about the issue of NRS and demanded a statement from the health minister. However, Health Minister

Ambarish Mukhopadhyay dismissed the allegations of the opposition parties.[168]

On April 12, 1983, Health Minister Ambarish Mukhopadhyay presented the annual health budget in the Legislative Assembly. At this point, the opposition party raised the question of the absence of the government's health policy. Dr. Sisir Kumar Bose, a Congress legislator and a noted pediatrician, stated that the information had been served in a sporadic manner in the health budget; there had been no specific strategy as to the health system. When the LF had been formed in the 1970s, it had emphasized the establishment of a scientific approach to policymaking. After coming to power, however, the LF government gave importance to 'unscientific' approaches such as ayurveda, unani, and homeopathy. In the health budget, the health minister spoke of 'Health for All by the year 2000.' According to Dr. Sisir Kumar Bose, both scientific health education and scientific health policy was needed to fulfil that goal. Yet there was a lack of scientific health education in West Bengal.[169] Health minister Ambarish Mukhopadhyay gave his opinion that ayurveda had an important role to play, because many people in Central Asia and India followed such methods. In addition, he laid the blame for the deterioration of the health system largely at the door of the union government.[170] One cannot ignore Sisir Kumar Bose's arguments as recent studies showed that the Left government failed to spread scientific temperament among the masses.[171] According to Bolan Gangopadhyay, a social activist, the Left Front used the science movement as a political weapon.[172]

The West Bengal government recruited health guides and health workers. It should be pointed out, however, that just such a scheme was introduced by the union government. On April 20, 1977, Raj Narain, then Union Health Minister of the *Janata Party Government*, announced the launching of the *Community Health Volunteer/ Worker* (CHV/CHW) scheme, of which the main objective was people's participation in primary health. It was planned that the CHW scheme would make people aware of disease prevention and that it would provide basic health services in rural areas. The scheme was implemented with modifications in selected districts of the states that agreed to participate in the program. However, the Raj Narain scheme was a failure.[173] Leftists criticized the CHW scheme. Dr. Gouripada Dutta argued that the seed of the *Community Health Practitioners* course was in the approach paper of 5th Five-Year Plan of 1971–1972 proposed by the Union Health Ministry. Those practitioners would have an academic qualification of class six to class eight and would have obtained training for six weeks in an integrated course of modern medicine, homeopathy, ayurveda and siddha. According to Dr Dutta, the RMP scheme of Dr Debi Prasad Chattopadhyaya, Union State Minister of Health (1971 to 1977), took a new shape in the *Raj Narain Scheme*, which emphasized that it was "as if the health protection of the people depends only on those half-educated ill trained village workers receiving a paltry sum of rupees sixty per month." He stated that Raj Narain wanted to put 'old wine in a new bottle.' The *Indian Medical Association* was also opposed to the scheme.[174] Astonishingly, the LF Government itself introduced just such a scheme. Bruno Jobert stated that "Marxists in Bengal felt it was not opportune to organize popular mobilization in the health sector. In Bengal, as elsewhere, the CHV programme was used first as a means of reinforcing the dominant political apparatus by distributing pseudo-jobs to the young unemployed."[175]

In 1985, at the budget session of assembly, Health Minister Dr Ambarish Mukhopadhyay mad the following observations:

> Health at 'Hamlet' should replace the concept of health at the hospital. Various schemes, like Multipurpose Health Workers' Scheme and Health Guide Scheme, aimed at achieving the above objective (health for all). The operation of the Multipurpose Health Workers' Scheme has, however, received a jolt because of an order of the honourable High Court. The Community Health Guide Scheme has made great strides and about 41,000 health guides have been trained and are working at the village level. We are going to cover each village of the state with one health guide in the very near future. They are serving as a link between the people, the community and the health institutions. We hope these programmes will have a tremendous impact on the health care of the rural population and spare many of them the pain of traversing long distances to reach a health centre for minor ailments.[176]

Ultimately, however, those health workers emphasized curative care instead of the prevention of disease. There was an allegation that health guides used to receive money from the poor rural people.[177] The government used to say that doctors did not want to serve in rural areas. As a result, this three-year *Community Medical Practitioners* course was introduced. It was anticipated that these *Community Medical Practitioners* would work in rural areas to serve the villagers. Through that course, the government launched a dual system of medicine. There were MBBS doctors for urban areas; in contrast, the qualified 'quack' doctors, with the name *Community Medical Practitioners*, were sent to treat rural people. It has to be recalled at this point that the Bhore Committee (1946) had spoken of abandoning the dual system of medical policy.[178]

A community health workers course was introduced during the period of the first Left Front government (1977–1982). The government argued that the poor people in the villages would receive benefits from the deployment of *Community Medical Services*; community medical practitioners would be recruited to supplement the system. Promode Dasgupta, the then chairman of Left Front, stated that, "A new medical team will be formed to serve the people of the village. They will not compete with the specialist but will help them."[179] Furthermore, the then health minister Nani Bhattacharya remarked that, "This is a completely new kind of medical course. Many people are thinking that 'half-doctors' will be created through this course. But this kind of thinking is not correct. The students have to acquire knowledge of medicine, which prevails in medical education systems."[180] The gazette notification, dated October 15, 1980, stated that those people who completed the three-year course would receive the Diploma CMC. They would also be given a registration number.[181] However, the government eventually closed that course, and they did not introduce any appropriate initiative for those who had done the course. Sisir Kumar Bose observed, "When the Left Front government introduced this course, I supported it because I thought that it could improve public health. But sadly, the course has been closed without any discussion in the assembly."[182]

The Left government stated that the colonial system should be abolished. According to the ministerial statement: "We are aiming to redesign the conventional westernized, urban-oriented, curative based health system."[183] But the government had not been able to bridge the gap between rural and urban health. In 1984, there were 381 government hospitals in the urban areas, where just one-quarter of the total population lived. In comparison, there were just 19 rural hospitals for the other three-quarters of the population. Although there were PHCs and SHCs in the villages, these were not sufficient to cater to the needs of rural people. According to Sisir Kumar Bose, there was one PHC for more than one lakh people in West Bengal, and there was one SHC for every 65,000 people. In terms of areas covered, there was only one primary health center in the geographical areas containing 278 sq. km and one subsidiary health center for every 108 sq. km. At the same time, the communication system in the countryside was also very bad. As a result, people living in the villages used to face serious problems in accessing treatment.[184]

There are some instances of the Left Front government acknowledged their failure, even if indirectly. Forward Bloc MLA Anil Mukherjee remarked that, "In the wake of population growth in Kolkata, patients are to stay on the verandahs of medical colleges or hospitals. It is not possible to give medicines etc. to the patients in many places. Health centres, hospitals, medical colleges are not able to cope with the pressure of the growing population. Although many patients have been admitted to the hospital, they are not being taken care properly."[185] Debaprasad Sarkar, a SUCI legislator, said that, in terms of the performance of the government health service, there was no difference between the period of the Congress government and that of the Left Front period. According to him, between 1970 and 1976, the number of health centers increased from 798 to 963. During this period, some 165 new health centers were established.[186] Next, between 1977 and 1983, the number of health centres increased from 984 to 1145; in other words, 161 new health centers were established during that period, which is a very similar rate of progress.[187] Amarendra Bhattacharya, an MLA from the opposition party, alleged that the condition of Dhubulia TB Sanatorium and Netaji Subhas Sanatorium gradually deteriorated.[188] At BC Ray Hospital, the death rate of patients was 12.28 per cent in 1976; by 1983, it had increased to 27.3 per cent.[189]

Prasanta Sur held the health portfolio in the cabinet of the third Left Front government (1987–1991). He recognized the miserable condition of health in the country (including West Bengal), but blamed the role of the union government in bringing about that condition.[190]

He vowed to restore discipline in government hospitals, making a series of surprise visits to several major hospitals. He received media coverage, but the situation did not improve.[191] He visited Maharashtra and Tamil Nadu to gain first-hand knowledge about the hospital services in those states. On his return, he staged a press conference at which he announced that doctors in the two states were responsible; these hospitals were run in a very disciplined fashion. He condemned the doctors of WB and blamed them for the deterioration of health services in that region.[192]

However, the government was silent about corruption in the medical education system and hospital deaths. In some cases, a departmental investigation was carried out at the hospitals, but the authorities did not release these reports. The *Petitions Committee* of the West Bengal Legislative Assembly had published several cases of malpractice in nursing homes, in which helpless common people were the victims of the misdeeds. But the government did no action to punish the culprits. The West Bengal *Vigilance Commission*, which had the responsibility for investigating corruption in government administration, identified those accused of corruption worth lakhs of rupees. Yet the commission regretted that those involved in corruption could not be punished due to the non-cooperation of the government.[193] In 1985, it was alleged that Chittaranjan Ghosh, a cashier of District family welfare department, Murshidabad, had misappropriated government cash amounting Rs. 30 lakhs.[194]

On boards which were displayed at government hospitals, it was written that "*Sabdhan, dalal ghurchhe, kono taka deben na. Kono kajer janya kono Karmacharike kono taka deben na, free bede vortir janya kono taka poysa lage na*" (Be careful, middlemen are roaming around, don't pay them any money. Don't pay any employee for any work; it doesn't cost any money to get admission to a free bed). Looking at that board, anybody could easily appreciate the degree of corruption in government hospitals.[195] Bribery was not a new issue in government hospitals. In January 1974, *Jugantar* reported that the activities of both political and non-political touts had recently increased in Berhampore Sadar Hospital.[196] Usually, at first, the touts made close contact with the poor and illiterate patients or their relatives coming from the villages for treatment in the hospital. They then took money by making promises of getting them admitted to the hospital and getting various pathological tests done. Most, but not all, incidents might happen without the knowledge of the doctors in the hospital. However, one part of the income of the touts was to be paid to different individuals as a commission.[197] About the hospital's condition under the LF government, a social worker said: "There are hospitals, but sincerely speaking, their doors are closed for the poor, despite being free. Poor people do not get a chance of admission without negotiating, without manipulating and paying black money."[198] In 1988, Sujit Kumar Das, a leader of the *Health Service Association*, also wrote about the failure of the health administration of the Left Front government in a well-known journal named *Economic and Political Weekly* (EPW).[199]

Allegations were made that substandard drugs were being supplied from the government hospitals. Three companies, the *Eastern Drug Company, Sumico Pharmaceuticals,* and *Bomikhal Pharmaceuticals*, produced adulterated drugs. As a result, the Orissa government blacklisted them and wrote a letter to inform the West Bengal government about the matter. Yet the West Bengal government did not revoke licenses of those companies, and they were strongly criticized by the opposition party.[200] The government tried to deflect that issue by blaming it on the policy of the union government.[201] The hospitals seemed to have turned into a kind of hell. There was an incident in which a baby was dragged away from the hospital by dogs. At this point even the Chief Minister was dissatisfied with the work of the health and electricity ministries. Chief Minister Jyoti Basu himself came back without getting treatment from *Seth Sukhlal Karnani Memorial Hospital* (SSKM) due to a problem with the medical instruments in the institution.[202] The state government repeatedly faced opposition party criticism over the safety of the female staff and patients at the hospitals.[203] Sumanta Banerjee, wrote "In the process, the CPI (M) leaders and their minion(s) destroyed the state's educational and health infrastructure, by usurping the administration of prestigious institutions like the Calcutta Medical College, appointing their own protégés (who often turned out to be totally incompetent)..."[204]

The tragic and shameful Bantala incident demonstrated the ultimate failure of administration. On May 30, 1990, a Red Cross-marked government vehicle was coming to Kolkata from Gosaba Rangabelia, carrying three ladies: Renu Ghosh, a UNICEF officer in New Delhi; and Anita Dewan and Uma Ghosh, two family welfare workers from the West Bengal government's health department. A group of youths stopped the vehicle near the CPI (M) party office on Bantala Road and dragged them out of the vehicle. They were raped brutally. Anita Dewan died. Asked about the incident, the then chief minister made the shocking remark that "*E rakam to katoi hoy*" (These kinds of incidents are quite common).[205]

In 1987, the *Subject Committee for Health and Family Welfare* was set up by the *Legislative Assembly* to scrutinize the government's activity in health care. Such a Subject *Committee* had been first introduced in Kerala in 1980; it was followed by the *West Bengal Legislative Assembly*.[206] The committee consisted of members of the government and the opposition party.[207] One of the members of that committee, CPI legislator Omar Ali, stated in the assembly that, "We have not been able to improve the condition of the hospital. The condition of the health centre is even worse. Hospitals could not be kept clean and dogs could not be stopped from entering hospitals."[208] But why would the condition of the government hospitals not be improved? The government argued that the chaotic situation at the hospitals was due not only to the lack of medicines, beds or other facilities, but also to the lack of service-oriented kindness of the doctors.[209] In its manifesto published before the West Bengal assembly election of 1982, the Left Front stated that: "New hospitals and health centres have been opened, but the health services continue to be affected by non-availability of doctors in villages. There is failure to improve the sense of duty among a section of medical and non-medical staff in urban hospitals."[210] According to the party in power, in the 1960s, the medical teachers taught students diligently. Later, however, that example was no longer visible.[211]

The government argued that those who were teachers could not invest time in what was needed for the students, patients, and research. They were associated with private practice.[212] It was for that reason that the government announced a pay scale of Rs 4500 and a non-practicing allowance of Rs 1000 in order to try and prevent the private practice of medical teachers. There was no benefit, however. According to the ruling party, doctors forgot their duty and simply tried to make money.[213] As a result, the government felt the need to make laws. It was thought that if medical teachers gave deeper or undivided attention to teaching, the medical system would improve.

The non-practicing system had already been introduced in some places in the hospitals of West Bengal. Making comparisons between among non-practicing and practicing hospitals, the ruling party showed that research works had been carried out more at the non-practicing hospitals than at practicing hospitals over the previous decade. According to government estimates, the average annual numbers of research work at the non-practicing School of Tropical Medicine were 15 to 20. At NRS Hospital, non-practicing doctors published an average of 14 research papers per year, while practicing doctors published only two per year on average. Over the period 1985–1988, two research projects were conducted: at the Calcutta Medical College and the National Medical College.[214]

The then health minister Prasanta Sur said, "It would be great if we could make all medical systems turn into 'non-practicing'. But it cannot be done in one step. So we first looked at the medical education system. If the medical education system is improved, medical students will be taught to treat with compassion in rural or urban areas. We are making laws to make this difficult task possible."[215] There was a uniform cadre in the West Bengal Health Service, which had been introduced in the reign of Bidhan Chandra Roy, which Roy made all the cadres non-practicing. However, according to Gauripada Dutt, Bidhan Roy did actually give the opportunity to practice to 40 doctors. For example, the vice-chancellor of Calcutta University Subodh Chandra Mitra got the opportunity to practice during the Congress government in West Bengal. As a result, the doctors of the well-known medical colleges also began to practice.[216] The new act introduced in 1990 divided *West Bengal Health Service* in two: 'practicing' and 'non-practicing.'[217] The wording of the act was as follows:

- The West Bengal Health Service shall include a cadre for Public Health-cum-Administration as a separate unit.
- The posts included in the cadre of West Bengal Medical Education Service shall be non-practising.
- No person appointed to the West Bengal Medical Education Service shall be transferred to the West Bengal Health Service.
- No person appointed to the West Bengal Health Service shall be transferred to the West Bengal Medical Education Service.
- The posts included in the cadre for public health-cum-Administration as a separate unit of West Bengal Health Service shall be non-practising.[218]

However, only medical teachers were made non-practicing as a result of the passage of the law. When the legislation was enacted, there were some 8000 cadres in West Bengal Health Service. Of these, 1400 were associated with education and 500 with the administration. This therefore indicates that the government made 1900 doctors non-practicing and tried to improve the health system.[219] The historian Amalesh Tripathi asserted that Jyoti Basu's efficient administration would be memorable. But he could not focus on education and health. Forbidding the private practice of medical teachers led to a further deterioration of the public health system, since no one had the knowledge that the experience and ability which a medical teacher developed through practicing.[220] Tripathi pointed out that Arun Mitra or Nagendranath Roychowdhury in the Department of Obstetrics and Gynaecology in the Medical College maintained a very high standard of teaching despite also carrying out their respective private practices. Similar views were expressed by Ashok Banerjee, a significant figure in surgery. According to him, good teachers could not have been found, even with a lot of allowances to close down the private practice. He also argued that in the health system during the LF government students had learned to memorize, but they had not been taught how to measure and treat diseases practically. In addition, the health system at the village level declined. The condition of urban government hospitals was also miserable.[221]

In its report, the chairman of the *Health Subject Committee*, Gouripada Dutta, demonstrated a real picture of the health system in the state. Some lines of the report were quoted by Manas Bhunia, Congress MLA, in the Assembly House in 1995, which stated:

> The Left Front Government in the last 18 years has instituted the remarkable qualitative and quantitative change in the concept and lifestyle of people of the state. This is unfortunate that in recent years during the third session of Left Front Government stagnation has become a marked phenomenon...The activities of different units of the department have become mechanical and uninspiring. The silver lining is, the department has agreed to almost all the recommendations of the committee in principle and recommended some major changes in the functioning of the department. In spite of this commendable effort by the department optimisation of the activities has not been achieved. It has rather slowed down and has distorted functioning in many situations. This is causing public grievance. The Committee apprehends that it may have a cumulative effect.[222]

A survey was conducted in 1993 in the pediatric department of the Calcutta Medical College Hospital. This ward was important in West Bengal as at this time the children's department in private or semi-government hospitals was relatively undeveloped. The pediatric ward of that hospital was larger. But the image of the hospital that emerged in the survey was a grim one.[223] The pediatric department had three sections: a nursery for new-borns; a pediatric medicine; and a pediatric surgery. According to the hospital data, the total number of beds in those three departments was just 160. In reality, however, the number was even lower. As a result, two or three children were often kept in the same bed.[224] It had been observed that there was no improvement in that department over the previous decade. The patients' admission rate across the whole pediatric department was very high. But the number of doctors and nurses was much lower than needed. There was no system of emergency pathological tests and most of the equipment was almost unusable. The IMR in the nursery department was 20–40 per cent per day, with the main cause of death being infections. In the wake of uncleanliness in the hospital, the level of infection through mosquitoes was increased. As a result, admitted children were often affected by malaria. In addition, only 32 medicines were available in the hospital, some of which were unsuitable for use by children. So, a lot of money had been spent by the people for medicines and conducting various tests.[225] Therefore, the government hospital declined dramatically. Owing to a lack of concern about the maintenance of health records, the state health department was unable to give the *Subject Committee* a detailed list of equipment of state hospitals, which were in working condition and which were in need of repair. In the mid-1990s, the committee found that the hospital authorities had no monitoring and supervision activities for maintenance, repairs, and supply of equipment, resulting in patient suffering; medical equipment such as X-rays and sterilizer in sub-divisional and district hospitals became useless due to a lack of minor repairs; and problems with the supply of electricity were also faced by district and subdivision hospitals; some rural hospitals did not even have an electrical supply.[226]

We refer here to a story of the plight of the rural health system in West Bengal from the memory of Dr. Aniruddha Sengupta. In 1990, he joined *Belpukur Health Center* in South 24 Parganas district as a doctor. In his memoir he wrote that the health center did not have the proper infrastructure for treatment. There was a lack of electricity, medical equipment, medicines, and trained health workers. Not only *Belpukur Health Center*, but also the sub-divisional hospital in Diamond Harbour had the same condition. The main problems of the villagers were stomach upsets, fevers, coughs, and itching. Since there were no doctors in the health center, they relied on the 'quack' doctors for treatment.[227] Dr. Parthasarathi Gupta's writing also painted a miserable picture of the government medical system.[228] He wrote that:

> Let me depict a rural health centre, located an hour's distance from a country town, which is run by two or three doctors, nurses and health workers. There is a pucca quarter soaked in rainwater. There is a tube well but no water. There is a facility of electricity but no power. The operation has to be done by lighting candles if the operation equipment is available.
>
> Near the hospital lies a large pond. Patients come from quite far by renting bullock carts. They nest under the tree beside the pond. They use that water body for morning pooping, bathing, cooking, drinking, and even cow washing. A huge poster, inside the hospital, reads water can spread intestinal diseases; do not use contaminated water.
>
> There are two or three medicine stores across the hospital. In two of them, two urban doctors practise twice a day. The government doctors helplessly see that the relatives of the patients are buying medicines from those

> stores with their last money and returning home in a bullock cart. That image implies that "Health for All" will be delivered in bullock carts.[229]

If there was a limited infrastructure of treatment in the health centers, it was occupied by the socially and politically influential groups in the villages. As a result, it was impossible to provide healthcare to all. Another doctor, Smarajit Jana, had a similar experience at two health centers, in Birbhum and Nadia districts.[230] This ill-condition was similar to that experienced in other states. Numerous studies, including a comprehensive study of 19 villages by D. Banerjee of Jawaharlal Nehru University, revealed that people all over the country were actively seeking the help of the government health system but were totally frustrated at its response. No one could be satisfied with having to walk to a PHC 5 km away and discovered that the doctor was almost never there; if he or she was present, the only thing that the patients were given was a piece of paper (the prescription). They then had to travel to the nearest town to buy the medicine. That disturbing situation was evident from the findings of the ICMR study of PHC services. According to the 1988 ICMR study on primary health care services, only 15 per cent of the PHCs in the country had the requisite ratio of one PHC to a population of 30,000. In addition, only a similar proportion had the requisite number of health personnel. The shortage of lady health visitors (LHVS) was particularly acute.[231] While discussing current trends in health care in India, O.P. Jaggi stated:

> Eighty per cent of the population in India lives in the villages and twenty per cent in the cities. Qualified doctors from medical colleges are available in these places in the reverse order: eighty per cent are in the cities while twenty per cent work in the villages. There is a surplus of doctors in the cities and a scarcity in the villages. As a result, unqualified practitioners of various healing arts such as bone-setters, boil-openers, snake charmers, witch doctors, etc., flourish in the villages.[232]

The *Bengal Initiative*, in its report titled *Health: A Critical Appraisal, 1999*, showed that 90 per cent of rural diseases would have been treated by the application of effective primary health care, and 8 per cent of patients might require coming to the second level. The remaining 2 per cent of patients would need to come to the medical college hospital.[233] In West Bengal, however, the opposite picture was noticed. Money was diverted from primary health care to the urban medical system. The weakness of the primary health system destroyed the foundation of the entire health system.[234] Toward the end of the Left Front regime, there was a significant shortage of health infrastructure in West Bengal.[235]

Shortfall of health infrastructure & health manpower of West Bengal as per 2001 population in India (as at March, 2008)

Health infrastructure & health manpower	*Required*	*In position*	*Shortfall*
Sub Centres	12,101	10,356	1745
Primary Health Centres (PHCs)	1993	924	1069
Community Health Centres (CHCs)	498	349	149
Health Worker [Female] / ANM at Sub Centres & PHCs	11,280	6051	5229
Health Worker [Male] at Sub Centres	10,356	4215	6141
Total Specialists at CHCs	1396	186	1210

Government of India, ***Bulletin on Rural Health Statistics in India***, March, 2008, New Delhi: Ministry of Health and Family Welfare, 2009

We have seen in the above table that the number of primary health centres was less than what was required even in the last phase of the Left Front government. In addition, the condition of those who had survived was very bad. In 1988, the *Health Subject Committee* of WB assembly reported that 200 out of 800 sub-centres in the state were not in operation. Additionally, the condition of another 200 was unsatisfactory. In 2000, Gauripada Dutta, chairman of the *Health Subject Committee*, wrote in a report that 400 of the 921 primary health centers were "completely useless." In the case of another 300, only the outdoors facilities were in operation. The government was hesitant about closing those useless health centers. It was a risk they could not take at the time.[236] If they were to take such action, this would harm the image of the government. There was deep inequality between rural and urban health services. In West Bengal, out of total number of deaths, 46 per cent died in hospitals. In rural areas, however, this figure was 14 per cent, which was lower than the national average (16 per cent). State government documents also stated that 50 per cent of villagers in the state would not have a doctor or a trained health worker by their side at the time of their death.[237] Another reference showed that when family members got ill, 60 per cent and 24 per cent of households in West Bengal used the private and public medical sector, respectively, for treatment. Another 16 per cent of households depend on home treatments, advice from medicine shops, and other sources of treatment. There was a difference between rural and urban households. 27 per cent of rural households and 15 per cent of urban households received public sector services. Public medical care users in West Bengal (24 per cent) were lower than the national average (29 per cent).[238]

Child deaths in government hospitals also revealed a picture of the poor quality of government health services. In the first four days in September, 2002, 18 children died at Bidhan Chandra Roy Hospital in Kolkata. These deaths were caused by a lack of proper infrastructure at the hospital. The building became overcrowded and there was a shortage of oxygen cylinders. The superintendent of the hospital, Dr. Anup Mondol, remarked that "we have been complaining to the State Government about the lack of infrastructure. But nobody has lent us an ear so far."[239] Surprisingly, however, the WB health minister Surjya Kanta Misra remarked that "ten deaths in a day is nothing new, nor unusual."[240]

Negligence of treatment in government hospitals also became a common occurrence in West Bengal. We may cite two incidents here. On 17 October2003, a 20-year-old young woman was taken to a government hospital. Despite the serious condition, the on-duty doctor did not agree to admit her. After a delay, she was finally admitted. But that was too late. She did not survive. A few days before that incident, a 6-month-old girl had been taken to a medical college by her parents. But they were told to deposit Rs. 1000 before treatment would be started. These poor parents did not have that much money with him. By the time they returned with the fee, it was too late to save the child.[241]

Jyoti Basu, the chief minister of West Bengal, inaugurated the *Garden Reach State General Hospital* on May 18, 2000. Minati Ghosh, the state minister for health and Mohammad Amin, the minister for minority development, spoke first, promising that the 10-bed hospital would soon be turned into a 100-bed facility. Then Jyoti Basu gave a speech. He said "How it would be turned into100-bed hospital? ...don't lie for votes. You should say what you can do." Hearing the speech, people clapped. Jyoti Basu regained the post of chief minister in 2000 and was succeeded by Buddhadeb Bhattacharya. In 2001, a few weeks after taking charge, Bhattacharya remarked that "the medical system in the state is very bad. People are not getting treatment in hospitals; they have become disgusted with government health services."[242]

In 2008, Mansi Shah conducted a survey at SSKM hospital. In her analysis, she showed that some 56 per cent of the patients had to wait for between one and four hours to consult with doctors in the out-patient department (OPD) of SSKM hospital. Some 44 per cent of patients said that they were unable to consult with the doctors. Even they could not get any treatment as they did not know the cause of their disease. Only 11 per cent of the critical patients got the chance to be admitted in the SSKM hospital. Many patients had to be referred to other hospitals, even in critical condition, due to the unavailability of beds. In teaching hospitals such as SSKM, R.G. Kar, NRS, and the National Medical College Hospital, patients had to also wait for several days to undergo surgery and even a variety of tests. Indeed, there was a huge gap between demand and facilities in public hospitals in Kolkata.[243] The state of health in West Bengal was also portrayed in all of India's newspapers.[244] For example, it was written in a leading newspaper in India,[245] that, among the many failures in the long period of rule of the Left Front in West Bengal, the most obvious were in the areas of health care and education. Due to bad health conditions in West Bengal, ministers would often travel to other states for treatment. No health minister had been able to stop the decay of this health system. Asok Sen, a noted researcher of social science, presented his view about the government health system in West Bengal, which is as follows:

> In the last few decades, the pressure of patients in government hospitals in Kolkata has reached such a point that the whole health or medical system is on the verge of collapse. From rural health centres to district hospitals—nowhere the proper health facilities exist. In case of sufficient doctors, arrangements for diagnosis, medicines, accommodation of the patients—crisis is everywhere.
>
> The disparity of demand and supply in medical system (government hospitals) did not happen overnight. It was a gradual process. Apart from this problem, the leadership of Left-Front government found that government hospitals have become the place of corruption.[246]

Public Spending on Health

I would like to investigate the fluctuations in spending on health in West Bengal. In 1985–1986, the share of health in the revenue budget of West Bengal was 8.9 per cent. From the early 1990s, however, expenditure on health services had been reduced gradually. The share of health stood at 5.23 per cent of the revenue budget of West Bengal in 2003–2004.[247] Public expenditure on health services in West Bengal was much less than India's national average (22 per cent). Another study found that during the period 1990–1991 to 2007–2008, spending on health services as a share of the *Net State Domestic Product* declined from 1.32 to 0.74 per cent, despite the growth in revenue.[248] West Bengal lagged behind many states in India in terms of per capita expenditure by the government on health: this included medical and public health; family welfare; water supply & sanitation; nutrition; child and handicapped welfare combined. In 1986–1987, West Bengal was ranked 10th out of 15 major Indian states with Rs. 40.76 expenditure per capita per year. Rajasthan (Rs. 71.44) and Kerala (Rs. 69.59) took first and second place, respectively.[249] While per capita health expenditure in West Bengal was Rs 206.90 in 2004–2005, it was Rs. 447.51, Rs. 418.42 Rs. 408.91, and Rs. 354.31 in Tamil Nadu, Haryana, Rajasthan, and Kerala, respectively.[250] Yet a report of the *Health Subject Committee* of the West Bengal legislative assembly, headed by Dr. Gauripada Dutta, stated that if theft, corruption, waste, and nepotism could be eradicated from the health sector and the administrative structure improved, better health services would be provided to the people, despite the relatively low level of public spending on health.[251]

In West Bengal, the revenue expenditure on hospitals and dispensaries in urban areas in 1998s showed a clear bias to the urban health service. One may find the picture by probing the following table.

Actual expenditure on allopathy in between Urban Health Services and Rural Health Services, Govt. of West Bengal

Year	*Actual expenditure (in 1000 of Rs.)*	
	Urban Health Services (Allopathy)	*Rural Health Services (Allopathy)*
1985–1986	1,040,395	329,415
1986–1987	1,232,127	366,336
1987–1988	1,313,314	365,042
1988–1989	1,446,603	423,346
1989–1990	1,619,110	436,104
1990–1991	2,220,394	589,638

Government of West Bengal, *Health on The March—1991*, Kolkata: State Bureau of Health Intelligence, Directorate of Health services, p. 34

Stepping Toward Privatization

Before the 2001 WB assembly election, the privatization policy with regard to healthcare of the union government was sharply criticized by the LF. The LF declared that they would not allow the country to be sold at all.[252] Following the election, new health minister of West Bengal, Surjya Kanta Mishra, in a letter to the Union health minister on September 18, 2001, categorically stated that:

> ...The Government of India...has followed the dictates of the World Bank, International Monetary Fund and World Trade Organization leaving people at the mercy of market forces even in the important social sector of health and education...The new policies of *Liberalization Globalization and Privatization* have led to showing down of growth rate, decline in per capita consumption of cereals, increasing poverty and adverse impact on health.[253]

Interestingly, the West Bengal government itself later emphasized the privatization of health care. In January 2002, the state government introduced polyclinics at government hospital premises, provided various services such as pathological and radiological tests on a paid basis. The government argued that "Charges at these polyclinics would be cheaper than in the private sector." But it was found that the outdoor ticket price for the evening clinic was Rs. 100, which was too high for poor people.[254] We have already seen that, in 1990, in enacting the law, the LF government made medical teaching non-practicing. As a result, many senior teaching doctors resigned from government service. In 2003, however, the government further brought an act "to make it mandatory for doctors of teaching hospitals (medical colleges and SSKM Hospital) to treat patients at polyclinics in their respective hospitals on a regular basis."[255] It was written in the *Times of India* that "Some senior teachers, who had left government jobs for a lucrative private practice, have been courted again through this quasi-private arrangement."[256]

The matter of privatization was also outlined in the 2001 annual budget of the Government of West Bengal. That was not the first instance, however. The privatization policy had been initiated by the Government of WB in the late 1980s and early 1990s.[257] While speaking at a conference of doctors in 1987, the then chief minister, Jyoti Basu, urged industrialists to take charge of a few 'sick' hospitals in West Bengal. The LF government then decided to hand over several state hospitals to the private sector. The government invited a few non-resident Indians (NRI) who were interested to invest foreign capital for modern sophisticated medical care. The health minister formed an expert committee to discuss with the entrepreneurs and to manage the handover of hospitals smoothly. A few NRIs, and a large number of industrialists, visited the proposed state hospitals, including a new-made building.[258] The minister's argument about the new policy was that the quality of medical care in West Bengal had declined; patients had to travel to Madras, Vellore, Delhi, Bombay etc. to get modern treatment and they had to spend a lot of money; so 'modern sophisticated diagnostic and therapeutic facilities' should be available in the state. As the government was unable to invest for such development, the private sector should be encouraged to invest.[259] In 1988, it was written in *India Today* that "After industry, it is now the turn of health services in West Bengal to go private. The CPI(M)-led Left Front Government which, a few years ago had thrown ideology to the winds by inviting capitalists to invest in the state, wants to hand over a few hospitals, managed by the state Government, to private entrepreneurs."[260] Additionally, it was also stated that: "The invitation to entrepreneurs amounts to an official admission of failure to improve the health services."[261]

In his inaugural speech to the 44th *National Conference of the Associations of Physicians* held in Kolkata in 1989, Jyoti Basu admitted the failure of the state to provide proper health care to its population. He pointed out that the breakdown of the state-funded health care infrastructure was principally due to the shortage of funds. As an alternative proposal, he had invited the private sector into health care to share the responsibility.[262]

West Bengal was one of the first three states in which the World Bank invested in the public health sector in the mid-1990s under the *State Health System Development Project-II* (SHSDP II). A report from the World Bank stated that:

> The project would be implemented in Karnataka, Punjab and West Bengal. It would be an investment loan with policy reform in areas of resource allocation for the health sector, capacity development for sector analysis and management strengthening, enhanced participation of the private and voluntary sectors in the delivery of health services, and implementation of user charges for those who can afford to pay.[263]

The total cost of the project was estimated to be around Rs. 16,691.4 million (US$416.7 million equivalent), including US$22.2 million in taxes and duties. The *International Development Association* (IDA) financed approximately US$350.0 million, or 88.7% of total project costs net of taxes. In West Bengal, the total project cost was US$174.2 million, of which the state government contributed US$25.3 million. It was stated in the financing plan that "Under current Government of India (GOI) policies and regulations, on-lending to Karnataka, Punjab and West Bengal takes the form of 30 per cent grant/70 per cent loan at 12 per cent interest per annum over 20 years."[264] SHSDP II opened up the public health sector to the market and introduced new management policies, such as the "outsourcing of non-clinical services, bringing in non-medical managerial posts in the secondary and tertiary hospitals, and filling in posts through contractual manpower."[265] That project provided a blueprint for the future reform of the health sector in West Bengal. The government had to spend a large portion of money for tertiary and secondary hospitals; consequently, it wanted to reduce public expenditure through the privatization of various services. West Bengal formulated its health care reform policy, and became one of the first states to formulate a *Public–Private Partnership* (PPP) policy for the health sector by 2004.[266] The National Health Policy 2002 also read that "In principle, this Policy welcomes the participation of the private sector in all areas of health activities—primary, secondary or tertiary".[267]

But now the question is: What does the PPP model mean? PPP is a policy in which the government makes infrastructure and delivers services in collaboration with private organizations. The government defined that *Public–Private Partnership* is:

> an arrangement between a government/statutory entity/government-owned entity on one side and a private sector entity on the other, for the provision of public assets and/or public services, through investments being made and/or management being undertaken by the private sector entity, for a specified period of time, where there is well-defined allocation of risk between the private sector and the public entity and the private entity receives performance-linked payments that conform (or are benchmarked) to specified and predetermined performance standards, measurable by the public entity or its representative.[268]

In the PPP model, the whole system is directed by the private partners; however, there is some surveillance on the part of the government. Although the profit is shared by only the private sector, losses are consumed by both. In this system, public money has to be spent twice—the first time when the infrastructure is built with taxpayers' money; the second time when charges have to be paid by people for the receipt of the service.

With the ideological shift in government policy in the 1990s, PPPs gained greater legitimacy. The global endorsement of such schemes by the WHO and multilateral organizations influenced the national and local levels of the planning and implementation of health policy. While there has been a longstanding history of collaboration between the public and private sectors within Indian health services, recent developments, particularly the rise of PPPs, have led to substantial transformations. Before the 1980s, most of the collaborations involved the non-profit sector and were restricted to National Health Programmes. Baru and Naundy has asserted that the distinction between the PPPs of the 1990s and the earlier forms of collaboration is that the former conceptualizes both partners as equal and is arbitrated through a formal memorandum of understanding (MoU) while the latter sees the role of non-state players as peripheral to the programme.[269] According to Bijoya Roy, a public health researcher, "The introduction of private providers within the public healthcare sector changes the legal basis, raises market related concerns of equity, cost of care, quality and health rights…PPPs offer little assurance in providing integrated and universal healthcare and act as means for the expansion of the private sector."[270] In this policy, private partners impose greater user fees for the provision of services. As a result, health care is no longer a publicly funded service. It becomes just like any other consumer product, and it can only be absorbed if the consumer is able to pay for it.[271]

Under SHSDP II 214, a number of medical facilities, including 18 district hospitals and two medical colleges, were brought.[272] The project was completed in March 2004.[273] Initiatives were taken to provide instruments for intensive care units (ICU), and the provision of equipment fo procedures such as endoscopies for government hospitals. In many hospitals, however, this valuable equipment was wasted due to a lack of maintenance. Expensive computers and fax machines were provided for diagnostic centers in each district; however, X-ray and ECG equipment, which was essential for diagnosis, was not provided.[274] Indira Chakravarthy wrote "Just like in other states, the funds under this HSDP were not utilized properly; procurement and supply of medical equipment without assessing their requirements has led to idle and dumped medical equipment worth at least Rs 55 lakhs in several hospitals in the state, and has thus led to wasteful expenditure of loan money that carried an interest burden."[275]

The government introduced a user-fee system in public hospitals. In 1992, government hospitals, including the Calcutta Medical College Hospital (CMCH), began to charge such fees at all levels. In the out-patient departments (OPDs), a fee of Re 1 began to be taken per patient for medical services. Although the cost of an OPD ticket was relatively small, this was contrary to the notion of 'Health for All' because it turned free medical services into a commodity. At that time, the 'paying bed' system was introduced through a reduction of 40 per cent in the number of free beds. District hospitals also began to charge for services. All of these were aspects of the *Structural Adjustment Programme* directed by the *World Bank*.[276] Based on PPP policy, X-rays, pathology, sonography, food supply, laundry, etc. of the several health centers were handed over to various private companies. CT scan, MRI, or dialysis services (for example Echo X-ray in CMCH, Suraksha in NRS, Mediclue in SSKM) were introduced in seven medical college hospitals in West Bengal on a paying basis.[277] However, before 1992, government health services were not completely free. About 10 per cent of the urban hospital beds were divided into a system of paying beds and cabin beds. The charges for paying beds and cabin beds were Rs. 6 and Rs. 8 per day, respectively. Patients in those beds had to pay for all services, with the exception of personal services and diet.[278] Services for 90 per cent of the beds, however, remain free as before.[279]

In 1992, the government took instant steps to increase user fees without issuing any notice or taking public opinion, which resulted in an emerging chaotic situation in public hospitals. Patients who were unable to bear the service charges were sent away without treatment. In some cases, after waiting a long time at the payment counter, many patients submitted their fees only to be told to return the next day because the counter for issuing health investigation tickets had closed for the day. Moreover, some of the service charges were higher than the market price. Therefore, a committee was formed to revise the price list.[280] There was a demand to withdraw the service charges and restoration of supply of 112 types of essential and life-saving medicines. A citizens' convention was organized in Kolkata.[281] One can see the growing increase of rate for different tests, conducted in government hospitals.

Rate of investigation fees of government hospital in Rs

Diagnostic test & bed	*1992*	*1998*	*Market rate (1999)*
X-ray	10	25–30	70
E.C. G	10	25	60
U.S. G	75	300	400
CT scan	500	800	1300
Endoscopy	0	200–250	400
Echocardiogram	0	150–200	500

Tarun Mondal, "Haspatale Chargebriddhi O Swasthyer Besarkarikaran", *Swastha Bikshan*, Vol. V, Issue 1, April–June 1999, pp. 2–8

The government promised that the introduction of user fees in government hospitals would improve the quality of health services. People need not go to private hospitals for treatment. Thus, it would be possible to close the booming market of the private healthcare sector. User fees would be taken only from those who can afford it. In the case of the poor, medical services would be provided free of cost. Those who were really poor would get free medical services on the basis of an 'Indigent Certificate' with monthly family income level of Rs. 1500 or less given by elected representatives, including the Panchayat Pradhans, urban board/municipalities' representatives, MLAs, and MPs.[282] The LF government argued that the ticket system in the outdoor department would stop corruption and reduce unnecessary crowding in the public hospital. The state government stated that the money collected in a hospital would be spent on the improvement of that hospital.[283] However, Dr. Margaret Chan, then director-general of the WHO, stated that "User fees for health care were put forward as a way to recover costs and discourage the excessive use of health services and the over-consumption of care. This did not happen. Instead, user fees punished the poor."[284] User fees created a barrier to universal access to health care. Studies from Uganda in Africa show that user fees hindered access to health care. In consequence of the abolition of user fees, however, the tendency of people to utilize health care services increased; in particular, poor people received more benefits.[285] In Andhra Pradesh, the peoples' movement was successful in forcing the state to abolish user fees. Kerala and Jharkhand also stopped their collection. However, the National Urban Health Mission (NUHM), in its draft mission document, called for the 'judicious' exercise of user fees as an effective mechanism for the mobilization of resources.[286]

In 1993–1994, and Advanced Medical Research Institute (AMRI) hospital was established based on the PPP model. The government handed over the house and land of Niramay Polyclinic, which had been established by Dr. Gunen Roy, to a private company owned by the Shrachi group. At that time the government's share was 51 per cent; by 1996, however, it had fallen to 26 per cent.[287] To establish KPC Medical College, the first PPP model medical college and hospital in West Bengal, the LF government provided land of the Dr. K.S. Roy TB Hospital at Jadavpur to a private company in return for an annual lease of Re 1.[288] In 1998, the West Bengal state government planned the involvement of non-governmental organizations (NGOs) to offer mobile (boat-based) health facilities to people in the Sunderbans region, as part of the *World Bank*'s health systems development project. Five NGOs were selected to provide mobile services. In 1999, the Government of WB tasked the Southern Health Improvement Samity (SHIS) with delivering river launch-based health services in four villages of South 24 Parganas. Since then, mobile health services were provided in 192 villages across two districts (North 24 Parganas and South 24 Parganas) of the state. The government contributed funding for boat maintenance, personnel salaries and operational expenses. The mobile health clinics got monthly medicine supplies for distribution free of cost. However, women complained about the level of the health services provided by NGOs.[289] They observed a number of flaws in the services, containing user fees, irregular camps, shortages of medicine, a lack of ambulance service during emergencies, and so on.[290] Baghajatin State General Hospital was set up in 1991 after a campaign by the people. The people of South 24 Parganas were heavily dependent on the hospital, as the nearest hospital, M. R. Bangur Hospital, was always over-crowded and could not provide the necessary levels of medical care. But the government of WB did not pay proper attention to Baghajatin State General Hospital. Finally, in 2011 the government signed an MoU with *Ashraya Charitable Trust* of Bangalore, allowing them to set up a private clinic at the main portion of the hospital.[291] The same PPP model was continued even after the change of power in the state.

Following the putting into practice of SHSDP II in 1996, the user fees were revised twice: once in December 1998, and again in 2002. In 2002, the fee for visiting the OPD was increased from Re. 1 to Rs. 2 and the monthly family income bracket for hospital fee exemption was raised from Rs. 1500 to Rs. 2000.[292] It was also stated in a government memo that "Thirty per cent (30 %) of the beds in all indoor patient departments of all the Teaching Hospitals, District Hospitals, Decentralised Hospitals, Sub-Divisional and State General Hospitals of the State shall be earmarked as paying beds by the Superintendents of the respective Hospitals w.e.f. 1st April 2002."[293]

The state government decided to hand over health care management to local agencies under an initiative called *People's Health in People's Hand*, which is a decentralized model. Cheema and Rondinelli defined decentralization as "the transfer of authority, responsibility, and resources through de-concentration, delegation, or devolution from the centre to lower levels of administration."[294] The government of West Bengal concentrated primarily on two aspects of decentralization: the de-concentration of power and resources to the district and lower levels of health administration; and the devolution of powers and resources to local bodies that are *Panchayats*.[295] However the government of WB experienced problems in staffing the PHCs. Therefore, initiatives were taken to implement the mode of PPP in health care. The government of WB established *District Health Committees* (DHCs) to plan and manage health programs and services at the district level. District health committees (DHCs) got permission from the Department of Health and Family Welfare to hire the services of private doctors on a contract basis.[296] In their annual budget, it was stated that "…serious attention has been given to achieving accountable decentralization by directly associating the *Gram Panchayats* in the management of health sub-centres, *Panchayat Samitis* in management of new Block Level Primary Health Centres and *Zila Parishads* in management of hospitals at district level."[297] However, while there was no hint regarding the handing over of health centers to private partners in the statement of the state's finance minister, that was clearly mentioned in the *Draft Policy for Public Private Partnerships in the Health Sector* published in 2004, which stated that: "The department of health, Govt. of WB may hand over management of health sub-centres, primary health centres, BPHCs/rural hospitals to private/NGO partners under lease agreements (with or without government staff)."[298] Analysing the draft, Achin Chakraborty wrote that "The whole document is overwhelmingly focused on the issue of managing health care facilities from a managerial perspective rather than with reference to population health goals."[299] In 2004, pay-based diagnostic services under the PPP framework was introduced in government hospitals in rural areas. In early 2010, the government introduced different user fees for the same medical services provided in the PPP mode and directly provided by the government in government rural hospitals.[300]

In 2006, the government of WB published a document on PPP which stated that it had been: ""encouraging establishment of *public private partnerships* (PPP) during last three years...PPP implemented by Department of Health and Family Welfare, Govt. of WB will be aimed at consolidating the strengths of public sector as well as private sector and at the same time addressing the weaknesses of both the sectors."[301] In relation to the background of introducing PPPs it was also stated that:

> ...India records a high private health spending, which is amongst the highest in the world...State governments do not have the adequate funds to invest in infrastructure development of hospitals...users of health services are still spending huge amount either directly or indirectly to avail the services...Out of Pocket expenditure health spending in West Bengal was equal to Rs 193.70 per capita in 1995. This was slightly less than the all-India average of Rs 222 per capita per year...The private sector is expanding but issues like quality assurance and pricing mechanisms are yet to be adequately addressed...Public Private Partnerships provide quality health care to the people at affordable and reasonable price.[302]

The PPP mode covered diagnostic services, including digitized radiology, CT and MRI scans, pathology, biochemistry, dialysis services, and other supportive services such as diet, security, and waste collection. Operations such as cataract surgery, and also the management of primary health care facilities, were also conducted through these channels. The WB government advanced an argument that "the private sector diagnostic centres being un-regulated have grown sporadically and high prices along with uncertain quality remain serious concerns not only for the referring doctors but also for the patients." Thus, the PPP mode was promoted by the government.[303] In 2001, the government of West Bengal took the initiative to introduce CT scan facilities in seven medical colleges in West Bengal under PPP. In 2008, the government decided to implement the same scheme across all district hospitals in the state.[304] A memorandum published by the Health and Family Welfare Department in February 2010 stated: "Administrative approval was accorded to set up Diagnostic Facilities under PPP in total number of 155 RHs/BPHCs from time to time since April 2004."[305] In 2005, the government of West Bengal put in place 133 ambulance services at the rural hospital (RH)/block primary health center (BPHC)/primary health center (PHC) level through PPPs in eight districts: Cooch Behar, Darjeeling, Jalpaiguri, Birbhum, Purba Medinipur, Paschim Medinipur, Purulia, and Bankura.[306] In 2010, the government of WB increased the rate of 44 diagnostic tests performed in the diagnostic units under PPP in RH/BPHCs,[307] which also increased the financial burden on the patients. On 3 December 2011, in a state-level consultative meeting of the government took decisions that:

- Overall, PPP is state-wide mandate and private partners are welcome. In the coming days they are sure to increase in number in the state.
- To ensure viable business opportunity Private Partner (PP), all the Medical Officers would have to refer all diagnostic cases to PP appointed under their jurisdiction.[308]

Due to the inadequacy of state-provided health services, common people were forced to buy private health services. Again, the people faced more problems as the government had no control over the private health system. In addition, rural masses who could not afford to buy treatment from large private nursing homes or hospitals have resorted to so-called 'quack; practitioners. In a study conducted in West Bengal by 'Future Health Systems: Innovations for Equity' in 2006–2007, it was found that the proportion of people going to unqualified medical practitioners (UMPs henceforth) for non-hospitalized treatment was 54 per cent in the rural areas of West Bengal.[309] As a result, 'quack' practices increased to a greater extent in rural areas. Therefore, the OOP expenditure of people also increased.[310]

In 1999–2000, approximately 32.5 million people (25.5 million in rural and 7 million in urban) in India went below the poverty line to pay for medical treatment. In terms of OOP expenditure in non-institutional care, West Bengal was one of the highest among the states of India.[311] Swadhin Mondal et al. conducted research on catastrophic medical expenditures in West Bengal. Catastrophic OOP expenditure for health services means that household spending on health is greater than 40 per cent of non-food expenditure.[312] They surveyed three districts (Malda, North 24 Parganas, and Bankura) in West Bengal during the period January–March 2007, showed that health care expenditure for illness and hospitalization was one of the major causes of the deteriorating economic condition or chronic poverty of the families in West Bengal.[313]

Thus, it can be said that, between 1977 and 2011, a number of initiatives were taken by the LF government but none of them were successful in delivering the desired level of quality health service. As a result, there was an erosion of the people's trust in government health services. According to Dr. Rezaul Karim, former president of the *West Bengal Doctors' Forum*, political changes in 1977 in West Bengal ushered in an outstanding prospect to improve the health care system. In addition to spending money to improve the health system, there was a need for a competent leader who could understand the demands for health care. Yet the health system worsened rather than improving.[314] In the year which marked the collapse of the LF regime, *The Telegraph*, the English daily newspaper, reported: "The 'sick wagons' chugging out of Howrah railway stations, packed with patients headed to south India, is a sorry statement on how the Left failed to channel investments into health care."[315]

2011 and After

In 2011, after 34 years of Left rule in West Bengal, the All India Trinamool Congress (AITC), led by Mamata Banerjee, came to power. This change was driven by the failure of the LF government in various sectors, including health. In Surjit S Bhalla's words, "Very few people seem to want to vote for her—but everyone wants to vote against the CPM. This means that Bengal does not love Mamata less, but that it hates the CPM more."[316] Before coming to power, Trinamool Congress (TMC) pledged that it would fulfil the social demands of the people. In the manifesto for the West Bengal assembly election 2011, AITC promised that: "the new health system will be built. As the days go by, the demand for medical infrastructure has become important. Common people of the state are not getting access to treatment. Our goal is to deliver life-saving treatment to the poorest people. Our journey is towards health for all."[317] But many were sceptical, saying that "despite Mamata Banerjee's promise of meeting these public demands, her government, being bound neo-liberal order, will have to make a right-about turn, and traverse the same trajectory that had been initiated by her predecessor—the Left Front."[318]

Mamata Banerjee was sworn in as chief minister. The people of West Bengal began to think that the government of *Ma-Mati-Manush* would come as a blessing for common people, as the health portfolio had been very badly neglected during the rule of the previous government. Moreover, the chief minister taking the health portfolio into her own hands set an example. We have already mentioned that Dr. B.C. Roy also held the health portfolio. Within a week of taking oath (May 24, 2011), the chief minister made an unannounced appearance at SSKM Hospital to inspect the infrastructure. She then made subsequent surprise visits to other hospitals. She talked to the patients and instructed the doctors and staff of the hospitals to perform their duties properly.[319] Over the period 1987–1996, the then health minister Prasanta Sur had made surprise visits to government hospitals. Mamata Banerjee adopted the same approach. She planned to reshape the state health system and to set up super-specialty hospitals in the districts, so that normal people would not have to travel to Kolkata for treatment. However, a large amount of money was required to implement those programs. To collect that money, she followed the policy of the Left, which means that she emphasized the PPP model, which could be regarded as a transitional phase toward the total privatization of health care.[320]

In 2011, a document was uploaded on the government's website seeking proposals from those who were interested to collaborate with the government in build health care infrastructure following the PPP model. In that document, the new government stated that: "This Concept Paper is initiated to draft a state policy for strengthening healthcare infrastructure in the state in *Public Private Participation* (PPP) mode. This is also to seek suggestions from interested market players to provide inputs to ensure success of the planned ventures."[321] The government decided to convert Ramrik Hospital and a maternity hospital, sited in Paikpara in Kolkata, from a government hospital to a PPP hospital. The government talked to Dr. Devi Sethi, a well-known corporate brand doctor in India, about the proposal. Dr. Sethi expressed his wish to build hospitals in PPP mode in 15 districts including Siliguri and Bolpur.[322]

The 200-day action agenda that was announced in the election manifesto of TMC did not materializes, however. The PPP model gained considerable attention from the government. Private enterprise was allowed in government-run hospitals from rural hospitals to urban super-speciality hospitals, and was also permitted to make profits. The government did not impose any conditions on the health traders participating in the PPP model, but it did ask them to inform the government about the conditions in these institutions. Indeed, there was nothing more than surprise visits and some symbolic announcements. There was no sign of improvement in medical services in rural health centers and district hospitals in the state during the first 200-day of Mamata Banerjee-led government.[323]

Thus, the policy of the LF government was continued in the health sector of West Bengal. The health care gap between rural and urban, the shortages of doctors and health workers, the inadequate infrastructures in hospitals, and the other shortcomings, all continued.[324] In the first half of September 2013, 49 children died at B.C. Roy Hospital.[325] West Bengal was still highest in the country in terms of the rates of diarrhoeal diseases among the states of India. 2,052,123 and 1,888,794 diarrhoeal cases were found in the state in 2016 and 2017, respectively.[326] A study conducted by the Springer group depicted the poor status of public health and health care in West Bengal. The authors wrote that "more than 78 per cent of inhabitants in Kolkata prefer the private medical sector over the public medical field, because of the poor quality of care service, the absence of nearby facilities and excessive waiting times at government health centres."[327]

A report of *The Economic Times*, an English daily, showed that "in India, there was one government doctor for every 10,189 people (the World Health Organization (WHO) recommends a ratio of 1:1,000), or a deficit of 600,000 doctors, and the nurse: patient ratio is 1:483, implying a shortage of two million nurses."[328] The situation in West Bengal also reflected that shortage. In accordance with the *National Health Profile 2018*, there was one government allopathic doctor in the state for every 10,411 people.[329] The data also showed that the bed and population ratio was 1:1170 in government hospitals in West Bengal.[330] But Mamata Banerjee, as had the LF government before him, blamed the policies of the union government for the shortage of doctors.[331] The state also argued that there were not enough doctors to recruit; CM said "we invited applications for 10,000 posts for doctors. We got only 4,000 applications."[332] Some doctors argued, however, that doctors did not want to work in government hospitals because of the lack of proper infrastructure and security. Moreover, the growth of private hospitals in the state ensuring jobs for doctors enhanced the problem of a shortfall of doctors in government hospitals.[333] Although the average number of doctors was relatively satisfactory at this time, government data showed that there was a distinction between rural and urban areas in terms of the numbers of doctors.

Population served per doctor in West Bengal, 1983–2015

Year	*Population served by doctor*		
	Rural	*Urban*	*Average*
1983	5386	808	2162
1990	5246	842	2191
1997	5192	815	2167
2004	4500	808	1974
2011	4581	773	1782
2012	4740	739	1739
2013	5781	676	1697
2014	5112	675	1651
2015	5100	673	1647

Government of West Bengal, *Health on the March 2005–06*, State Bureau of Health Intelligence, Directorate of Health Services, Kolkata, https://www.wbhealth.gov.in/other_files/2005/10_6.html, retrieved on October 21, 2020; Government of West Bengal, *Health on the March 2015–16 (Draft)*, State Bureau of Health Intelligence, Directorate of Health Services, Kolkata, p. 247

Total number of registered allopathic medical practitioners having recorded their address in the state

Paramedical staff also play a crucial role within the health care system. A report published by the union government in 2012, *From Paramedics to Allied Health Professionals: Landscaping the Journey and Way Forward*,[334] has pointed out that, over the past decade, there has been a significant transformation in health care delivery primarily driven by advancements in science and technology. There is now a greater acknowledgment than ever before that the provision of health services is not solely the responsibility of doctors and nurses. Instead, it is now a team effort, drawing upon the expertise of both clinicians and non-clinicians. Historically, these professionals or health service providers have been referred to as 'paramedical staff,' 'paraprofessionals,' or 'health technicians.' K.S. Reddy, the dean of the Jawaharlal Institute of Post-Graduate Medical Education and Research (JIPMER), noted that "during the process of cardiac surgery, the functions of the heart are taken over by a machine. The person who handles this machine literally holds the life of the person. Any mistake can be life-threatening. This is why we now insist on trained staff to handle such machines."[335] It is also very important to develop trained paramedic personnel for emergency treatment. They can provide support to critical patients before they are admitted to hospital. Staff trained as 'emergency medical technicians' are regarded as an essential part of hospital treatment in Western countries. Their role in saving the lives of patients injured in accidents, or those who suddenly fall ill, is recognized and appreciated. This service is not given less importance in the mainstream of the medical system in India. There is a tendency in this country to confine medical services to hospital premises. Ambulance facilities are available outside the hospital to provide emergency services. But most of the ambulance drivers and their assistants know little more than carrying patients and putting on oxygen masks. The report revealed that there was an "overall national shortage of approximately 64 lakh AHPs (Allied Health Professionals), with the highest deficiencies being in the states of Uttar Pradesh, West Bengal, Maharashtra, Bihar and Andhra Pradesh".[336] The national level estimates of the shortfall of the various categories of AHPs included the dearth of ophthalmology professionals, rehabilitation-related professionals, surgical and intervention-related technicians, medical laboratory technicians, healthcare workers specializing in the fields of radiology and imaging, audiology and speech-related professionals, medical technologists, dental technologists, health care professionals helping in surgery and anaesthesia, and miscellaneous technologists. According to the report, the huge shortage of well-qualified human resources in the health services is one of the major reasons for the high rates of morbidity and mortality in India. A report by *The Telegraph*, published in March 2018, stated that government-run healthcare facilities in West Bengal had a shortfall of around 2500 paramedics. This has led to the emergence of a significant number of untrained personnel who masquerade as medical professionals and prey on people's desperation. A senior official from *Swasthya Bhawan*, the headquarters of the state health department, stated that "government hospitals and smaller health care centers have 9,000 sanctioned posts of paramedics, but 28 per cent of these are vacant."[337]

In India, patients' relatives often complain that they have to pay extra to get timely and better services at government hospitals; the attitudes of doctors and other paramedical staff are unsympathetic and rude; they have to endure long waits at hospitals and are harassed by hospital staff. Hence, people are forced to look for alternatives and these are becoming increasingly expensive. Members of patient families in Orissa have stated that "they avoided going to government hospitals because the 'staff there behaves rudely, abuses us, and refers to us here and there to extort money'."[338] This scenario also exists in West Bengal. One of the reasons for this suffering of patients is the lack of human resources. Temporary staff at hospitals justified their acceptance of bribes by stating that their salaries are very low and that it is difficult to feed their families. Some hospital staff are also alleged to be involved in various forms of corruption. Even worse things also occur: On August 8, 2024, a female PG intern was brutally raped and murdered at R.G. Kar Medical College Hospital in Kolkata. This heinous act, along with the subsequent efforts to conceal the evidence, has brought to the fore the persistent issues of corruption and lawlessness within the health care system. One significant aspect of this corruption pertains to biomedical waste management. At the heart of this issue is a booming 'black' market in the unauthorized commercial reuse of biomedical waste. This is not a new problem, however. In 1998, a report by *The Economic Times* stated that biomedical waste was being smuggled out of a total of 272 hospitals, nursing homes, and clinics in Kolkata and back to the same hospitals and clinics where they were sold back and reused. The All India Institute of Hygiene and Public Health conducted a survey on the biomedical waste business from April 1996 to September 1997. The survey found that the staff of various hospital wards used to collect hospital waste twice a day. Syringes, saline bottles, blood and urine bags, medicine foil, rubber tubes, gloves, and other materials were all stored behind the hospital. It was alleged that those objects were subsequently sold to local purchasers separately. Materials would then be sent to the manufacturer through brokers. Furthermore, objects that could be reused were preserved in the wards rather than being thrown away. According to a survey carried out at the *Calcutta Medical College* in 1998, a sweeper's daily earnings from selling hospital waste were 16 rupees 43 paise.[339] The illegal reuse of such biomedical waste might lead to the spread of many infectious diseases.

On October 22, 2014, the chief minister of the state announced that all people, irrespective of whether they were Above Poverty Line (APL) or Below Poverty Line (BPL), would get treatment, diagnostic tests, and medicine free of cost in government hospitals. The next day, however, the revised announcement stated that free beds would be provided in all government hospitals with the exception of medical colleges/super-specialty hospitals. In 2015, the chief minister again announced that all of the services of government hospitals would be available free of cost.[340] However, by virtue of the huge gulf between demand and supply in government hospitals, patients had to wait for a long time to receive free medical care, which compelled them to go to private hospitals.[341] Therefore, the patient's OOP expenditure and suffering for health care continued. Most of the spending on the health of people was for pathological tests and medicines.[342] But there was a dearth of medicines at hospital outlets. In addition, PPP model-based diagnostic centers did not allow people for pathological testing free of cost.[343] Mention should be made here that, after assuming power in December 2012, the AITC government scheduled the rate for digital X-ray (digital X-ray CR Rs. 70 and digital X-ray DR Rs. 100) for different government hospitals in West Bengal.[344] In 2014, another government document stated that "fifty per cent of beds in CCU/HDU will be designated as 'paying' and the rest would be 'free'. Free beds should be made available to poor patients to be identified by the *Rogi Kalyan Samity*/MSVP/ Superintendent of the Hospital…Charges for paying beds may be collected as per Memo No. HF/O/MS/121/W-10/2001 dated: 18.03.2002 till the Government publishes the revised rates for CCUS/HDU beds."[345] It is important to note that medical care was also announced as being free for those who could afford the expense of medical care. The tragedy was created because the chief minister had announced a policy of free medical treatment without taking into account monetary provision.[346]

But now the question is: Were the medical services really available for free of cost in the government hospitals? In this context, we may mention two incidents. On the first occasion, a patient was admitted to the burns unit of MR Bangur Hospital. When he was released from the hospital, seven months later, his family's expenses for treatment stood at Rs. 1.5 lakh. The patient's family literally had to sell their land to access the expensive antibiotics![347] Another incident occurred in Purulia. A patient admitted to the gynaecology department of Deben Mahato Hospital there. She needed an operation on her uterus. The combined cost of medicine and various diagnostic tests of her family were 8000 rupees![348] There were more examples of that kind. According to an official of the health department (*Swasthya Bhaban*) in West Bengal, at an earlier stage, when there had been free beds in government hospitals for Below Poverty Line (BPL) patients, some tests, minor surgeries, and certain medicines were all free of charge. All other expenses related to healthcare had to be borne by the patients. It would be the same in the future.[349] Besides this, most of the people for outpatient care did not visit government hospitals because of poor accessibility/long distance and long waiting times.[350] Montu Bose and Arijita Dutta conducted a comparative study on health spending in three Indian states: Tamil Nadu, Rajasthan, and West Bengal. They found that in 2014, the OOP expenditure on medicine during hospitalization in public hospitals was highest in West Bengal (INR. 1917), followed by Rajasthan (Rs. 1516). During 2014, Tamil Nadu (Rs. 150) had the lowest

OOP spending on medicine during hospitalization in public hospitals. In 2014, West Bengal (Rs. 5603) accounted for the highest total medical expenditure in public institutions, followed by Rajasthan (Rs. 3629) and Tamil Nadu (Rs. 451). In West Bengal, poor people spent Rs. 3438, the highest amount, on public hospitalization in 2014, compared to other groups, while in Tamil Nadu the poorest class spent the least (64.72). In 2014, the benefit shares in overall public subsidies of the poorest in Tamil Nadu and West Bengal was 54.17 and 31.30, respectively.[351] They came to the conclusion, saying that the "Tamil Nadu model has been successful in achieving its health goals after implementing various health financing strategies. Following the same strategies, Rajasthan is also reaping the benefit. However, West Bengal has failed to achieve its goals."[352]

After 2011, the level of government hospital beds was still inadequate, whereas the number of beds in private hospitals increased greatly. A statistic of *Frontline* showed, "in 2010, the total number of beds in a government hospital in West Bengal stood at 55,942, which increased to 62,665 in 2015—a growth of 11 per cent; in the same period the growth in private health care establishments was around 26 per cent (from 34,281 beds to 43,564)."[353] Apart from this, one statistic that also has to be noted is that, in 2017, there were around 48 government-run hospitals in Kolkata, whereas the number of private hospitals stood at nearly 370.[354]

We may mention here a brutal incident which took place at a corporate hospital in Kolkata. Sanjay Roy, a resident of Dankuni, was seriously injured in a road accident near Baltikuri in Howrah on February 16, 2017. He had been admitted to *Apollo Hospital* in Kolkata on the same day. Surprisingly, the hospital bill for his treatment stood at Rs. 7.23 lakh on February 23. As a result, his family members decided that the patient should be moved to the state-run SSKM Hospital. But the authorities in the *Apollo* stated that the patient would not be released if the amount due was not paid in full. But it was difficult for a middle-class family to pay the bill; the patient's family did not have that amount. Finally, Sanjay Roy was shifted to Seth Sukhlal Karnani Memorial Hospital (SSKM) on February 23 after his family deposited a fixed deposit receipt as security. Tragically, he died in SSKM the next day.[355] After that incident, many intellectuals condemned the government health policy. Bolan Gangopadhyay, a human rights activist, asserted that because of the lack of government monitoring infrastructure, government health care facilities did not reach the people.[356]

Private hospitals are only for the rich; they are not available to poor people. Before the 1990s, there were only two big private hospitals in

Kolkata.[357] We have already discussed the changes that took place in the 1990s, when the LF government encouraged the corporate sector. After 2011, the private medical market in West Bengal grew even further. Common people have knowledge about the exploitative character of private hospitals. Additionally, some doctors shared their experiences about private medical care. Dr Goutam Mistry, a senior cardiologist of Kolkata, wrote:

> ...I joined a major hospital and worked there for seven years...In order to benefit the hospital and meet its commercial needs, one has to do things like keeping patients in the hospital longer than necessary, and doing unnecessary investigations and procedures (including angioplasty) since there was pressure from the management of the hospital. My conscience began pricking me, and left that hospital.[358]

Similarly, a general practitioner in Kolkata, Dr. Parthapratim Das, observed that "unnecessary procedures are advised because there is pressure on the cardiologist from the multi-speciality hospital to meet their targets."[359] As mentioned earlier, parents' relatives also complained against private hospitals.[360] According to Uttan Bandopadhyay, a health activist, "...in most cases, harassment of patients in private hospitals happens in the form of inflated bills...In most cases, the poor and the general masses go to private hospitals not out of choice, but out of compulsion." In 2012, the West Bengal government formed a multidisciplinary Expert Group (EG) to "assess the status of the patent care services" provided by government institutions and to submit a report. The chairman of this EG was Dr. Subrata Maitra.[361] In 2015, in respect of the health system of West Bengal he stated that the cost and quality of service in the private health care sector is not regularized. At the same time, it is impossible for the government to provide service to all, considering the population. The state is, however, developing a number of projects that follow the PPP model.[362]

During the LPG (Liberalization, Privatization, Globalization) era, technology-based treatment and the privatization of health care has broken the previously cordial relationship between doctors and patients. The concept of a family physician has declined. Solomon R. Benatar et al. commented "Over the past 150 years, health care delivery has expanded from what was largely a social service provided by individual practitioners, often in the home, to include a complex system of services provided by teams of professionals, usually within institutions and using sophisticated technology."[363] The concept of public health has also changed. In the present day, health means medical care. The fear of disease—'risk factor'—always affects people in this era.[364] This is why, "so called 'master health check-ups' have become an unregulated commercial activity in India, sometimes causing significant harm to physical and mental wellbeing of individuals."[365] As discussed earlier (see Chap. 1), Ivan Illich described this trend as the "medicalization of life," in which medicine increasingly dominates everyday experiences and creates iatrogenic illnesses—health problems which are caused by medical treatment itself. Rather than repeating his full argument, it is worth noting that this idea remains relevant today, especially as commercialized healthcare continues to blur the line between healing and sickness.[366] A study carried out by Dr Barbara Stanfield showed clear statistics of deaths due to iatrogenic disorders in America.[367] Similarly, in the case of India, it is estimated that about 5,000,000 people die every year as a result of medical negligence.[368] Sabyasachi Chatterjee also focused on 'iatrogenic' diseases in an article.[369] In this light, he questioned the operation of the air conditioner-based hospital system (both private and public) in West Bengal. The fire at AMRI Hospital in Kolkata on December 9, 2011 was an example of corporate negligence. In that accident, 92 people died because of 'asphyxia' after the fire began in the basement of the five-story building. As the building was centrally air-conditioned, the walls were completely sealed, with no ventilation. The central air-conditioning system sprayed toxic smoke from the basement into the building. Dense smoke gathered in the patient wards, causing low visibility and smothering those who were trapped in wards.[370]

In other incident, a former chief minister of West Bengal was infected with the "nosocomial infection" from the hospital. He was admitted to a corporate hospital at Salt Lake in Kolkata suffering some senile conditions and a shortness of breath. In the hospital, three germs—*Klebsiella, Pseudomonas*, and *Acinetobacter*—which lived in the hospital equipment, clothes, and dust, entered his body. When he was first admitted to the hospital, these germs had not been present. He was readmitted even after returning from the hospital and eventually died from the infection.[371]

The exploitation of private hospitals increased to such an extent that the West Bengal government was forced to bring in a new law. The state government enacted *The West Bengal Clinical Establishments (Registration, Regulation, and Transparency) Act, 2017*,[372] to regulate private hospitals. However, this new law differed little from *The West Bengal Clinical Establishments (Registration, Regulation) Act*, which had been passed by the Left Front government on July 29, 2010. It is to be noted that in 2010 the AITC opposed the bill because there was no regulation issued by the union government. However, the act of 2010 could not be implemented properly. Accordingly, there were doubts regarding changing the exploitation of health traders by this law. It is pertinent to note here that the licence of AMRI Hospital was revoked in 2011 after a fire broke out in the hospital, at Dhakuria in Kolkata. However, the hospital authority was allowed to run their business again. When it did so, there was no shortage of business.[373]

The *West Bengal Clinical Establishments (Registration, Regulation, and Transparency) Act, 2017* reads "any clinical establishment which has received land or other facility from the Government during initiation and in course of continuance of their projects shall be responsible to provide completely free treatment to 20 per cent of Outdoor Patient Department patients and 10 per cent of Indoor Patient Department patients..."[374] The WB government stated this endeavor of private hospitals should be viewed as part of their "Corporate Social Responsibility."[375] We must remember, however, that it is foolish to expect social responsibility from those who understand nothing but making money. It is also pertinent to note that the same instruction was mentioned in the *Clinical Establishment Rule in 2003*, which was based on the *West Bengal Clinical Establishment Act of 1950.*[376] Shantanu Sen, national president (2018–2019) of the *Indian Medical Association* (IMA), stated that "There are several private medical establishments in the State which have taken concessions from the State government, but none of them fulfil their part of the agreement."[377] One crucial allegation against the *West Bengal Clinical Establishments Act 2017* was that hospitals or health centers run by the union government, state government, municipalities, *panchayats*, etc. were kept outside the scope of this act, at a time when the government health service was getting worse.[378]

To 2018, the state government had established 42 super-specialty hospitals. Some of these were in remote areas, like Salboni in West Midnapore.[379] In most cases, however, there were only glossy buildings; the infrastructure and services did not improve.[380] It is a matter of great regret that, though Salboni super-specialty hospital had been initially run successfully by the government, the responsibility to manage it was given to the Jindal Group, a private company, at the end of 2018. An agreement was also signed in September 2018.[381] Mamata Banerjee stated that Salboni Super-Specialty Hospital would henceforth be run by the Jindal

Group. They would provide better healthcare there.[382] It has been found in our discussion that the LF government advanced the same arguments before launching such projects. After 1977, people gained knowledge about the party system in West Bengal. During the period 1977–2011, the people understood that the party meant CPI (M). Partha Chatterjee, a prominent social scientist, wrote "…the party and its local functionaries are the principal arbitrators in all social, family and personal disputes and the principal facilitators when individual villagers need help in matters of health, education, finances, employment or travel."[383]

This trend of dominance carried on even after 2011. The dominance of party leaders over hospital officials did not come to an end. The party's doctors controlled the non-political doctors by exploiting their fear of being transferred to remote areas. Administrative decisions in the hospitals, such as patient admissions, pathological tests of patients, and equipment sanctioned for various departments were taken by the party's doctors.[384] We may observe that the health policy of Mamata Banerjee-led government is, to reuse an old phrase, 'putting old wine in new bottles.' A professor of a government-run leading medical college in West Bengal has observed that "Healthcare is not a 100-metre dash but more of a marathon towards excellence. If the Left ran in the direction opposite to the other runners during its three-decade stay, the new government hasn't yet taken off."[385]

Instead of emphasizing primary and preventative care, the West Bengal government has been promoting an insurance-based health care approach. In 2020, the AITC-led government extended the *Swasthya Sathi*[386] health insurance scheme to provide citizens with access to secondary and tertiary health care up to Rs 5 lakh per annum per family. It appears that the ruling party introduced this program simply in order to gain political advantages in the 2021 Legislative Assembly Elections.[387] However, Mampi Bose, a researcher associated with National Health System Resource Centre, assumed that *Swasthya Sathi* might put the population of the state at the risk of being exposed to high medical expenses in the absence of a sound public health system.[388] Leftist academician and former CPI(M) M.P. Malini Bhattacharya has argued that "be it Ayushman Bharat or *Swasthya Sathi*, these are targeted schemes, which means the expenses will go from the existing general health care system. Unfortunately, in such targeted schemes, those who need the services most are often excluded. Instead, if the general health care system is improved, then almost everybody will enjoy the benefit of government services equally."[389]

We can conclude that, even after several decades of independence, the government of this country has not recognized the people's 'right to health.' The state government has just followed the policy of the union government. As a result, corporate power has grown; after the 1990s, a large number of corporate hospitals came into being in West Bengal. The state's people have become slaves to corporate power. They were repeatedly deprived of proper health services. However, in order to achieve 'Health for All,' mass movements must be launched.

Notes

1. World Health Organization, "Health policy", https://www.who.int/topics/health_policy/en/, retrieved on December 3, 2019.
2. Michael Marmot, *The Health Gap: The Challenge of an Unequal World*, United Kingdom: Bloomsbury Publishing, 2015, p. 20.
3. Ibid., p. 309.
4. Alok Mukhopadhyay (ed.), *Report of the Independent Commission on Health in India*, New Delhi: Voluntary Health Association of India, 1997, p. 36.
5. Dipesh Chakrabarty, "Sharir Samaj o Rashtra", in Goutam Bhadra (ed.), *Nimnabarger Itihas*, Kolkata: Prativas, 1998, pp. 165–166.
6. Kabita Ray, *History of Public Health: Colonial Bengal 1921–1947*, Kolkata: K.P. Bagchi & Co., 1998.
7. Anil Kumar, *Medicine and the Raj: British Medical Policy In India, 1835–1911,* New Delhi: Sage Publications, 1998.
8. J.C. Hume. "Colonialism and Sanitary Medicine: The Development of Preventive Health Policy in the Punjab, 1860–1900", in *Modern Asian Studies*, Vol. 20, No. 4, 1986, pp. 703–724.
9. V.R. Muraleedharan, "Malady in Madras: The Colonial Government's Response to Malaria in the Early Twentieth Century", in Deepak Kumar (ed.), *Science and Empire: Essays in Indian Context (1700–1947*), New Delhi: Anamika Prakashan, 1991, pp. 101 12; V.R. Muraleedharan, "Rural health care in Madras Presidency: 1919–39", in *Indian Economy and Social History Review*, Vol. 24, No. 3, September 1, 1987, pp. 323–334.
10. Arabinda Samanta, *Rog Rogi Rashtra: Unish Shataker Bangla* (*Disease, patient, state: Nineteenth-century Bengal*), Kolkata: Progressive Publishers, 2004, p. 28.
11. Imrana Qadeer, *Public Health in India: Critical Reflection*, Delhi: Danish Book, 2011, pp. 82–83.

12. Debabar Banerji, "Landmarks in the Development of Health Services in India", in Imrana Qadeer et al. (eds.), *Public Health and the Poverty of Reforms: The South Asian Predicament*, New Delhi: SAGE Publications, 2001, pp. 42–43.
13. "Presidential address of the 51st session of the Indian National Congress at Haripura February 19, 1938," in *Selected Speech of Subhash Chandra Bose*, Delhi: Publication Division, Government of India, 1962, pp. 72–94.
14. K.T. Shah (ed.), *Report of Sub-committee on National Health* (Sokhey Committee), National Planning Committee, Bombay: Vora & Co, 1948.
15. Ibid., pp. 141–142.
16. Sunil S. Amrith, *Decolonizing International Health India and Southeast Asia, 1930–65*, New York: Palgrave Macmillan, 2006, p. 57.
17. Government of India, *Report of the Health Survey and Development Committee (Bhore committee)*, Volume I to IV, Delhi: Manager Publication, 1946.
18. Ibid., Vol. I.
19. Ibid., Vol. II, chapter-III, pp. 17–32.
20. Roger Jeffery, *The Politics of Health in India*, Berkeley: University of California Press, 1988, p. 112.
21. Alok Mukhopadhyay (ed.), *Report of the Independent Commission on Health in India*, op. cit., p. 36.
22. Meera Chatterjee, *Implementing Health Policy*, New Delhi: Manohar, 1988, p. 7.
23. Government of India, *Health Survey and Planning Committee* (Mudaliar Committee), New Delhi: Ministry of Health, Government of India, 1961.
24. Ravi Duggal, "Historical Review of Health Policy Making", in Leena V Gangolli et al. (ed.), *Review of Healthcare in India*, Mumbai: CEHAT, 2005, pp. 28.
25. Ibid.
26. Radhika Ramasubban, "History of public health in modern India 1857–2005", in Milton J. Lewis and Kerrie L. MacPherson (eds.), *Public Health in Asia and the Pacific: Historical and Comparative Perspectives*, London: Routledge, 2008, pp. 87–105.
27. Government of India, *Health Survey and Planning Committee (Mudaliar Committee)*, op. cit.
28. Sandy Caimcross et al., "Vertical health programmes", *The Lancet*, Vol. 349, June 1997.
29. Imrana Qadeer, "Continuities and Discontinuities in Public Health: The Indian Experience", in Amiya Kumar Bagchi & Krishna Soman (eds.), *Maladies, Preventives and Curatives: Debates in Public Health in India*, New Delhi: Tulika, 2005, pp. 79–94.

30. Debabar Banerji, "Landmarks in the Development of Health Services in India", in Imrana Qadeer, Kasturi Sen and K R Nayar, *Public Health and the Poverty of Reforms: The South Asian Predicament*, New Delhi: Sage Publications, 2001, p. 44.
31. Debabar Banerji, "The battle for total health care", in *India International Centre Quarterly*, Vol. 14, No. 3, Forty Years, India, 1987, pp. 119–128; Debabar Banerji, "The People and Health Service Development in India: A Brief Overview", *International Journal of Health Services*, Volume 34, Number 1, 2004, pp. 123–142.
32. Leela Visaria and Rajani R. Ved, *India's Family Planning Programme Policies, Practices and Challenges*, UK, USA: Routledge, 2016, p. 47.
33. Government of India, Ninth Five Year Plan, 1997–2002, New Delhi: Planning Commission, Government of India, Vol. II, p. 246.
34. Alok Mukhopadhyay (ed.), *Report of the Independent Commission on Health in India*, op. cit., p. 48.
35. Debabar Banerji, "Landmarks in the Development of Health Services in India", op. cit., p. 45.
36. K. Sujatha Rao, *Do We Care? India's Health System*, New Delhi: Oxford University Press, 2017, pp. 12–13.
37. Ibid.
38. Ibid.
39. Rama Vaidyanathan Baru, *Some Aspects of the Private Sector in Medical Care and Its Inter-relationship with the Public Sector: A Study of Hyderabad-Secunderabad*, unpublished PhD thesis, Centre of Social Medicine and Community Health School of Social Sciences, Jawaharlal Nehru University, New Delhi, 1992, p. 56.
40. Achintya Kumar Dutta, *Trauma in Public Health: Tuberculosis in Twentieth-century India*, Kolkata: K.P. Bagchi & Company, 2018, p. 87.
41. Debabar Banerji, "The battle for total health care", op. cit.
42. Skylab Sahu, State, *Civil Society and the Politics of Health: Exploring Gender, Sexuality and HIV/AIDS in India*, London: Taylor & Francis, 2024.
43. Kabita Ray, *History of Public Health: Colonial Bengal 1921–1947*, Kolkata: K.P. Bagchi & Company, 1998, p. 191.
44. Ibid., p. 192.
45. Madhvi Gupta and Pushkar, *Democracy, Civil Society, and Health in India*, London: Palgrave Macmillan, 2015, p. 43.
46. Health for All: an Alternative strategy, report of a study group set up jointly by Indian Council of Social Science Research (ICSSR) & Indian Council of Medical Research (ICMR), Pune: Indian Institute of Education, 1981, p. 10.

47. Mudaliar Committee (1959), Chadha Committee (1963), Mukherjee Committee (1965), Jungalwalla Committee (1967), Kartar Singh Committee (1973), Shrivastav Committee (1975). Full reports of these committees are available at: https://www.nhp.gov.in/miscellaneous/committees-and-commissions.
48. Government of India, *Report of the Working Group on Health for All by 2000 A.D.*, New Delhi: Ministry of Health and Family Welfare, 1981.
49. Address By The Right Honourable Mrs Indira Gandhi, Prime Minister of India, in Thirty-Fourth World Health Assembly, Geneva, 4–22 May 1981, Verbatim Records of Plenary Meetings Reports of Committees (World Health Organization Document No. WHA34/1981/REC/2), pp.73–76.
50. Government of India, *National Health Policy*, New Delhi: Ministry of Health and Family Welfare, 1983.
51. Ibid.
52. Ibid.
53. Alok Mukhopadhyay (ed.), *Report of the Independent Commission on Health in India*, op. cit., p. 38.
54. Ibid., pp. 38–39.
55. Ibid., pp. 39–42.
56. Ashok Kumar Mukhopadhayay, "Udarnitir Rashtratatwa", in Dipak Kumar Das (ed.), *Rajnitir Tatwakatha*, vol-1, Ekushe, Kolkata, second edition 2006, pp. 81–114; Jan Swasthya Abhiyan, *Whatever Happened to Health For All by 2000 AD!*, Chennai: National Coordination Committee, 2000, p. 15.
57. Biplab Dasgupta, *Globalisation: India's Adjustment Experience*, New Delhi: Sage Publications India Pvt Ltd, first edition 2005, cited edition 2006, pp. 15–26.
58. Jan Swasthya Abhiyan, *What Globalization does to People's Health!*, Delhi: National Coordination Committee, 2006, pp. 12–18.
59. Debabar Banerji, "A Simplistic Approach to Health Policy Analysis: The World Bank Team on the Indian Health Sector", *International Journal of Health Services*, Vol. 24, No. 1, 1994, p. 153.
60. Juan Carlos Verdugo, "The Failures of Neoliberalism: Health Sector Reform in Guatemala", in Meredith Fort, Mary Anne Mercer, and Oscar Gish (eds.), *Sickness and Wealth the Corporate Assault on Global Health*, Cambridge, Massachusetts: South End Press, 2004, p. 57.
61. World Bank, *Financing Health Services in Developing Countries: An Agenda for Reform* (A World Bank Policy Study), Washington, DC: World Bank, 1987.
62. World Bank, *World Development Report 1993: Investing in Health*, Washington, DC: World Bank, 1993.

63. World Bank, *Financing Health Services in Developing Countries: An Agenda for Reform*, op. cit., pp. 25–48.
64. Juan Carlos Verdugo, "The Failures of Neoliberalism: Health Sector Reform in Guatemala", op. cit.
65. Rama V Baru, "Privatisation of Health Services: A South Asian Perspective", *Economic and Political Weekly*, Vol. 38, No. 42, October 18–24, 2003, pp. 4433–4437.
66. Jan Swasthya Abhiyan, *Health System in India: Crisis & Alternatives,* Delhi: National Coordination Committee, 2006, pp. 19–28.
67. Ibid.
68. Imrana Qadeer and Indira Chakravarthi, "The Neo-liberal Interpretation of Health", *Social Scientist*, Vol. 38, No. 5/6, May–June 2010, pp. 49–61.
69. Amrita Bagchi, *Health Care in Crisis: The Changing Pattern of Private Health Care in Post-Independence Kolkata*, PhD thesis, Department of History, Jadavpur University, Kolkata, 2010, pp. 102–129.
70. Alok Mukhopadhyay (ed.), *Report of the Independent Commission on Health in India*, op. cit., pp. 252–258.
71. Rama V. Baru, "Medical–Industrial Complex Trends in Corporatization of Health Services", in Purendra Prasad and Amar Jesani (eds.), *Equity and Access Health Care Studies in India*, New Delhi: Oxford University Press, 2018, pp. 80–81.
72. Amrita Bagchi, "Metamorphosis of Health Care: The Transformation of 'Private' to 'Corporate' Health Care In Post 1947 India", *Proceedings of the Indian History Congress*, Vol. 71, 2010–2011, pp. 1223–1232.
73. Sarah Hodges, "'It All Changed after Apollo' and Other Corporate Hospital Myths", in Sarah Hodges and Mohan Rao (eds.), *Public Health and Private Wealth: Stem Cells, Surrogates, and Other Strategic Bodies*, New Delhi: Oxford University Press, 2016, pp. 139–164.
74. Anu Rai, *Medical Tourism in Kolkata, Eastern India*, Switzerland: Springer International Publishing, 2019.
75. Government of India, *National Health Policy-2002*, New Delhi: Ministry of Health and Family Welfare, 2003.
76. Ibid.
77. Biswanath Pariya, "Jatiya Swasthyaniti 2002: Besarkarikaraner Joralo Padakshep", in *Swasthya Bikkhan*, January–June, 2003, pp. 38–47.
78. Government of India, *Report of the National Commission on Macroeconomics and Health*, New Delhi: Ministry of Health & Family Welfare, 2005.
79. Ibid., pp. 15–17.
80. Ibid., p. 7.
81. Ibid., p. 5.

82. Government of India, *National Rural Health Mission (2005–2012)*, Mission document, New Delhi: Ministry of Health & Family Welfare, available from: https://www.wbhealth.gov.in/uploaded_files/nrhm/nrhm.pdf.
83. Framework of Implementation: Meeting people's health needs in rural areas, National Rural Health Mission (2005–2012), Ministry of Health and Family Welfare, Government of India, 2005.
84. Kalpana Sharma, "Viewing Health as an Inalienable Right", *India Together*, 7 October 2005, http://www.indiatogether.org/health-op-ed retrieved on 03.04.2019.
85. Ibid.
86. K. Srinath Reddy, *Making Health in India*, Hyderabad: Orient Blackswan, 2019, pp. 48–54.
87. Planning Commission of India, *High Level Expert Group Report on Universal Health Coverage for India*, New Delhi: Planning Commission of India, 2011.
88. Ibid., p. 56.
89. Ibid., pp. 15–51.
90. Government of India, *Twelfth Five Year Plan (2012–2017)*, Social Sectors, Volume III, Planning Commission, pp. 18–19.
91. Rama V Baru, "A Limiting Perspective on Universal Coverage", *Economic and Political Weekly,* Vol. 47, No. 8, February 25, 2012, pp. 64–66.
92. Vikas Bajpai, "National Health Policy, 2017: Revealing Public Health Chicanery", *Economic and Political Weekly,* Vol. 53, No. 28, July 14, 2018.
93. Government of India, *National Health Policy, 2017,* New Delhi: Ministry of Health & Family Welfare.
94. Ibid.
95. T Sundararaman, "Opinion: Modicare is more an election gimmick than a real solution to India's health needs", *Scroll*, February 5, 2018, https://scroll.in/pulse/867524/modicare-is-more-an-election-gimmick-than-a-real-solution-to-indias-health-needs retrieved on April 17, 2020.
96. Kenneth J. Arrow, "Uncertainty and Welfare Economics of Medical Care", *The American Economic Review*, Vol. 53, Issue 5, December 1963, pp. 941–973.
97. Ibid.
98. Government of India, *Rashtriya Swasthya Bima Yojana Guidelines*, March 13, 2008, available in http://www.nrhmhp.gov.in/sites/default/files/files/RSBY_Guidelines_13_3_08.pdf, retrieved on February 26 2021.
99. Soumitra Ghosh & Nabanita Datta Gupta, "Targeting and Effects of Rashtriya Swasthya Bima Yojana on Access to Care and Financial

Protection", *Economic and Political Weekly*, Vol. 52, No. 4, January 28, 2017, pp. 61–70.

100. Jackie Range, "India's Poor Get Health Care in a Card", *The Wall Street Journal*, August 26, 2008, https://www.wsj.com/articles/SB121971773721671817, retrieved on February 26, 2021.
101. K. Sujatha Rao, "The Government's Previous Health Insurance Schemes Failed. Why Should the New One Work?", *The Wire*, February 5, 2018, https://thewire.in/health/the-governments-previous-health-insurance-schemes-have-failed-why-should-the-new-one-work retrieved on April 17, 2020.
102. Ibid.
103. "NDA's crop insurance scheme bigger scam than Rafale: P. Sainath", *Business Standard*, November 3, 2018, https://www.business-standard.com/article/news-ians/nda-s-crop-insurance-scheme-bigger-scam-than-rafale-p-sainath-118110300875_1.html, retrieved on November 24, 2021.
104. Jean Drèze and Amartya Sen, *An Uncertain Glory: India and Its Contradictions*, op. cit., pp. 150–155.
105. Healthcare Access Quality Index based on mortality from causes amenable to personal health care in 195 countries and territories, 1990–2015: a novel analysis from the Global Burden of Disease Study 2015, *Lancet*, Vol. 390, 15 July 2017 (online published May 18), pp. 231–266.
106. Ibid.
107. Jean Drèze and Amartya Sen, *An Uncertain Glory: India and Its Contradictions*, op. cit., pp. 143–146.
108. Dilip Ghosh, "Bhumikar Paribarte", in Punyabrata Goon (ed.), *Swasthya A-byabastha*, Kolkata: Guruchandali Publication, first edition 2017, pp. ii–viii.
109. Monica Das Gupta et al., "How Might India's Public Health Systems Be Strengthened? Lessons from Tamil Nadu", op. cit., pp. 46–60.
110. Amartya Sen, "Foreword", in Samiran Nundy et al. (eds.), *Healers or Predators?: Healthcare Corruption in India,* New Delhi: Oxford University Press, 2018, pp. ix--xiii.
111. "India: extreme inequality in numbers", Oxfam, https://www.oxfam.org/en/india-extreme-inequality-numbers, retrieved on April 18, 2020.
112. *Anandabazar Patrika*, September 21, 2019. https://www.anandabazar.com/business/modi-government-slashes-corporate-tax-1.1048617, retrieved on April 18, 2020.
113. Jean Drèze and Amartya Sen, *An Uncertain Glory: India and Its Contradictions*, USA: Princeton University Press, 2013, pp. 177–182.

114. NGO response to Jakarta Declaration: Report of the NGO Briefing held at the World Health Assembly Geneva, 13 May 1998, World Health Organization, WHO/HPR/HEP/98.10, pp. 5–6.
115. Indian Constitution, Seventh Schedule, Article 246.
116. Amrita Bagchi, *Healthcare in Post-Independence India: Kolkata and the Crisis of Private Healthcare Services*, New York & London: Routledge, 2023.
117. Assembly Proceedings, West Bengal Legislative Assembly, Vol. 2, No. 1, Second Session, from 10th February to 30th March 1948.
118. Sekhar Bandyopadhyay, *Decolonization in South Asia: Meanings of freedom in post-independence West Bengal, 1947–52*, London/New York: Routledge, 2009, pp. 30–31.
119. Government of West Bengal, Directorate of Health Services, *Annual Report on the Health of the Population of West Bengal: For the Year 1950* (by B. C. Das Gupta Director of Health Services, West Bengal), Kolkata: Superintendent, Government Printing, West Bengal Government Press, 1953, pp. 1–2.
120. Ibid.
121. Ibid.
122. Government of West Bengal, Directorate of Health Services, *Annual Report on the Health of the Population of West Bengal: For the Year 1951* (by B. C. Das Gupta Director of Health Services, West Bengal), Kolkata: Superintendent, Government Printing, West Bengal Government Press, 1954, p. 1.
123. Nitish Sengupta, *Builders of Modern India*, New Delhi: Publication Division, Government of India, 1st edition 2002, reprint 2016, pp. 14–15.
124. Myron Wiener, *State Politics in India*, USA: Princeton University Press, 2015, pp. 309–310.
125. Ibid.
126. Gouripada Dutta, *Janaswasthya Bhabana*, Kolkata: Banglar Mukh Publication, 2011, p. 121.
127. Tapas Kumar Bhattacharya, "Sarkari Swasthya Byabastha—Patan, Abhyuday, Bandhur Pantha", *Doctors' Dialogue*, Vol. 2, No. 4, December 2004, pp. 5–9.
128. Government of West Bengal, Department of Health, *The Health Service (Cadre, Pay and Allowance) Rule 1958, with Some Important Government Orders, Corrected up to 1st September 1966*, Kolkata: Superintendent, Government Printing, West Bengal Government Press, 1967, pp. 1–3.
129. Ibid., preface page.
130. Gouripada Dutta, *Health Care in India: An Appraisal*, published by P K Choudhuri (secretary of the Journal of IMA), Kolkata, 1987, p. 1.

131. Speech of Suman Chattopathyay, in a debate-meeting at Medical College Hospital on West Bengal Clinical Establishment Act 2017 organized By Health Services Association, August 10, 2017; Punyabrata Goon, "Corporate Haspataler Biruddhe Chikitsakrao", in *Nirantar*, Vol. V, No. 2, May 2015, pp. 19–21.
132. Balay Chakraborty, "Rajyer Chikitsa O Swasthya-parishebar Bartaman O Bhabisyat", https://ritambangla.com/health/state-hospital-scenario/, retrieved on April 18, 2020.
133. Kabita Ray, *History of Public Health: Colonial Bengal 1921–1947*, op. cit., p. 187.
134. Meenakshi Gautham and K M Shyamprasad, "The 'Basic' Doctor for Rural India: A Failed Promise?", *Economic and Political Weekly*, Vol. 45, No. 38, September 18–24, 2010, pp. 25–29.
135. S.C Dutta and Pravash Chandra Sengupta, "Patients & Hospitals", *Amrita Bazar Patrika*, Annual Puja Number, 1956, p. 91.
136. Ibid.
137. *Mukti* (Weekly), Vol. 23, No. 31, August 13, 1962, pp. 1–2.
138. Apurba Mukhopadhyay, "The Left in West Bengal: Government and Movement, 1967–1982", in Rakhahari Chatterji (ed.), *Politics in West Bengal: Institutions, Processes and Problems*, Calcutta: The World Press Private Limited, 19885, pp. 83–84.
139. *Jugantar*, May 5, 1967, p. 3.
140. *Jugantar*, May 4, 1967, p. 3.
141. Speech of Timir Baran Bhaduri (16th March), in Assembly Proceeding, Fifty-Sixth Session (from February to May 1974), Vol. 56, No. 2, published by Authority of Legislative Assembly, West Bengal, pp. 322–326.
142. Ibid.
143. Speech of Satya Ghosal (16th March), in Assembly Proceeding, Fifty-Sixth Session (from February to May 1974), Vol. 56, No. 2, Published by Authority of Legislative Assembly, West Bengal, pp. 327–337.
144. West Bengal's Approach to Fifth Five-Year Plan (1974–1979), State Planning Board, Government of West Bengal, 1972.
145. *Jugantar*, January 2, 1974, p. 8.
146. Anil Biswas, "An Overview", in Jyoti Basu et al. (eds.), *People's Power in Practice: 20 Years of Left Front in West Bengal*, Kolkata: National Book Agency, 1997, pp. xix–xl.
147. Rajesh Bhattacharya, "Bam-front O Bam-Bikalpa", in Prabrit Dasmahapatra & Rajesh Bhattachariya (eds.), *Bamraj: Tattwa O Charchay*, Kolkata: Charchapada Publication, 2013, pp. 51–59.
148. M.S Jayalakshmi, "National Policy and Programmes in Family Planning: The Impact and Challenges", in Alex Vadakumthala (ed.), *Reproductive*

Health: Catholic Ethics and Praxis in India, New Delhi: Health Commission, Catholic Bishops' Conference of India, 2007, p. 125.

149. Assembly Proceedings, West Bengal Legislative Assembly: Vol. 58, No. 1, Fifty Eighth Session, February–May 1975; Vol. 62, Sixty Second Session, 11 October to 19 October 1976; Vol. 66, No. 2, Sixty Six Session, August to October 1977; Vol. 66, No. 5, Sixty Six Session, August to October 1977.
150. Assembly Proceedings, West Bengal Legislative Assembly, Vol. 66, No. 2, Sixty Six Session, 25 August to 5 October 1977.
151. Bidyut Chakrabarty, *Left Radicalism in India*, London/New York: Routledge, 2014, p. 64.
152. Speech of Nani Bhattacharya, in *Data India 46*, published by Press Institute of India, November 14–20, 1977, pp. 733–734.
153. Speech of Satya Ranjan Bapuli (28th February 1979), in Assembly Proceedings, 70th session of West Bengal Legislative Assembly (February to April, 1979), Vol. 70, No. 2, published by Authority of Legislative Assembly, West Bengal, pp. 125–130.
154. Speech of A K M Hasanuzzaman, 6th March 1979, 70th session of West Bengal Legislative Assembly (February to April, 1979), Vol. 70, No. 2, pp. 492–495.
155. Speech of Debaprasad Sarkar (6th March 1979), in Assembly Proceedings, 70th session of West Bengal Legislative Assembly (February to April, 1979), Vol. 70, No. 2, pp. 495–503.
156. "Printed Speech of Nani Bhattacharya on Demand No. 36, 37 & 38" (6th March 1979), in Assembly Proceedings, 70th session of West Bengal Legislative Assembly (February to April, 1979), Vol. 70, No. 2, pp. 469–491.
157. Ibid.
158. Shaibal Gupta, "Chikitsateo Durniti", *Desh*, Vol. 63, No. 13, 20 April 1996, p. 36.
159. Speech of Debaprasad Sarkar (6th March 1979), in Assembly Proceedings, 70th session of West Bengal Legislative Assembly (February to April, 1979), Vol. 70, No. 2, pp. 495–503.
160. "Lest we forget", *The Telegraph*, May 14, 2011, https://www.telegraphindia.com/india/lest-we-forget/cid/392276, Consulted on July 6, 2020.
161. Partha Sarathi Banerjee, "Power and Political Violence in West Bengal", *Economic & Political Weekly (EPW)*, Vol. 46, No. 6, February 5–11, 2011, pp. 16–18.
162. Assembly Proceedings, West Bengal Legislative Assembly, Seventy-Eight Session (from 1st September, 1982 to 8th October, 1982), Vol. 78, No. 2, 1982.

163. Sujit Kumar Das, *Chikitsar Katha: Rajniti Arthaniti Prayukti O Janagan*, Kolkata: Drug Action Forum, West Bengal, 2006, pp. 37–38.
164. Sujit Kumar Das, *Chikitsar Katha: Rajniti Arthaniti Prayukti O Janagan*, op. cit.
165. Government of West Bengal, *Report of Administrative Reforms Committee*, Home (Personnel and Administrative Reforms) Department, 1983, pp. 21–22.
166. Speech of Manas Bunia and Debaprasad Sarkar, in Assembly Proceedings, West Bengal Legislative Assembly, Seventy-Ninth Session (from 11th April, 1983 to 23rd April 1983), Vol. 79, No. 3, 1983, pp. 42–43.
167. Speech of Satyaranjan Bapuli and Abdus Sattar, in Assembly Proceedings, West Bengal Legislative Assembly, Seventy-Ninth Session (from 11th April to 23rd April 1983), op. cit., pp. 44, 45, 51.
168. Speech of Ambarish Mukhopadhyay, in Assembly Proceedings, West Bengal Legislative Assembly, Seventy-Ninth Session (from 11th April to 23rd April 1983), op. cit., pp. 146–148.
169. Speech of Dr. Sisir Kumar Bose, in Assembly Proceedings, West Bengal Legislative Assembly, Seventy-Ninth Session (from 11th April to 23rd April 1983), op. cit., pp. 192–202.
170. Speech of Dr Ambarish Mukhopadhyay, in Assembly Proceedings, West Bengal Legislative Assembly, Seventy-Ninth Session (from 11th April to 23rd April 1983), op. cit., pp. 258–268.
171. Sabyasachi Chatterjee, "Comrade, Nabajug Anle Na?", *Anandabazar Patrika*, December 1, 2018, p. 4.
172. Bolan Gangopadhyay, "Chhabita Kato Anyrakam Chhilo", *Anandabazar Patrika*, July 10, 2019, p. 4.
173. Mark Nichter, "Community Health Worker Scheme: A Plan for Democratisation", *Economic & Political Weekly*, Vol. 15, No. 1, January 5 1980, pp. 37–43.
174. Gouripada Dutta, *Health Care in India: An Appraisal*, published by P K Choudhuri (secretary of the Journal of IMA), Kolkata, I987, pp. 65–66.
175. Bruno Jobert, "Populism and Health Policy: The Case of Community Health Volunteers in India", *Social Science & Medicine*, Volume 20, Issue 1, 1985, pp. 1–25.
176. Speech of Dr. Ambarish Mukhopadhyay (12th April), in Assembly Proceedings, West Bengal Legislative Assembly, Eighty-Third session (from 11th March to 10th May 1985), Vol. 83, No. 3, 1985, pp. 211–230.
177. Speech of Dr. Hoimi Basu, in Assembly Proceedings, West Bengal Legislative Assembly, Seventy-Ninth Session (from 11th April to 23rd April 1983), op. cit., pp. 202–206.
178. Ibid.

179. Speech of Dr. Sukumar Roy (12th April), in Assembly Proceedings, West Bengal Legislative Assembly, Eighty-Third session (from 11th March to 10th May 1985), op. cit., pp. 255–257.
180. Ibid.
181. Ibid.
182. Speech of Dr. Sisir Kumar Bose (12th April), in Assembly Proceedings, West Bengal Legislative Assembly, Eighty-Third session (from 11th March to 10th May 1985), op. cit., pp. 230–234.
183. Speech of Dr. Sisir Kumar Bose (17th April), in Assembly Proceedings, West Bengal Legislative Assembly, Eighty-First session (from 16th April to 27th April 1984), Vol. 81, No. 4, 1984, pp. 173–180.
184. Ibid.
185. Speech of Anil Mukherjee (12th April), in Assembly Proceedings, West Bengal Legislative Assembly, Eighty-Third session (from 11th March to 10th May 1985), op. cit., pp. 242–246.
186. Speech of Debaprasad Sarkar (12th April), in Assembly Proceedings, West Bengal Legislative Assembly, Eighty-Third session (from 11th March to 10th May 1985), op. cit., pp. 246–249.
187. Government of West Bengal, *Economic Review: 1988–89 (Statistical Appendix)*, Kolkata: Govt. of WB, p. 193.
188. Speech of Amarendra Bhattacharya (12th April), in Assembly Proceedings, West Bengal Legislative Assembly, Eighty-Third session (from 11th March to 10th May 1985), op. cit., pp. 262–264.
189. Speech of Ajit Panja (17th April), in Assembly Proceedings, West Bengal Legislative Assembly, Eighty-First session (from 16th April to 27th April 1984), Vol. 81, No. 4, 1984, pp. 184–191.
190. Speech of Prasanta Kumar Sur (5th June), in Assembly Proceedings, West Bengal Legislative Assembly, Eighty-eight session (from May to June 1987), Vol. 88, No. 2, 1987, pp. 331–354.
191. Sujit K. Das, "Left Front's Health Circus", *EPW*, Vol. 23, No, 21, May 21, 1988, pp. 1056–1058.
192. Ibid.
193. Ibid.
194. Speech of Amarendra Bhattacharya (12th April), in Assembly Proceedings, Eighty-Third session (from 11th March to 10th May 1985), op. cit., pp. 262–264.
195. Swati Bhattacharya, "Kono Oshudhei Swasthya Fereni", in *Desh*, January 6, 2001, p. 38.
196. The term "political touts" referred to intermediaries close to ruling political groups, while "non-political touts" indicated independent brokers without connection with any political party.
197. *Jugantar*, January 5, 1974, p. 2.

198. Ross Mallick, *Development Policy of a Communist Government: West Bengal since 1977*, New York: Cambridge University Press, 1993, p. 97.
199. Sujit K Das "Left Front's Scheme for Modernising Health Care: Ill-Conceived", *EPW*, April 2–9, 1988, Vol. 23, No. 14/15, April 2–9, 1988, pp. 690–691.
200. Speech of Dr Hoimi Basu (12th May), in Assembly Proceedings, Ninety-Second session (from February to May 1989), West Bengal Legislative Assembly, Vol. 92, No. 4, 1989, pp. 545–549.
201. Speech of Prasanta Sur (12th May), in Assembly Proceedings, West Bengal Legislative Assembly, Ninety-Second session (from February to May 1989), op. cit., pp. 579–586.
202. Speech of Satya Ranjan Bapuli (12th May), in Assembly Proceedings, West Bengal Legislative Assembly, Ninety-Second session (from February to May 1989), op. cit., pp. 554–556.
203. Speech of Dr Hoimi Basu (12th May), in Assembly Proceedings, West Bengal Legislative Assembly, Ninety-Second session (from February to May 1989), op. cit.
204. Sumanta Banerjee, "West Bengal's Next Quinquennium, and the Future of the Indian Left", *Economic & Political Weekly*, Vol. 46, Issue No. 23, 04 Jun, 2011, pp. 14–19.
205. Derek O'Brien, "Aro Anek Path Baki", *Anandabazar Patrika*, June 21, 2013, p. 4; Srikanta Ghosh, *The Indian Mafia*, New Delhi: Ashish Publishing House, 1991, pp. 64–65.
206. G. C Malhotra, "Parliamentary Committee with Special Reference to Departmentally Related Standing Committee", in *The Journal of Parliamentary Information*, Vol. XLIV, No. 3, September, 1998, pp. 236–264.
207. Speech of Dr Gouripada Dutta on the West Bengal State Health Service (Amendment) Bill 1990 (20th August), in Assembly Proceeding, West Bengal Legislative Assembly, Ninety-Sixth Session (from 14th August to 31st August 1990), Vol. 96, 1990, pp. 43–45.
208. Speech of Dr Omar Ali on the West Bengal State Health Service (Amendment) Bill 1990, in Assembly Proceeding, Ninety-Sixth Session (from 14th August to 31st August 1990), op. cit., pp. 48–50.
209. Speech of Tarapada Ghosh on the West Bengal State Health Service (Amendment) Bill 1990 (20th August), in Assembly Proceeding, West Bengal Legislative Assembly, Ninety-Sixth Session (from 14th August to 31st August 1990), op. cit., pp. 47–48.
210. Manifesto of the Left Front—West Bengal Assembly Election published on April 10, 1982, p. 7.
211. Speech of Satyendra Nath Ghosh on the West Bengal State Health Service (Amendment) Bill 1990 (20th August), in Assembly Proceeding, West

Bengal Legislative Assembly, Ninety-Sixth Session (from 14th August to 31st August 1990), op. cit., pp. 45–47.

212. Speech of Dr Gouripada Dutta on the West Bengal State Health Service (Amendment) Bill 1990 (20th August), in Assembly Proceeding, West Bengal Legislative Assembly, Ninety-Sixth Session (from 14th August to 31st August 1990), op. cit., pp. 43–45.
213. Speech of Satyendra Nath Ghosh on the West Bengal State Health Service (Amendment) Bill 1990 (20th August), in Assembly Proceeding, West Bengal Legislative Assembly, Ninety-Sixth Session (from 14th August to 31st August 1990), op. cit.
214. Speech of Gouripada Dutta on West Bengal Health Service Bill, 1990 (17th April), in Assembly Proceeding, West Bengal Legislative Assembly, Ninety-Fifth Session (from march to May 1990), West Bengal Legislative Assembly, Vol. 95, No. 1, 1990, pp. 1001–1004.
215. Speech of Prasanta Sur on the West Bengal State Health Service (Amendment) Bill 1990 (20th August), op. cit., p. 50.
216. Speech of Gouripada Dutta on West Bengal Health Service Bill, 1990 (17th April), in Assembly Proceeding, Ninety-Fifth Session (from March to May 1990), op. cit.
217. Speech of Dr. Gouripada Dutta on the West Bengal State Health Service (Amendment) Bill 1990, in Assembly Proceeding, West Bengal Legislative Assembly, Ninety-Sixth Session (from 14th August to 31st August 1990), op. cit.
218. West Bengal Act VII of 1990, The West Bengal State Health Service Act, 1990, Passed by the West Bengal Legislature, in the Calcutta Gazette, Extraordinary, 16th May, 1990.
219. Speech of Tarun Adhikari on West Bengal Health Service Bill, 1990 (17th April), in Assembly Proceeding, Ninety-Fifth Session (from March to May 1990), op. cit., pp. 998–1001.
220. Amalesh Tripathi, *Swadhinatar Mukh*, Kolkata: Ananda Publishers, 2010, p. 46.
221. Ibid.
222. Speech of Manas Bhunia (21st July), in Assembly Proceeding, Hundred and Sixth Session (from march to August, 1995), West Bengal Legislative Assembly, Vol. 106, No. 4, 1995, pp. 522–532.
223. "Sarkari Swasthya—Ekti Samikkha", *Bijnan O Bijnan-Karmi*, Vol. XVI, No. 1, January–March, 1994, pp. 29–32.
224. Ibid.
225. Ibid.
226. Bijoya Roy, *Private Investment in Public Sector Medical Care Institutions: A Study of Processes in Tertiary and Secondary Level Care in Six Districts of West Bengal*, unpublished PhD thesis, Centre of Social Medicine and

Community Health, School of Social Sciences, Jawaharlal Nehru University, 2007, pp. 115–116.
227. Aniruddha Sengupta, *Ek Ganyer Daktarer Galpo*, Kolkata: Gurchandali Publication, 2019.
228. Parthasarathi Gupta, *Chikitsa O Apachikitsa*, Kolkata: Foundation for Health Action, first published 2000, cited second edition 2019, pp. 38–40.
229. Ibid., p. 40.
230. Smarjit Jana, *Rogir Jonya Chikitsa Na Chikitsar Jonya Rogi*, Kolkata: Ganabijnan Sathira, 2018, pp. 15–17.
231. Alok Mukhopadhyay (ed.), *State of India's Health*, New Delhi: Voluntary Health Association of India, 1992, pp. 63–64.
232. O.P. Jaggi, *History of Science, Medicine in India: Modern Period* (General Editor: D.P. Chattopadhyay, Philosophy and Culture in Indian Civilization, Volume IX, Part 1), New Delhi: Oxford University Press, first edition 2000, cited edition 2011, p. 299.
233. Bengal Initiative, *Health: a Critical Appraisal*, Kolkata, 1999.
234. Swati Bhattacharya, "Kono Oshudhei Swasthya Fereni", op. cit.
235. Government of India, *Bulletin on Rural Health Statistics in India*, March 2008, New Delhi: Ministry of Health and Family Welfare, 2009.
236. Swati Bhattacharya, "Kono Oshudhei Swasthya Fereni", op. cit.
237. Ibid.
238. International Institute for Population Sciences (IIPS), *National Family Health Survey (NFHS-2) India 1998–99: West Bengal*, Mumbai: IIPS, 2001, pp. 202–203.
239. Suman K Chakrabarti, "18 Babies Die in Four days in Kolkata's Bidhan Chandra Roy Hospital for Children", in India Today, September 16, 2002, https://www.indiatoday.in/magazine/indiascope/story/20020916-18-babies-die-in-four-days-in-kolkatas-bidhan-chandra-roy-hospital-for-children-796314-2002-09-16.
240. Ibid.
241. Achin Chakraborty and Subrata Mukherjee, "Health Care in West Bengal: What Is Happening?", *Economic and Political Weekly*, Vol. 38, No. 48, November 29–December 5, 2003, pp. 5021–5023.
242. Swati Bhattacharya, "Kono Oshudhei Swasthya Fereni", op. cit.
243. Mansi Shah, "Waiting for Health Care: A Survey of a Public Hospital in Kolkata", https://ccs.in/internship_papers/2008/Waiting-for-Healthcare-A-survey-of-a-public-hospital-in-Kolkata-Mansi.pdf retrieved on December 11, 2020.
244. "What is ailing Bengal hospitals?", *Times of India,* November 6, 2011, https://timesofindia.indiatimes.com/What-is-ailing-Bengal-hospitals/articleshowprint/10626408.cms, retrieved on September 16, 2019.

245. Ashis Chakrabarti, "Now for the Booster Dose", *The Telegraph*, October 16, 2001, https://www.telegraphindia.com/opinion/now-for-the-booster-dose/cid/916678, retrieved on June 27, 2020.
246. Ashok Sen, *Itihaser Thikthikana*, Kolkata: Seriban, 2005, pp. 67–68. (Indent lines have been translated from Bengali to English.)
247. Government of India, *Report of the National Commission on Macroeconomics and Health*, New Delhi: Ministry of Health & Family Welfare, Government of India, 2005, p. 72.
248. Indranil Mukhopadhyay, *Public Health Care Expenditure in India a Study of Kerala, Tamil Nadu and West Bengal*, an unpublished PhD thesis, Centre of Social Medicine and Community Health, Jawaharlal Nehru University, New Delhi, 2011, p. 82.
249. K. N. Reddy and V. Selvaraju, *Health Care Expenditure by Government in India: 1974–75 to 1990–91*, New Delhi: National Institute of Public Finance & Policy, 1994, p. 35.
250. M. Govinda Rao & Mita Choudhury, *Inter-State Equalisation of Health Expenditures in Indian Union*, New Delhi: National Institute of Public Finance and Policy, 2008, p. 11.
251. Medical Service Centre, *Sarkari Maranphande Janaswasthya*, Kolkata: Medical Service Centre, 1992, pp. 27.
252. "Editorial", *Swastha Bikshan*, Vol. VII, Issue 2 & 3, April–September 2001, pp. 2–3.
253. The letter has been quoted by Tarun Mondal in his article titled "PHC Tule Debar Parikalpana Swasthya Byabsa Briddhi Korar Swarthei", *Swastha Bikshan*, Vol. X, Issue 3, July–September, 2004, pp. 11–17.
254. "Polyclinics at Hospitals to Herald Year", *The Telegraph*, December 31, 2002, https://www.telegraphindia.com/india/polyclinics-at-hospitals-to-herald-year/cid/904692, retrieved on July 2, 2020; "Low turnout at new polyclinics", *The Times of India*, January 2, 2002, https://timesofindia.indiatimes.com/city/kolkata/Low-turnout-at-new-polyclinics/articleshow/216995229.cms, retrieved on July 2, 2020.
255. "Bill will bring doctors back into pay clinics", *The Telegraph*, July 12, 2003, https://www.telegraphindia.com/west-bengal/bill-will-bring-doctors-back-into-pay-clinics/cid/1091927, retrieved on July 2, 2020.
256. "Govt. Lifts Ban on Doctors' pvt Practice", *The Times of India*, July 24, 2003, https://timesofindia.indiatimes.com/city/kolkata/Govt-lifts-ban-on-doctors-pvt-practice/articleshow/92583.cms?from=mdr, retrieved on July 2, 2020.
257. "Editorial", in *Swastha Bikshan*, Vol. VII, No. 2 & 3, April–September, 2001, pp. 2–3.
258. Sujit K Das "Left Front's Scheme for Modernising Health Care: Ill-Conceived", op. cit.

259. Ibid.
260. "Health services in West Bengal to go private", *India Today*, March 31, 1988, https://www.indiatoday.in/magazine/states/story/19880331-health-services-in-west-bengal-to-go-private-797112-1988-03-31, retrieved on March 2, 2022.
261. Ibid.
262. Amrita Bagchi, *Healthcare in Post-Independence India: Kolkata and the Crisis of Private Healthcare Services*, New York & London: Routledge, 2023, p. 100.
263. World Bank, *India Health Systems Project II, Report No. 15106-IN*, Washington DC: World Bank, 1996, p. v.
264. Ibid., pp. 26–29.
265. Bijoya Roy, "Public Private Partnership in Healthcare: Trajectories and Experiences from West Bengal", in Imrana Qadeer (ed.), *India: Social Development Report 2014: Challenges of Public Health*, New Delhi: Oxford University Press, 2015, pp. 191–204.
266. Ibid.
267. Government of India, *National Health Policy-2002*, New Delhi: Ministry of Health and Family Welfare, 2003.
268. Government of India, *National Public Private Partnership Policy: Draft for Consultation*, New Delhi: Department of Economic Affairs Ministry of Finance, 2011.
269. Rama V. Baru and Madhurima Nundy, "Blurring of Boundaries: Public–Private Partnerships in Health Services in India", *Economic and Political Weekly*, Vol. 43, No. 4, January 26–February 1, 2008, pp. 62–71.
270. Bijoya Roy, "Why Public–Private Collaboration is Bad News for Healthcare in India", *The Wire*, March 20, 2017, https://thewire.in/health/ppp-healthcare-health-policy, retrieved on June 5, 2021.
271. Mampi Bose, "Bengal's Healthcare Has Become Dysfunctional: Here's How We Can Fix It", *The Wire*, June 27, 2019, https://thewire.in/health/west-bengal-doctors-strike-healthcare, retrieved on June 5, 2021.
272. "Editorial", *Swastha Bikshan*, Vol. VII, Issue 2 & 3, April–September 2001, pp. 2–3.
273. Government of West Bengal, *Economic Review: 2004–2005*, Kolkata: Government of WB, p. 194.
274. Interview with Dr Hiralal Konar, a former secretary of Health Service Association, Kolkata, February 13, 2020.
275. Indira Chakravarthy, "Public health privatisation in Bengal", August 29, 2008, available at: http://sanhati.com/excerpted/946/, retrieved on Augist 4, 2023.
276. Siddhartha Gupta, *Swasther Byabsa Chikitsar Rajniti*, Kolkata: Bodhisattva, 2018, pp. 72–73.

277. Ibid.
278. Sujit K. Das, "Public Health: A Question of Entitlements", *EPW*, Vol. 27, No. 39, September 26, 1992, pp. 2095–2096.
279. Ibid.
280. Ibid.
281. "Privatization of Health Care?", *EPW*, Vol. 27, No. 19, May p, 1992, pp. 977–978.
282. Ibid.
283. *Sarkari Maranphande Janaswasthya*, Kolkata: Medical Service Centre, 1992, pp. 27.
284. Margaret Chan, "The Impact of Global Crises on Health: Money, Weather and Microbes", World Health Organization. https://www.who.int/dg/speeches/2009/financial_crisis_20090318/en/, retrieved on September 16, 2020.
285. Juliet Nabyonga et al., "Abolition of Cost-sharing is Pro-poor: Evidence from Uganda", *Health Policy and Planning*, Vol. 20, No.2, April 2005, pp. 100–108.
286. Oommen C. Kurian et al., *Mapping the Flow of User Fees in a Public Hospital*, Mumbai: CEHAT, 2011, p. 1.
287. Sajal Biswas, "Public Private Partnership (PPP) Policy Ebang Swasthya Khetre Tar Prabhab", *Swastha Biskhsan*, Vol. XVIII, Issue 1, January, 2013, pp. 14–20.
288. Ibid.
289. A. Venkat Raman & James Warner Björkman, *Public–Private Partnerships in Health Care in India: Lessons for Developing Countries*, London and New York: Routledge, 2009, pp. 68–69.
290. Ibid.
291. "Baghajatin State Hospital in South Kolkata—The Privatisation of Healthcare in West Bengal", *Sanhati* archive, March 6, 2011, http://sanhati.com/articles/3290/, retrieved on September 16, 2019.
292. Government of West Bengal, *Memo No HF/O/MS/121/W-10/2001 Dated 18th March, 2002, Fixation of Rates of Hospital Charges for Hospital Services*, Kolkata: Health and Family Welfare Department.
293. Ibid.
294. G. Shabbir Cheema, Dennis A. Rondinelli (eds.), *Decentralizing Governance Emerging Concepts and Practices*, Washington, DC: Brookings Institution Press, 2007, p. 1.
295. Government of West Bengal, *Health Sector Reforms 2003–2007*, Department of Health and Family Welfare, Government of West Bengal.
296. Ramesh Bhat, "Issues in Health: Public-Private Partnership", *EPW*, Vol. 35, No. 52/53, December 30, 2000–January 5, 2001, pp. 4706–4716.

297. Budget Statement by Asim Kumar Dasgupta, Minister-in-Charge, Finance, Government of West Bengal, June 2, 2001, p. 38.
298. Achin Chakraborty, "Confused Policy for Public–Private Partnership", *EPW*, Vol. 40, No. 5, January–February, 2005, pp. 351–353.
299. Ibid.
300. Bijoya Roy and Siddharta Gupta, "Public–Private Partnership and User Fees in Healthcare: Evidence from West Bengal", *EPW*, Vol. XLVI, No 38, September 17, 2011, pp. 74–78.
301. Government of West Bengal, *Policy for Public Private Partnerships in the Health Sector*, Kolkata: Department of Health and Family Welfare, January 2006, p. 4.
302. Ibid., pp. 4–9.
303. Government of West Bengal, *Establishing Diagnostic Services in Block Primary Health Centres/Rural Hospitals through Public Private Partnerships*, Kolkata: Department of Health and Family Welfare, January 2010, p. 3.
304. Government of West Bengal, *Scheme for Establishing C.T. Scan Facilities under Public Private Partnerships*, Kolkata: Department of Health and Family Welfare, 2008, p. 4.
305. Government of West Bengal, *Memo No HF/PPP/11/2009/ Dated: February, 2010*, Kolkata: Public Private Partnerships Branch, Department of Health and Family Welfare.
306. Government of West Bengal, *Ambulance Services at Rural Hospitals/ Block Primary Health Centres/Primary Health Centres through Public Private Partnerships*, Kolkata: Department of Health and Family Welfare, November 2006, p. 3.
307. Government of West Bengal, *Memo No HF/PPP/13 /2009/ 15 Dated: January 28, 2010,* Kolkata: Public Private Partnerships Branch, Department of Health and Family Welfare.
308. Government of West Bengal, *Memo No HFIPPP/247/2008/68, Dated: 13th February, 2012,* MS Branch, Kolkata: Department of Health and Family Welfare.
309. Manabesh Sarkar, *Unqualified Medical Practitioners: Unavoidable for the Health Care of Rural People?*, Pratichi Occasional Paper No. 5, Pratichi (India) Trust, Kolkata, 2017, p. 8.
310. Krishna Soman, "Rural Health Care in West Bengal", *Economic and Political Weekly*, Vol. 37, No. 26, June 29, 2002, pp. 2562–2564.
311. Charu C. Garg and Anup K. Karan, "Reducing Out-of-Pocket Expenditures to Reduce Poverty: A Disaggregated Analysis at Rural–Urban and State Level in India", *Health Policy and Planning*, Volume 24, No. 2, March 2009, pp. 116–128.

312. Swadhin Mondal et al., "Catastrophic out-of-pocket payment for health care and its impact on households: Experience from West Bengal, India", *Economics Bulletin*, 2014, Vol. 34 No. 2 pp. 1303–1316. http://www.chronicpoverty.org/uploads/publication_files/mondal_et_al_health.pdf, retrieved on November 12, 2020.
313. Ibid.
314. Rezaul Karim, "Swasthya, Swasthya Byabastha, Sarkar-2011", in the *Souvenir of Health Service Association published on the Occasion of 38th annual Conference*, January 23, 2011, pp. 5–7.
315. "Lest we forget", *The Telegraph*, May 14, 2011, https://www.telegraphindia.com/india/lest-we-forget/cid/392276, retrieved on July 6, 2020.
316. Surjit S Bhalla, "Change is finally here", *The Indian Express*, May 13, 2011, http://archive.indianexpress.com/story-print/789815/, retrieved on August 20, 2020.
317. West Bengal Assembly Election Manifesto 2011 of Trinamool Congress, Kolkata, 2011, p. 11.
318. Sumanta Banerjee, "West Bengal's Next Quinquennium, and the Future of the Indian Left", op. cit.
319. Siddhartha Gupta, "Paschimbange Swasthya Khetre PPP Model: Kar Lav Kar Kshati?", *Aneek*, Vol. 48, No. 5, November, 2011, pp. 16–20.
320. Ibid.
321. "Concept Paper cum Suggestion Solicitation Paper for Health Care Infrastructure builds up in Public Private Participation (PPP) Mode", Kolkata: Department of Health and Family Welfare, Government of West Bengal, https://www.wbhealth.gov.in/uploaded_files/notice/ppp_hosp.pdf, retrieved on August 20, 2020.
322. Uttan Bandopadhyay, "Swasthye Panyayan: Ekhon", *Bijnan O Bijnan-Karmi*, January–December, 2011, pp. 54–59.
323. Amitava Chakraborty, "Paschimbange Swasthya: Paribartan Ki 'Pratyabartan'-er Pathae?", *Swasthyer Britte*, Vol. 1, No. 3, February–March, 2012, pp. 35–37.
324. Punyabrata Goon, "Paschimbange Sarkari Chikitsa Parisheba: Ghoshana O Bastabata", *Swasthyer Britte,* Vol. 4, No. 1, October–November, 2014, pp. 18–20.
325. "49 Infants Die in B C Roy Hospital in Last 7 days", *The Economic Times*, September 9, 2013, https://economictimes.indiatimes.com/news/politics-and-nation/49-infants-die-in-b-c-roy-hospital-in-last-7-days/articleshow/22438278.cms, retrieved on August 20, 2020.
326. Government of India, *National Health Profile 2018*, New Delhi: Central Bureau of Health Intelligence, Ministry of Health & Family Welfare, 2018, pp. 91–92.

327. Giovanna Tavecchi and Andrea Rebecchi, "The Current Indian Healthcare System and West Bengal's Health Status", in Stefano Capolongo & Marco Gola Andrea Rebecchi (eds.), *Healthcare Facilities in Emerging Countries The Challenge for India*, Italy: Springer, 2018, pp. 13–31.
328. "India Facing Shortage of 600,000 Doctors, 2 Million Nurses: Study", *The Economic Times*, April 14, 2019.
329. Government of India, *National Health Profile 2018*, op. cit., p. 221.
330. Ibid., p. 260.
331. "Mamata Blames Centre for Doctor Shortage", *The Statesman*, July 28, 2018, https://www.thestatesman.com/cities/mamata-blames-centre-doctor-shortage-1502666210.html, retrieved on February 27, 2020.
332. Kerean Watts, "CM Banerjee Calls Attention to Doctor Shortage in West Bengal", *Health Issue in India*, July 3, 2019, https://www.healthissuesindia.com/2019/07/03/cm-banerjee-calls-attention-to-doctor-shortage-in-west-bengal/, retrieved on June 5, 2021.
333. Siddhartha Gupta, *Chikitsak Rogir Sangharsher Uutsa Sandhane*, a booklet published by author from Kolkata, 2019, pp. 3–23.
334. *From Paramedics to Allied Health Professionals: Landscaping the Journey and Way Forward*, A report commissioned by the Ministry of Health and Family Welfare, Government of India, New Delhi: Public Health Foundation of India, 2012.
335. Ibid., p. 5.
336. Ibid., pp. 84–85.
337. Rith Basu, "Paramedics short, touts prosper", *The Telegraph*, March 21,, 2018, https://www.telegraphindia.com/west-bengal/paramedics-short-touts-prosper/cid/1413163, retrieved on October 31, 2024.
338. Nirmala Murthy and Alka Barua, "Non-medical Determinants of Maternal Death in India", *Journal of Medical Management*, Vol. 6. No. 1, 2004, pp. 47–61.
339. *The Economic Times*, February 21, 1998.
340. Punyabrata Goon, "Paschimbange Swasthya Niye Mamata Banerjee-r Udyog: Sabar Janya Swasthya Ki Ei Vabe Hobe?", in Punyabrata Goon (ed.), *Swasthya Abyabastha*, Kolkata: Guruchandali Publication, 2017, pp. 30–40.
341. Speeches in a discussion meeting on "In Search of Origin Violence in the Health Sector" organized by Doctors' Dialogue on 22 April, 2022.
342. Government of India, *Health in India, National Sample Survey (NSS) 71st Round*, January–June 2014, Report No. 574 (71/25.0), New Delhi, 2016, pp. 42–43.

343. Sajal Biswas, "Mukhyamantrir 'Free' Chikitsa-r Ghosana Ebang Sadharan Manusher Pratyasha", *Swasthya Bikshan*, Vol. XXI, Book Fare Issue, January 2017, pp. 26–31.
344. Government of West Bengal, *Memo No. HF/O/MS/735(4)/W-86/12 Dated: 3rd December 2012*, Medical Services Branch, Kolkata: Department of Health and Family Welfare.
345. Government of West Bengal, *Memo No. HF/SPSRC/321/1(123) Dated: 11.08.2014*, Strategic Planning & Sector Reform Cell (SPSRC), Kolkata: Department of Health & Family Welfare, 2014.
346. "Free-r Thela Samlate Jadukathir Khonj", *Anandabazar Patrika*, November 24, 2015.
347. Soma Mukhopadhyay, "Free Kintu Free Noy, Bolchhe Haspataler Aviggata", *Anandabazar Patrika*, 23 September 2015.
348. Ibid.
349. Ibid.
350. Government of India, *West Bengal Development Report*, New Delhi: Academic Publication, 2010, p. 125.
351. Montu Bose and Arijita Dutta, "Health Financing Strategies to Reduce Out of-Pocket Burden in India: a Comparative Study of Three States", *BMC Health Services Research*, Vol. 18, November 2018, https://doi.org/10.1186/s12913-018-3633-5.
352. Ibid.
353. Suhrid Sankar Chattopadhyay, "Systemic ills", *Frontline*, April 14, 2017, https://frontline.thehindu.com/cover-story/systemic-ills/article9604230.ece, retrieved on September 7, 2020.
354. Ibid.
355. "Apollo Patient's Death: Hospital's Regional Director Steps Down over Medical Negligence Case", DNA, March 2, 2017, https://www.dnaindia.com/india/report-apollo-patient-s-death-hospital-s-regional-director-steps-down-over-medical-negligence-case-2340403, retrieved on August 20 2020.
356. Bolan Gangopadhyay, "Sarkari Byabasthay Astha Ferano Ki Khub Kathin?", *Ei Samay*, Kolkata, March 22, 2017, p. 10. (The quoted lines have been translated from Bengali.)
357. Punyabrata Goon, "Corporate Hasopataler Biruddhe Chikitsakrao", op. cit.
358. Arun Gadre & Abhay Shukla (ed.), *Dissenting Diagnosis*, India: Penguin Books, 2016, p. 50.
359. Ibid., pp. 52–53.
360. Amitabha Bhattashali, "Kolkata-r Besarkari Haspatal Niye Eto Avijog", March 2, 2017, https://www.bbc.com/bengali/news-39137688, retrieved on March 13, 2019.

361. Government of West Bengal, No HF/SPSRC/08/2012/28, dated March 16, 2012, Kolkata: Strategic Planning & Sector Reform Cell, Health & Family Welfare Department.
362. Lecture delivered by Dr. Subrata Maitra in August 6, 2015 at the Calcutta Chamber of Commerce. The text of it is available from: https://www.calcuttachamber.com/major-events2014-15.php, retrieved on June 10, 2022.
363. Solomon R. Benatar et al., "A Shared Statement of Ethical Principles for Those Who Shape and Give Health Care", *British Medical Journal*, Vol. 318, No. 7178, January 23, 1999, p. 249.
364. Jayanta Bhattacharya, *Bio-medicine Theke Najardari Medicine: Clinical Medicine Foucault Ebang Tarpar*, Kolkata: Hawakal, 2017, pp. 32–33.
365. Sreenivasa Raju, "The Good and The Bad about 'Master Health Check-Up' in India", *The Times of India*, September 10, 2012, http://timesofindia.indiatimes.com/articleshow/16333659.cms?utm_source=contentofinterest&utm_medium=text&utm_campaign=cppst, retrieved on July 28, 2022.
366. Ivan Illich, *Medical Nemesis: The Expropriation of Health,* New York: Pantheon Books, 1976.
367. Barbara Starfield, "Is US Health Really the Best in the World?", *Journal of American Medical Association*, Vol. 284, No. 4, July 26, 2000, pp. 483–485.
368. "India's Medical Error Deaths, Nearly 5 mn a Year, Can Be Cut by 50%: Expert", in *Business Standard*, October 28, 2018, https://www.business-standard.com/article/current-affairs/india-s-medical-error-deaths-nearly-5-mn-a-year-can-be-cut-by-50-expert-118102800193_1.html, retrieved on January 6, 2020.
369. Sabyasachi Chatterjee, "Haspataler Byadhi Niye Amra Katata Sachetan?", *Ei Samay*, January 24, 2020, p.8.
370. Smita Chakraburtty, "The Fire at AMRI: Need for Legislation on Corporate Culpability", *Economic & Political Weekly*, Vol. 52, No. 34, August 26, 2017, pp. 15–17.
371. Siddhartha Gupta, "Haspataler Asukh", in *Swasthyer Britte*, Vol. 2, No. 2, December 2012–January 2013, pp. 27–29.
372. Government of West Bengal, *The West Bengal Clinical Establishments (Registration, Regulation and Transparency) Act, 2017*, in the Kolkata Gazette, March 17, 2017.
373. Prabir Gangopadhyay, "Stent-baji o Anyanya Bhoj-baji", *Swasthyer Britte*, Vol. 6, No. 4, April–May, 2017, pp. 5–9.
374. Government of West Bengal, *The West Bengal Clinical Establishments (Registration, Regulation and Transparency) Act, 2017*, op. cit., p. 9.
375. Ibid.

376. Suhrid Sankar Chattopadhyay, "Systemic Ills", op. cit.
377. Ibid.
378. A debate-meeting at Calcutta Medical College Hospital on West Bengal Clinical Establishment Act 2017 organized By Health Services Association, August 10, 2017.
379. Arkamoy Dutta Majumdar, "JSW Cement to Take Management Control of a Govt. Hospital in West Bengal's Salboni", January 15, 2018, https://www.livemint.com/Companies/6gwTlsKGuJTeiJxme7ebRL/JSW-Cement-to-take-management-control-of-a-govt-hospital-in.html, retrieved on February 2, 2020.
380. "Natun Swapna Salbanir: Jindal-sparshe Hal Firbe Haspataler", *Anandabazar Patrika*, January 16, 2018, https://www.anandabazar.com/district/midnapore/jsw-group-to-take-charge-of-salboni-super-speciality-hospitals-1.740706, retrieved on February 2, 2020.
381. *Swasthyer Britte,* Vol. 8, No. 3, February–March, 2019, pp. 52–53.
382. "Natun Swapna Salbanir: Jindal-sparshe Hal Firbe Haspataler", op. cit.
383. Partha Chatterjee, "The Coming Crisis in West Bengal", *Economic and Political Weekly*, Vol. 44, No. 9, 28 February, 2009, pp. 42–45.
384. Swati Bhattacharya, "Nijabhume Bahiragat", *Anandabazar Patrika*, June 21, 2019, p.4.
385. Drimi Chaudhuri, "Bengal's public healthcare needs to be rescued from Apathy", *DNA India*, February 28, 2018, https://www.dnaindia.com/analysis/column-bengal-s-public-healthcare-needs-to-be-rescued-from-apathy-2589195, retrieved on September 17, 2019.
386. The scheme was officially launched by Hon'ble Chief Minister of West Bengal on December 30, 2016.
387. Mampi Bose, "Healthcare Financing in West Bengal", *Indian Journal of Human Development*, Vol. 16, No. 1, 2022, pp. 194–201.
388. Ibid., p. 200.
389. Sudarshana Chakraborty, "Swasthya Sathi will now include Bengal's entire population: Mamata", *Down To Earth*, November 30, 2020, available at: https://www.downtoearth.org.in/news/health/swasthya-sathi-will-now-include-bengal-s-entire-population-mamata-74458, retrieved on March 1, 2024.

CHAPTER 4

Healing the Health System: An Alternative Activism

The united struggle of people freed India from the grip of British rule. After independence, the common people hoped that the new government would bring stability and prosperity to their lives. Their dreams, however, were not fulfilled. In the wake of this, discontent began to increase among the population. Sumit Sarkar, a noted historian, wrote that "…many of the aspirations aroused in the course of the national struggle remained unfulfilled—the Gandhian dream of the peasant coming into his own in Ramrajya, as much as Left ideals of social revolution."[1] Historian Ranajit Guha argued that, by the end of the 1960s, the plight of the poor and the unemployed was so acute that latent anger could erupt at any time. He stated that the ground for a movement was ready, but that what was needed was a little bit of gunpowder. This charge was supplied by the peasant movement of Naxalbari (1967). This movement started as a protest of the peasants against the zamindars. Later, however, it spread to different areas, reflecting broader structural inequalities in Indian society. By the late 1970s, the resonance of the movement extended beyond the political sphere, influencing literature, art, history, and the social sciences. This intellectual ferment contributed to the rise of Subaltern Studies, a historiographical approach led by Guha and others that sought to recenter the voices of the marginalized in historical narratives.[2] While Subaltern Studies did not directly affect the nature or intensity of activism, it did offer a framework for rethinking oppression, resistance, and voice. Although

© The Author(s), under exclusive license to Springer Nature Switzerland AG 2025

N. Malakar, *Historicising the People's Health Movement in West Bengal, India*, https://doi.org/10.1007/978-3-032-02696-5_4

Subaltern Studies itself was not a political movement, it contributed to shaping the discourse and strategies of activism by providing intellectual tools that challenged dominant narratives and highlighted people's struggles. Subaltern historians argued that, although colonial rule in this country came to an end in 1947, colonial culture did not disappear. The machinery of the state remained thoroughly colonial. In the wake of these events, it was not possible to alleviate the suffering of the common people.[3]

Likewise, it was impossible to heal the health system radically. There was a colonial legacy in the health system. Under colonial rule, the people of this country were deprived of adequate health facilities, and this continued after independence. The health system was unable to accommodate every citizen. Furthermore, people who were able to obtain this facility were subjected to some intrinsic malpractices within the health care system itself.[4] Debabar Banerji wrote that "a large number of 'seeds of hope' emerged when the leaders of the freedom movement dreamed of the health actions that would take place after India gained independence. These, however, remained mere dreams in the changed political conditions of the post-Independence period."[5] As a result, the people's health movement emerged. Amar Jesani, a researcher of public health, holds the view that a new phase of 'health activism' began in the late 1960s, when the breakdown of the planning became apparent and an immense movement of the rural masses hit the country. That epoch was marked by the unrest not only in India, but also in the international arena. In developed countries such as France, Leftist students and working people took to the streets to change the world.[6]

What is the health movement or the people's health movement? According to Dr. Abhay Shukla and Dr. Anant Phadke, health activists' "activities initiated to counterpoise the current health system, attempting to collectively influence health determinants, health care and health-related ideology in a democratic, may be regarded as the health movement in our country."[7] Anant Phadke also wrote that "Those environmental movements which are aimed at improving the environment of human habitat are launched with the explicit aim of improving the health of the people can also be seen as health movements. The occupational health movement is one such movement."[8] The main objectives of the broad-based people's health movement were:

- To struggle for developing social determinants of health (pollution-free environment, proper sanitation, nutrition, pure drinking water, psychosocial factors, etc.).
- To make movements to create people-oriented medical systems and to create small alternative model health care systems.
- To make the people aware of healthcare's commercialization and the exploitative nature of healthcare and to create pressure for change in health policies and policies related to essential drugs.[9]

As part of the popular movement, this movement strives for a just and democratic society in which the slogan of "health for all" would become a reality and health would become a right for all Indians. It is noteworthy that "the struggle for health was part of the overall struggle against colonial rule."[10] It prompted a number of internally originated movements aimed at developing ways to enhance people's health.[11] In independent India, the struggle for health was inextricably linked to the struggle for a more compassionate social, economic, and political order. According to Lawrence O. Gostin and Lindsay F. Wiley, "The public health community takes it as an article of faith that health must be society's overarching value. Yet politicians do not always see it that way…What is needed is a clear vision of, and rationale for, healthy populations as a political priority."[12] However, political parties put a greater focus on curative medicine rather than preventive medicine. To improve people's health, however, the priority should be on disease prevention, which can help to minimize hospital overcrowding. As a result, those in need of medical treatment would be able to receive it properly. However, neither the West Bengal state government nor the union government took the matter seriously. Thus, people became infected with diseases, and hospitals became overcrowded.[13] In a true sense, initiatives for improving public health may not be visible. By contrast, the offering of medical treatment is easily visible. In view of this, the government might have placed a greater focus on insurance-based health care. Kumar Rana, a researcher and social activist, expressed the opinion that "political leaders decide what to be stressed on, and in poor areas they put pressure on the administration to concentrate on such schemes that involve visible benefit to the people."[14] In his thesis, he also quoted the statement of a political leader of Birbhum district, who stated

> Ours is a poor district. So, we cannot but take up some schemes which give immediate relief to the people…Toilets can be built up later on, we have

> time for that. What is needed now is to transfer some money to the hands of the people from government treasury. So, our emphasis is on schemes like *Janani Suraksha Yojana* (JSY), which helps enhance institutional delivery on one hand and give some money in the hands of people on the other.[15]

Thus, people's expectations of 'health for all' failed to materialize. At different times, ordinary people organized movements with various demands, among which the food movement of the 1960s was a prominent example. The people organized movements for various issues, but did not organize any mass movement demanding a decent public health and health care system. The fact is that people could not acknowledge a lack of a proper health system until they became ill, because they were unaware of the socio-economic causes of the diseases. That is why the people's health movement aimed to unite the people to struggle for the betterment of public health and to awaken the people to fight for 'Health for All.' This movement, in fact, aspired to do what the mainstream political parties could not. In this scenario, Kerala was an exceptional example. People there protested when they were deprived of health care. Moni Nag wrote[16]

> ...when a primary health centre in Kerala was short of a physician or para-medical personnel, there was a strong public demand for immediate replacement...My observation in West Bengal villages in the 1970s led me to feel that a similar situation there would not have elicited any protest either.

Sunil S. Amrith asserts that Kerala developed a rights-based approach to public health in the period after independence. In Kerala, the 'universal' campaigns for disease control and eradication were accompanied by a sustained and highly politicized effort to strengthen local institutions. During the mid-twentieth century, health was promoted as a 'people's right' in a manner that was nearly unparalleled in the region. Rooted in nineteenth-century social reform traditions in Travancore and Cochin, this culture was reinforced by a strong communist movement and the People's Science Movement, which promoted health awareness and activism. The widespread politicization of public health issues engendered a heightened consciousness among the poor that 'health services were their right and not a boon conferred upon them.' The People's Science Movement has played a crucial role by conducting health camps, campaigning against unsafe drugs, and spreading public health awareness through its publications, *Sastragathy* and *Sastra Keralam*. Furthermore, Kerala's high literacy rates and active popular press—especially women's magazines and newspapers—played a pivotal role in circulating ideas about health and rights. Significant participation of women in the workforce also contributed to a more informed and health-conscious society.[17]

Following Amartya Sen, we can state here that inequity in health care access was significantly lower in Europe since there had been numerous political movements demanding equality for a long time; old leftist and Marxist ideas also had a strong influence there. However, the leftist movement in West Bengal and India had been weakened.[18] In reality, no political party bothered about the health movement because it might have taken time to secure the political benefits of the movement. According to Moni Nag, "to raise the awareness of people about their right to demand and use health facilities has never been an important agenda of any Indian political party, but such awareness should be considered as one aspect of what may broadly be called political awareness."[19] Mahesh Rangarajan, a political analyst and historian, said "…the idea of political rights is more established in India than social rights. However, the latter has had greater currency in southern and western India, due to reformists who took up health and education as key priorities."[20] He also remarked that "…because of acute poverty, and the sheer struggle for survival faced by millions of people, something like access to food gets greater political attention than access to health care in this country."[21]

In states where health care became an electoral issue, however, political parties demanded improvements in order to win polls. For example, the *Rajiv Aarogyasri Scheme*, state-funded health insurance, seemed to have contributed to the Congress's success in the assembly election of Andhra Pradesh in 2009. The Governments of Tamil Nadu and Karnataka also launched programs: the *Kalaignar Insurance Scheme* and the *Yeshasvini Cooperative Farmers Health Care Scheme*, respectively.[22] Even the union government launched *Ayushman Bharat Pradhan Mantri Jan Arogya Yojana* before the Lok Sabha election of 2019.[23] In West Bengal the access to healthcare also became an electoral issue.[24]

However, in the late 1970s and early 1980s, the people of West Bengal became increasingly aware of their right to health, assisting in organizing the people's health movement. After World War II, as medical research advanced, the cost of modern medical treatment was enhanced, resulting in an increase in people's demand for government medical services. People grew to believe that receiving government health care is their right, and they blamed the government when they were denied access to public health services. This is applicable throughout the world.[25] The Alma-Ata Conference, which opened a new horizon in the health movement, was held in 1978 to cope with that pressure coming from below.[26]

Impact of Left Ideology

India experienced an emergence of radicalism after the potential of economic growth through the Nehruvian model became exhausted by the 1970s. Various anti-establishment groups with different ideologies had a resurgence. Initially, this kind of opposition was primarily located in the political sphere. However, gradually some educated younger people opted out of mainstream politics and went into the fields of alternative rural development, health, education, and 'science popularization.' Some of them forged new politics through struggles on the issues of caste, gender, and the environment. In each of these new groups, there was a mixture of people belonging to different ideologies—from Gandhians to Marxists or humanists of various hues; some had been part of a political organization earlier and hence had a clear political perspective, whereas many had no such background.[27]

In West Bengal, the Naxals (Naxalites) wanted to demolish the old ideas and bring about changes in the world of ideas. Moreover, people understood that good times would not be brought about by political changes alone; rather, a cultural revolution was needed as Mao had brought about in the case of China. The Naxalites claimed that social change would be brought about by armed struggle, with peasants as the main force. Many youths who believed in that ideology went to the villages to make the ordinary people involved in the movement. However, the movement gradually slowed down in the 1970s because of their practice of violence. The questions raised by the Naxalites, however, were not resolved. Those who were influenced by the Naxalite ideology wanted to come to the people. Thus, they became activists of various organizations who aimed to work for the people.[28]

Sabyasachi Chatterjee, who has investigated the history of the people's science movements, pointed out that after the Naxalite movement failed to achieve its goal, it was realized that scientific temper should be spread among people in order to promote the 'Cultural Revolution.' As a result, the people's science movement (PSM) was in full swing in West Bengal. Those who had been active in the political movement for so long turned to various new fields of movement, including group theatre, little magazines, and the fold of the PSM.[29] The people's health movement in West Bengal was just such a movement. Indeed, it is not even possible to separate the people's health movement from the PSM. Anwar Jaffry et al. wrote that "Evolving a people's health movement should form one of the most important elements of a People's Science Movement. This was the unanimous opinion of all the groups."[30] This article also stated that four areas, health, education, the environment, and the use of art as important mediums of communication with the people, were identified for future programmes for initiating a people's science movement in India.[31] Venni Venkata Krishna wrote:

> PSM groups have also initiated programs relating to people's health in the literacy movement. The main objective is to make people aware of their fundamental right(s) to demand access to health facilities. PSM groups are extending the concept of people's health to include health care, nutrition, safe drinking water, sanitation, employment and basic housing rather than equating health with disease, doctors, hospitals and drugs.[32]

Now the questions are: What was the nature of the people's health movement? Did it want to bring reformatory or revolutionary changes? According to Abhay Bang and Ashvin Patel, there were two schools of thought in the arena of people's health. One school was confident that the alternative approach to health care delivery, which often involved the use of non-professionals (village health workers) and 'appropriate technology' in health care, would be a 'panacea' for people's health problems. Another school believed that the contemporary economic system was the main cause of health problems and that nothing could or should be done to remedy these problems unless the contemporary economic-political system was changed by revolution.[33] The health movement in Dalli-Rajhara, a town in Chattisgarh, India, focused on "alternative construction," which was a revolutionary approach. Another writer, Shankar Guha Niyogi, thought that "alternative construction" would make the exploited people aware of their rights on the one hand and intensify the conflict with the exploiting class on the other.[34] In addition, according to Zafrullah Chowdhury, the leading figure in *Gonoshasthya Kendra* in Bangladesh, "it may be impossible to bring about a revolution till reformist measures significantly improve the health and nutrition of the masses and make them receptive to political education conductive to revolutionary upsurge."[35] So, it may be stated that the role of the people's health movement is to pave the way for bringing revolutionary changes in the field of health and health system.

The people's health movement in West Bengal was primarily initiated by the efforts of some science activists, physicians, medical students, and junior doctors. However, the history of the participation of doctors in the movement of common people is not a recent phenomenon. In his presidential speech at *All-India Medical Conference* in Lahore in 1929, Bidhan Chandra Ray stated

> Gentlemen, I have very definite views on this question. In India we never regarded the various affairs of life as watertight compartments: politics, technically so-called, is intermixed with economic, social and medical problems. If politics means the science of organization for the purpose of securing the greatest good for the greatest number, I declare, we members of the profession dare not keep away from politics.[36]

During the pre-independence period, some doctors in Bengal were associated with the revolutionary movement. Narayan Roy (1903–1973), a meritorious student of the Calcutta Medical College, took part in the freedom struggle after becoming a doctor. He had close ties with the revolutionary groups and was later imprisoned after being convicted in a political case (the Mechua Bazar Bomb Case) in 1930–1931. In addition to joining the revolutionary movement, he also gained a reputation as a doctor.[37] In the mid-1930s, the *All India Students Federation* attracted a number of medical students, including Sisir Bose. In 1940–1941, he took a leading role in the attempt to establish a *Students Congress.* In August 1942, the students marched in support of the Quit India movement.[38]

I have mentioned earlier that doctors associated with the *People's Relief Committee* stood by the common people during the famine of 1943 and a variety of other disasters. Dr. Purnendu Ghosh, who was known as *Ranga Daktar*, was one who helped the people during the *Tebhaga Movement* at Kakdwip (an area of South 24 Parganas district).[39] In the post-independence era, some doctors and medical students joined the mass movement for society. One of them was Dr. Jnanabrata Sil, the pioneering person of the *Norman Bethune Janaswasthya Andolan.* He participated in the food movement and was injured by a police baton.[40] He was a member of *Bengal Provincial Students' Federation* (BPSF) and *Communist Party of India* (CPI). He also led the *Medical College Hostel Students' Association* at 217 Bowbazar Street in Kolkata.[41]

Although some scattered incidents did take place, there was no organized movement of medical students at that time with people's health demands. Neither the left parties nor the doctors made any attempt to build a health movement. Dedicated doctors did, however, use their medical knowledge to help people. They were either sympathizers of the party or members of the party. From the 1980s onward, the health movement in West Bengal started to take on a wider dimension.[42] But the development of organized people's health movements should really be traced back to the 1970s.

We have already mentioned that the Naxalite movement was the inspiration for organized resistance. They used to say that students, youth, and intellectuals would be unable to revolutionize if they could not unite with the workers and peasants.[43] Thus, many medical students or junior doctors also tried to work with the workers-farmers. Many young doctors from West Bengal rushed to Chhattisgarh to join the movement led by Shankar Guha Niyogi. One medical student wrote in his diary that:

> In 1970, I was admitted to R.G. Kar Medical College Hospital as a student. The wave of Naxalite movement then hit Kolkata hard. On the first day of my arrival in Kolkata, Vidyasagar hostel was raided. Kanu Sanyal was probably arrested that day. Every day there were clashes between students and the police. It was written on the walls of North Kolkata that 'Turn the seventies into the decade of liberation'. Stencil pictures of Chairman Mao were very common. The influence of the Naxalite movement was enormous. Every medical student was trying to enrich the daily life of the common people. Apart from the Naxalite movement, their socio-economic background had influenced the medical students.[44]

Since the 1970s, a tendency was noticed among medical students to get involved with the concept of social justice.[45] Giving up their lucrative career, they committed themselves to the cause of equity and justice. Dr. Sthabir Dasgupta (Binod), a student at R.G. Kar Medical College, discontinued his studies in 1970 and went to villages with the dream of making a new world through an armed revolution. He worked with people in several villages for six years. His dream was not fulfilled, however, and he returned to Kolkata in 1976.[46] Similarly, Jayanta Bhattacharya, a second-year medical college student, took part in the Naxalite movement in 1970–1971. He dropped out of medical college and left Kolkata determined to participate in the peasant struggle. When Naxalites were being suppressed, Bhattacharya was arrested in the Gaya district of Bihar before being imprisoned in Kolkata. There he was severely tortured. In 1983–1984, he was released from prison. Meanwhile his classmates became doctors. Many of them, who were involved in student politics, joined the leftists in power. Jayanta re-entered the medical college as a third-year student. During this period, he became very popular with the *Medical College Democratic Students Association* (MCDSA).[47]

In India, during the 1970s, the union government's policy was criticized. The declaration of a "Total Revolution" by Jayaprakash Narayan against the misrule in Bihar and the union government played a leading role in building the human rights movement.[48] Jayaprakash Narayan said that people have the right to protest against any government if it fails to perform its duties. He put a greater focus on the power of the people. According to him, people associated with the mass movement should not be associated with any political party.[49] There were many similarities between the Naxalite movement and JP's movement.

In the 1960s and 1970s, the flow of an alternative movement began. The new genre of Subaltern Studies was developed within the field of history. In the 1960s, Rachel Carson's book, *Silent Spring*,[50] gave impetus to the environmental movement. Around the same period Ivan Illich wrote *Medical Nemesis*,[51] in which he attacked the Western medical system for its over-emphasis on 'medicalization.' Both of these books encouraged people to think in new ways and to raise questions.

Similarly, the Naxalite movement and the movement of Gandhian leader Jayaprakash Narayan also inspired many ideological youths in India to look for alternatives. As a result, various human rights organizations and non-political state-level city-based groups were formed in the 1970s.[52] Following the end of two years of state emergency in 1977, India witnessed an explosion of new human rights and socio-economic movements.[53] Those movements were called the "New Social Movements," and one of them was the people's health movement.

In this light, mention can be made of the *Medico Friend Circle* (MFC), which was influenced by the movement of Janata Wave led by Jayaprakash Narayan. MFC arose as a platform for health professionals from different geographical areas and socio-political backgrounds, who were dissatisfied with the elitist nature of the existing health system.[54] MFC was initiated by visionaries of an alternative society in 1974. It is an organization that has operated for forty years as a 'thought current' without allegiance to any specific ideology. Its only commitment has been to intervene in and understand the debates, policies and health practices in an independent India.[55] "MFC wanted to be a body to provide deeper analysis of the health situation and its relation to socioeconomic-political factors." "It wanted to experiment in alternative health approaches at micro level informed with critical analysis of the health system. MFC wanted to promote philanthropic health services."[56] MFC shared its view through the *Medico Friend Circle Bulletin*, which was first published in 1976.[57] In the first issue of the *MFC Bulletin*, it was written that "This monthly bulletin hopes to continue to provide a common forum for the exchange of experience and views among those who are genuinely concerned with health and health related problems."[58] MFC organized annual meetings to discuss health problems in the country. The doctors of West Bengal participated in the meetings of MFC at different times. All across India, other initiatives in community health in that era were the *Comprehensive Rural Health Project* (CRHP)[59] at Jamkhed (Maharashtra), *Lok Biradari Prakalp*,[60] the *Integrated Rural Health Project* at Pachod (Maharashtra), the *Catholic Health Association of India* (CHAI), the *Christian Medical Association of India* (CMAI), *Kerala Shashtra Sahitya Parishad* (KSSP), the *Voluntary Health Association of India* (VHAI) etc.

CHAI was founded by Dr. Mary Glowrey, an Australian sister-doctor, in 1943 along with 15 sisters with the goal of providing curative care to people, especially to the poor, women, and children.[61] In the 1970s, it worked together with other organizations. KSSP, which was founded in 1962 as a forum of science writers and which evolved into a people's science movement in the 1970s, promoted a people-oriented approach to health. Led by a dedicated band of doctors, health workers, and activists, the organization conducted village-level classes and discussions on common health problems and scientific and cost-effective solutions. Additionally, it campaigned to expose the role of multinational corporations and big business in promoting and perpetuating ill-health. The KSSP developed an alternative people's health policy after critically analysing the health policies of the union and state governments.[62] VHAI had begun in 1969 as the Coordinating Agency for Health Planning (CAHP), when 25 leaders of Christian hospitals across the country met to discuss the problem of delivering health care to millions of rural people. By 1974, VHAI had emerged as a federation of State Voluntary Health Associations that was geared toward promoting the community health movement.[63]

West Bengal Voluntary Health Association (WBVHA) was established in 1974 as a state organization of VHAI.[64] Aim and objectives of the organization were:

- To do works or charity and service aimed at improving the health or the people irrespective of race, religion, caste or community.
- To promote greater cooperation among voluntary as well as government health agencies by undertaking joint coverage of community health work.
- To collaborate with other health agencies working in the area to ensure conservation of resources and as wide public health coverage as possible.
- To collect, exchange and disseminate health information as well as to do research in the area.
- To conduct seminars, workshops and conferences.[65]

The enthusiasm of voluntarism in the 1970s was not entirely based on a medical perspective, but rather on social, political, and economic environments in India[66] in which young, newly graduated doctors sought to "change the world."[67] Two major networks, the *All India Drug Action Network* (AIDAN) (1980) and the *All India People's Science Network* (AIPSN) (1988) were organized in the 1980s.

The *Tamil Nadu Science Forum*, established in 1980, initially concentrated on promoting literacy, much like the People's Science Movement in Kerala. By the 1990s, however, it had expanded its focus to include public health. Its health initiative, the *Arogya Iyakkam*, was active in around 500 villages, working to raise awareness and provide education on key public health issues.[68]

An important periodical, named the *Socialist Health Review* (SHR), started its journey in 1984 and continued to be brought out until 1988. It functioned as a platform for propagating and developing a Marxist approach to health (i.e. determinants and dynamics of health and disease) and medicine (i.e. medical technology as well as systems of medical care). SHR, being a periodical devoted to theoretical aspects of health and medicine, did not attempt to become an action-oriented periodical in the sense of an organizer of an action group. It believed that the formulation and clarification of these theoretical issues were essential for successful, politically relevant action and that, in that way, the periodical would facilitate effective health action.[69] SHR stated that "we feel that the very fact of the need for such a periodical having been felt indicates that the health movement within the broad left movement has reached a stage of maturity…"[70] SHR started publishing again in 1995 under the new name *Radical Journal of Health.*

Organizations of Medical Students and Doctors

Since its very beginning, the people's health movement in West Bengal was initiated by members of the medical fraternity. Thus, the role of doctors' organizations needs to be analysed. *Indian Medical Association* (IMA), the oldest doctors' organization, was established on January 1, 1928 as a part of India's freedom movement, especially in Bengal. From its inception, the IMA drew the attention of the governments of both the center and state levels regarding the problems of health care, medical education, drug policy, and the problems of industrial health hazards.[71] This organization used to publish its views on the medical system and medical education system in the country and overseas in the *Journal of the Medical Association.* When the United Front (1967) was established in West Bengal, the Left-wing doctors organized a health fair in Kolkata for seven days. In 1972, at the IMA's all-India conference in Bombay, delegates from West Bengal demanded that a national health policy should be made by the union government. The conference was attended by many political leaders, including E.M.S. Namboodiripad.[72] In Kolkata, those doctors started a movement to improve the Employee State Insurance (ESI) system. The doctors spent a night in front of the Raj Bhavan in an effort to secure their demands. They sent a memorandum to the then Governor Shanti Swaroop Dhavan (1969–1971) demanding improvement in the labour-health system. However, the IMA could not involve the general public in their movement.[73] According to Dr Hiralal Konar, "it was an organization of the elite class of physicians."[74] They had not been able to form people's health movement literally. Furthermore, it is worth noting that no powerful organization of government doctors existed in West Bengal till 1972.[75]

The first organization of government doctors in West Bengal was established during the 1970s. The state's health services were not fully engaged in public service due to government mismanagement and the absence of people's health movements. That organization of doctors came out in protest against the government's neglect of the health sector.[76] The *Health Service Association* (HSA) of West Bengal, the organization of government doctors, was established in 1972. Initially, the organization began to run a movement focusing on the field of service discrimination to address issues like salary, rank etc. They also demanded that the health system should be created to serve the common people. They said that public health care should not be aimed to serve the rich only; it should be run in the service of the ordinary people. They organized cease-work 46 days in 1974 and 34 days in 1976 to improve health service, although they simultaneously arranged alternative outpatient facilities for the common people. The HSA also launched a long-standing movement aimed at establishing the right to health. They categorically pointed out that health is not a consumer product. In that movement, HSA gained the support of the medical students. As a result, the *Students and Doctors Social Services & Survey Association* and the *People's Health Service Association* were established.[77]

At that time Siddhartha Shankar Roy was the chief minister of West Bengal and the state's health minister was Ajit Panja. According to Asim Sarkar, a senior doctor, a cease-work had started to draw attention to the lack of infrastructure of the hospitals. The theme song of that movement in 1974 was "*ay re ebar korbo ebar eksathe larai/ e larai banchar larai/ banchate chai banchteo chai*" (Come on, we will fight together in this time/ this fight is a fight to survive/ we want to save, we want to be saved). The song was composed by Asim Sarkar himself.[78] In their agitation against the then Congress government, they received widespread support from the Leftists.[79] It was quite natural for the leftists to join the movement against the established power.

In 1974, doctors of HSA received support from engineers in launching a strike to establish the importance of technicians instead of bureaucrats in health policymaking. That movement affected medical students. In 1975, medical students participated in relief work in drought-affected Bankura.[80]

The influence of the Naxalite movement shook the whole of West Bengal during that time, which also motivated the medical students. Medical students raised questions about the luxurious lifestyle of senior doctors. They also questioned the colonial curriculum in medical education because the books written by foreign writers were based on curative medicine. These books did not talk about the prevention of diseases of poor farmers or labourers. The middle-class, lower-middle-class and medical students were well aware of the health problems of the common people. Before the late 1960s, it had been only the students from 'elite' families who used to study medicine.[81]

Poor people were regularly deprived of medical services in public hospitals. That problem was addressed by the Naxalite medical students.[82] Therefore, by 1972–1973, medical students, house-staffs, and senior doctors at Calcutta Medical College formed the *Central Action Committee* (CAC). This body had a number of demands: that the proper hospital services should be available for 24 hours; that there should be a blood bank; that the X-ray system should be kept open for 24 hours; and that medicines would be provided free of cost. They also stated that their demands should be addressed within a given time limit. They threatened that if their demands were not resolved, they would launch an outdoor strike. In such circumstances, however, they always made alternative outdoor options for the ordinary people. Then, from 1974 to 1977, medical students tried to reach common people through cultural and social activities.[83]

There was a protest against autocracy during the emergency era (1975–1977) in India. This led to the formation of a number of democratic organizations. Within that context, on March 21, 1977, an organization called the *Medical College Democratic Students Association* (MCDSA) was formed at the Calcutta Medical College.[84]

In the beginning, all Leftist student organizations with affiliation to different Leftist parties in power acted in collaboration with MCDSA. But when the MCDSA opposed the Left Front government's anti-student policies, the student wing of *Communist Party of India (Marxist)* [CPI-M], *Student Federation of India* (SFI), emerged from the MCDSA in 1978. During that period, organizations such as MCDSA were established at various medical colleges, but they each had different names. The name of the organization was given as MCDSA in the Calcutta Medical College and the R.G. Kar Medical College and DSU in the Nil Ratan Sircar Medical College. Although the names were different, their thinking was along the same lines.[85] The medical students had chosen the ideal of humanitarian doctors such as Norman Bethune (1890–1939) and Dwarkanath Kotnis (1910–1942). With their ideal and the dream of creating a new society, the members of the *Democratic Students Association* (DSA) planned to work amongst the laborers and the peasants, as they were the real revolutionary forces of the society. They sincerely believed that the common people bore the cost of making a doctor. The government gives subsidies in medical education from taxpayers' money. Thus, the doctors have the responsibility to serve the interests of the common people. Punyabrata Goon, an activist of the peoples' health movement, offered recollections of his memory of those 'memorable days.'[86]

In 1977, the Left Front government came to power in West Bengal. However, the conditions of the government hospitals did not improve significantly. Patients observed that the hospitals did not have a sufficient supply of life-saving drugs and essential equipment. The authorities were not in a position to provide required services in government hospitals. The superintendent of the Nil Ratan Sircar Hospital had given notice that "Due to non-availability of essential life-saving drugs and equipment the emergency rooms are temporarily closed and admissions are stopped until further order."[87] In this way, the patients continued to be deprived of the medical services of the government hospital. Repetitive deprivation began to cause resentment. Ultimately, they wanted to express their anger against the doctors.

In 1979, MCDSA tried to identify the problems of the health services at the Medical College Hospital. Their investigation exposed the poor conditions within the hospital. In a bid to change the situation, in 1979 medical students and junior doctors launched a movement named 'Hospital Movement' at Calcutta Medical College Hospital. A similar movement was begun at R.G. Kar Medical College Hospital. This was the preparatory phase of the greater junior doctors' movement of 1983.[88]

Junior Doctors' Movements

The 'junior doctors,' an indispensable part of the medical community of the state, are a force that always plays an active role in the improvement of medical service in the state. Their movements have been highlighted in the newspaper on a number of occasions It is important at the very outset to clarify the term 'junior doctors,' After graduating from medical college, students have to work for one year as an intern in the hospital from where they have passed. Following the completion of the internship, one may be registered with the Medical Council of India (MCI). After that, they may join as house-staff in a specialized department of a teaching hospital. Some of them enter the diploma or degree courses for postgraduate education through the entrance examination. The interns, house-staff and postgraduate trainees are all termed junior doctors.[89]

Junior doctors did not push for any greater movement before 1983. Until this time they believed that the promises given by the government might be fulfilled at a later stage. However, the situation remained the same. That's why junior doctors from different medical colleges began to form organizations like the *House Staff-Intern Association* and the *Junior Doctors Association*. In January 1982, such organizations from seven medical colleges in West Bengal came together under the umbrella of the *All Bengal Junior Doctors' Federation* (ABJDF),[90] which was influenced by Naxalite ideology with the dream of ending anarchy in hospitals.[91] During the movement of 1983, their demands were divided into two categories: action demands and basic demands.[92]

Action Demands

- The supply of life-saving and essential drugs, other equipment from rural health centers and city hospitals should be regularized and be made available. Antibiotics must be supplied.
- X-ray, ECG, blood, and other necessary tests should be made available for 24 hours.
- All the willing junior doctors will have to be employed in a government job after the completion of the house staff period.
- The stipend of junior doctors should be increased.
- Work hours should be specified as 48 hours a week.
- The draconian Hospital Bill should be nullified.
- The hospital management system should be developed democratically. This management system should have representatives from all levels of staff including doctors.
- The actual safety of all levels of health workers, including hospital doctors, must be ensured. Illegal houses and people should be removed from the hospital.

Basic Demands

- The government must take initiative to formulate a public-oriented scientific national health policy, recognizing the right to every human health service as a 'fundamental right' and to implement it effectively.
- There should be one primary and three subsidiary health centres per block so that there is one doctor for 1000 people.
- Scientific drug policy should be formulated. To ensure life-saving and essential drug availability and distribution, medicines should be prepared at a low cost under state control.
- Health sector allocation should be increased in the central and state budgets.

- For the prevention of disease, a public health system (improved drainage, safe drinking water, vaccination, adequate nutritious food supply) should be developed.
- The scientific and public-oriented education system should be developed instead of unscientific medical education.[93]

In January 1982, the first convention of the ABJDF was held at Nil Ratan Sircar Medical College and Hospital and their demands were specified. Thereafter, through demonstrations and rallies, they repeatedly presented their charter of demands to the government. Except for a verbal promise of the government, however, nothing was gained. On March 23, 1983, the ABJDF held its second convention at Calcutta Medical College and Hospital. The ABJDF started a campaign at outpatient departments by distributing leaflets outlining their demands. They held 67 rallies in and around Kolkata to put their demands before the public. On April 8, the ABJDF handed over a memorandum to the hospital superintendent and the principal. They informed them that they would boycott all the hospitals outdoors on a gradual basis from April 25 to 30 if their demands were not fulfilled.[94] But the position of the hospital authorities and the government remained unchanged. Then junior doctors met the health minister on May 3, 1983. However, having no hope, they began to boycott outdoors of different hospitals from May 9, according to their plan.[95]

Junior doctors protested when two of the house staff, Tapas Bhoumik and Naren Mukherjee of Burdwan Medical College, were dismissed before the completion of their terms. They demanded that the government should overturn the dismissal order. As a protest, they began to boycott the outdoor and indoor departments of hospitals from June 15, 1983. However, emergency squads were created to facilitate the patients.[96] Chief Minister Jyoti Basu held a meeting with junior doctors on June 17 to resolve the problem.[97] Shyamal Chakraborty wrote about the meeting with the Chief Minister in the *Rabibasariya* of *Anandabazar Patrika*.[98]

They had talks with Health Minister Ambearish Mukherjee, but the government refused to accept their demands.[99] As their movement continued, the situation became even more chaotic. One woman died soon after reaching the Nil Ratan Sircar Hospital (NRS) and doctors were assaulted by relatives of the patient. As a result, ABJDF called cease-work in the hospital's outpatient departments for seven days beginning on September 21, 1983. However, they still continued the alternative clinic so that patients' interests were protected. The alternative clinics became overcrowded.[100] Health Minister Ambarish Mukherjee commented that "Some multinational companies are helping the doctors. Otherwise, where would they get such unlimited supplies of costly drugs that they distributed free at their parallel clinics which they ran during their seven-day cease-work?"[101]

At that time, Chief Minister Jyoti Basu was in Kashmir and Benoy Choudhury was the acting government chief. He called on senior doctors to mediate the problem. But junior doctors rejected this offer. As a result, Choudhury stated that, "The government will not bow to any pressure." Although the Leftists were silent, filmmaker Mrinal Sen was not. He criticized the government, saying "What has the government done to improve the condition of the hospitals?"[102]

In 1983, when the LF government consistently refused to hold talks with the agitating junior doctors, the Health Service Association (HSA) intervened with a package which was accepted by both parties. But the health minister made a sudden volte-face.[103] The government demanded a written statement from the agitating junior doctors regarding the circumstances in which they had abstained from the service during the cease-work in several government hospitals. The government also decided to defer the payment of stipends to junior doctors for September and the issuing of internship completion certificates to those who had completed their training on September 30, or earlier. The junior doctors refused to present a written explanation, presenting an ultimatum to several hospital authorities for the unconditional payment of the stipends and the issuance of completion certificates.[104]

The situation became more complicated when junior doctors gheraoed the principals or superintendents in different medical colleges and hospitals. On October 4, junior doctors gheraoed the Superintendent Dr. Sujit Mitra and Principal Dr. Haren Ghosh of the National Medical College, Kolkata, protesting against non-receipt of stipends and internship completion certificates. A similar situation was created in the NRS, SSKM and R.G. Kar medical college hospitals. In that situation, junior doctors were beaten by police. Many doctors were injured. Junior doctors from SSKM alleged that one of the junior doctors' shoulder bones had been badly damaged. Blood clotted on the backside of another's head. On the night of the attack by the police, doctors had to leave the entire compound of the Nil Ratan Sirckar Hospital for their own safety. Police also brought a van to arrest the doctors. The main roadside gate was closed by the police.[105] The next day, on October 5, 1983, the first page of *Anandabazar*

Patrika, published news with the caption, "*5 Haspatale Ghearao, Lathi Daktar Ahato*" (Gheraoed in 5 hospitals, doctors were injured by lathi-charge).[106] The agitating junior doctors came on the streets that night and shouted "***daktarder rakta habe na ko byartha***" (the blood of doctors will not go in vain).[107]

The LF government wanted to suppress the health right movement by deploying the police. In this regard, we may mention Nilanjan Dutta's comment:

> It is not that the Left parties in West Bengal, including the CPI (M), did not understand the importance of the rights issue. They knew that they rode to power after the people of the state suffered massive violation of human rights in the hands of the previous Congress regime, which they had promised to restore. But even if they had restored the rights, they failed to protect them because of their exigencies of staying in power in a system that feels constantly threatened by the people's exercising of their rights. Not only that, they responded to the people's repeated protests against this failure with further restriction and repression.[108]

Benoy Choudhury spoke on behalf of the government, stating that the police had to make a lathi-charge in order to rescue the gheraoed officials.[109] In a protest against the brutal attacks by the police on junior doctors, the HSA called cease-work in the emergency and outdoor departments of all major hospitals in West Bengal for an indefinite period from October 7. The West Bengal branch of the *Indian Medical Association* (IMA) supported the call to strike. After the return of Jyoti Basu from Kashmir, negotiations with the government took place on October 11, but the first round was unsuccessful.[110] The negotiations were resumed on October 13. The government accepted several more demands and requested that the junior doctors withdraw their strike. On October 14, HSA and IMA decided to withdraw the strike and, at night ABJDF decided to re-join the work.[111]

To check the progress of the junior doctors' movement, the CPI (M) formed the *All Bengal Junior Doctor Council* (ABJDC), a separate organization. The *Association of Health Service Doctors* (AHSD), a parallel organization with party patronage, was also formed, in the presence of several ministers and three members of the party secretariat. Thus, the people of West Bengal perceived the AHSD to be an organization of government employees directly sponsored by the ruling party, and which naturally owed open allegiance to the ruling party. To increase the membership of the new organization, about 300 new doctors were recruited on an ad hoc basis, by-passing the *West Bengal Public Service Commission* (WBPSC). The health minister told the press that they had been appointed to serve as a 'strike-breaking force' in future.[112] For the loyalty of the party, arrangements were also made to award hospital officials or doctors in several ways such as accelerating promotion, gainful appointments, financial incentives, etc.[113] In contrast, the doctors of the AHSD argued that

> In early 1983, in the wake of the unjustifiable movement of junior doctors in Burdwan Medical College and Hospital, a chaotic situation arose in the medical colleges and hospitals across the state. The crisis was exacerbated when some leaders of the then *Health Service Association* (HSA) shamelessly supported the movement, ignoring the views of most members of the organization, and urged the service doctors to cease work, which created an anarchy in medical services across the state. All decisions were taken without the consent of the then president of HSA, Bhaskar Roychowdhury (eminent neurologist). Consequently, he was forced to resign from his post…In such an unusual situation; several members started thinking of forming a separate organization. On June 24, 1984, in a conference at the Moulali Youth Centre, in the presence of the then Chief Minister of West Bengal Jyoti Basu and 451 members, the *Association of Health Service Doctors* (AHSD), West Bengal, started its way. Some doctors in service, such as Dr. Gauripada Dutt, Dr. Monindra Banerjee, Dr. Naresh Banerjee et al., assisted in forming the organization.[114]

On the AHD website, it was also written that "the organisation was born in 1984 amidst a turbulent period of chaos and attempts to jeopardise the government health care system, with a vow to protect, promote and improve it, under the banner of Science, Service & Society."[115]

However, in addition to the HSA and the IMA, junior doctors received support from the *Medical Services Centre*, the *General Practitioners' Associations*, the DSO (Democratic Student Organization), the DYO (*Democratic Youth Organization*), *Krishak O Khetmajur Federation* (Federation of Farmers and Farm Workers), UTUC (*United Trade Union Congress*), *Mahila Sanskritik Sangha* (Women's Cultural Association), *Sampradayik Sampriti O Ganatantrik Adhikar O Byakti Swadhinata Raksha Committee* (the Committee for the Protection of Communal Harmony and Democratic Rights and Individual Freedom), the *University Students Cultural Forum, Sramik Sangram Committee* (Labour Struggle

Committee), the *Federation of Association of Unit Jadavpur University*, the *Junior Advocate Association*, the *All Engineering and Technological Officers*, the *Juvenile Diabetic Foundation*, and other organizations.[116]

Intellectuals also supported the movement. Noted Bengali writer Premendra Mitra stated that, "In a civilized country, this condition of the hospital cannot be continued—there is a great need for better treatment of ordinary people. This movement has made people aware of the condition of the hospital— it is not a small gain."[117] In support of the movement, writer and social activist Mahashweta Devi commented, "Their movement has no comparison. They are doing well. That should be. I have been supporting them from the beginning. If this is the medical condition in Kolkata, then the state of the village can be easily estimated. This movement is not a war against the patient but an oath to approach them."[118] Birendra Chattopadhyay, noted Bengali poet, held the pen in support of the junior doctors' movement and wrote a poem titled "Haspital Mane" (Hospital Means).[119]

It was not only the support of intellectuals, but also the movement of the junior doctors gained widespread support from the common people because, besides the professional demands, the movement spoke of people's health. They were able to say in front of the chief minister and the health minister that "Health is not a matter of charity; the right to health is our fundamental right."[120] Dr. Debashish Dutta of R.G Kar Medical College, the first president of the ABJDF, said: "…the spontaneous support of the public has helped us to direct the movement in the right way…We feel that people's health movement can be fulfilled only by ensuring the direct participation of the people. Doctors or health workers may have played some role in initiating the movement, but after a stage, the people should organize and take the initiative."[121] Dr. Ashok Samanta, secretary of the *Medical Service Centre*, similarly wrote: "The CPI (M)-led state government has tried to dilute the mass movement to gain the support of the capitalist class in West Bengal. The government has been somewhat successful, but the historical junior doctors' movement developed on a solid base which has been created by the language movement, bus-tram-train fare increased resistance movement."[122]

In the late 1980s, the PIX group,[123] with some financial support from ABJDF, made a documentary named *Swasthya Aamar Adhikar* (Health is my right) about the movement of junior doctors. It was screened several times to full house audiences at the Muslim Institute auditorium and in

All Bengal Student Association (ABSA) programs all across Bengal. That documentary attracted considerable acclaim.[124]

With the movement of junior doctors in 1983, the government immediately gave some attention to the hospitals. But it kept few of its promises. Therefore, the movement started up again. The Left Front government claimed that the outlay on health care had increased substantially. According to a booklet issued by the State Information and Cultural Affairs Department, the per capita expenditure on health care was Rs. 15.90 in 1976, but had increased to Rs. 37.07 by 1985 during the Left Front regime. According to the ABJDF, these funds were still inadequate; the per capita allotment for hospital patients was Rs. 4 for food and only Re 1 for medicines.[125]

A letter from the health minister, Ambarish Mukherjee, gives a pathetic picture of the state of the hospitals of West Bengal during the 1980s. Health Minister Ambarish Mukherjee wrote in a letter sent on November 11, 1986 to the Superintendent of R.G. Kar Medical College Hospital that "Smt. Parul Champa Banik is reported to be an O.P.D patient of your hospital, who was advised for an X-Ray sometime in the month of July 1986. During these months she was requested occasionally to turn up in your hospital for her X-Ray, but the same has not yet been done. I would request you to look into the case so that the X-Ray is done at an early date."[126] It is not known whether or not the X-ray of Parul Chapa was carried out at all. However, a genuine picture of the hospital can be inferred from the contents of that letter. Perhaps more significant is that it is likely to be impossible for an ordinary person to receive a letter from the health minister.

Debashish Dutta argued, "we expected the government would keep its promise, but our hopes did not come true. We had hoped that, as at R.G. Kar, other hospitals too would have round-the-clock X-ray and biochemistry test facilities. That, however, had not materialized. Hospital facilities remained inadequate, and and the living arrangements for junior doctors were extremely poor. Furthermore, no regular recruitment of doctors through the West Bengal Public Service Commission (WBPSC) had been arranged. Consequently, we had no choice but to agitate again."[127]

In August 1986, the ABJDF submitted a 13-point charter to the government. This contained four basic demands, including the improvement of public health facilities in the hospitals. But the government ignored the demands.[128]

Nabarun Ghoshal, one of the leaders of the junior doctors' movement in 1987, wrote from his memory that:

> In 1987, we were house staff. The junior doctors of SSKM made a movement for a salary hike. The police came and beat them. Then Samir, our friend, also was house staff there. Entering the stick in his mouth, Sultan Singh, a police officer, said *Kha shala daktar, lathi kha* (take this stick in your mouth bloody doctor). As a result of that incident, a new movement of junior doctors in West Bengal was started. In all the colleges, junior doctors spontaneously joined the movement. Consequently, in the area adjacent to R.G. Kar, Laxmi Sen, a heavyweight leader of CPI (M), lost the election. In retaliation, goons of CPI (M) attacked us in the campus.
>
> ...We went on a hunger strike and gheraoed the principal (for not taking the appropriate step to fulfil their demands). Police charged tear gas at the hospital campus unprecedentedly and took the junior doctors into the police van. The girls laid down on the front of the van.[129]

In January 1987, junior doctors opted on a novel way to achieve their aims. They began to use their left thumb impression (LTI) instead of signing, at the time of receiving their monthly stipends. They argued that since their stipend was actually lower than that of illiterate employees, such a gesture was appropriate. The news of their actions spread to different hospitals. The government instructed the hospital superintendents that junior doctors should not be paid based solely on their LTI. On January 31, the management at SSKM hospital refused to allow its junior doctors to sign for their allowances in this manner. The young doctors then squatted in front of the cash counter and proceeded to chant slogans. At this point, a large police presence, led by two deputy commissioners, entered swinging sticks and made a random lathi-charge without warning.[130] Twenty doctors were injured, some of them seriously; five of them, including a woman, were admitted to hospital; and some eight to ten doctors were arrested. The news rapidly spread to all government hospitals. From the afternoon of January 31, 1987, the ABJDF called for a cease-work, with only emergency services being maintained. On February 2, in protest at the police action, the HSA called for a day's strike, although emergency departments would be kept operational. The *All-India Association of Junior Doctors* called a nationwide token cease-work on March 12 and also pressed for an investigation into the police actions. The *All India Medical Association* (AIMA) also protested.[131]

Jyoti Basu was in Bangladesh at that time. The LF government had claimed that the junior doctors harassed the female super, so the police were compelled to lathi-charge.[132] After returning from Bangladesh, the chief minister threatened the agitators with severe punishment. This only served to intensify the movement. It is surprising to note that CPI (M) and the CITU both extended support to junior doctors' strike in Bihar, Uttar Pradesh, Delhi, whereas the Left Front government of West Bengal justified police action and condemned cease-work by junior doctors in West Bengal. Junior doctors meanwhile had been running alternative clinics, which were also joined by many senior doctors. The government declared that such illegal alternatives must be stopped immediately.[133]

Junior doctors stated that they had no allegiance to any political party and that their movement was not politically motivated. They invited various mass organizations including government employees' associations and coordination committees, to participate in the rally held at Esplanade East (Kolkata). CPI (M) state secretariat member Sailen Dasgupta opposed the junior doctors' statement saying—"of course since the beginning of this movement, the Congress, SUCI, the Naxalites were involved. That was not just a movement against the health department—at the same time it was a war against the patients."[134] When allegations were made that the party leaders, ministers, and high-ranking employees were being given access to medical courses in government colleges for their sons and daughters, he said that "out of 800 seats in the state, 10 seats are filled under the Chief Minister's quota. Admission under that quota is carefully regulated. The Chief Minister is ready to answer any question in this context. However, the quota in this state is very low compared to other states."[135] It is therefore clear that the claims made by junior doctors were not without foundation.

Junior doctors stepped up their propaganda campaign through street rallies, hunger strikes and the formation of citizens' committees. They wanted to reach the people, and so they organized a blood donation program. They put their posters everywhere in the form of protest. One of the ABJDF's posters read "We do not want police in hospital, we want drugs."[136] In describing the outcomes of the junior doctors' movement in 1987, Nabarun Ghoshal stated:

> That movement made too many humanitarian doctors, most of whom treat patients without commission yet. At least they take care of the patients. In some cases, they still protest against social injustice. So, I think the time I

> spent in that movement was the best use of my life. That movement had taught me to think for people, made me free from superstition, and made me dream of being a revolutionary.[137]

The situation improved for a while following the actions of the movement in 1987. Over time, however, the conditions in hospitals returned to their previous state. As a result, the movement restarted. So, in 1991, junior doctors had chosen the path of movement in the same way as was in 1987. On September 1, 1991, a 26-year old patient, Tarak Das, who was suffering from copper sulfate poisoning, was brought to the Calcutta Medical College Hospital. Doctors arranged emergency treatment for the patient, but it was found that the hospital had no stock of the drug required for metallic poisoning. Nevertheless, the doctors tried their best to treat the patient with alternative methods. Despite these efforts, the relatives of the patient assaulted the doctors, including the deputy superintendent of the hospital, Dr. S Sinha, on the pretext of 'medical negligence.'[138] The junior doctors of the hospital then resorted to a 'wildcat' strike under the banner of ABJDF.[139] They said junior doctors would not work in hospitals if the Health Minister's statement was not withdrawn.[140] The junior doctors stated that they would refuse to work in hospitals unless the Health Minister withdrew his statement. They alleged that the Minister's remark—that "junior doctors do not work in hospitals"—was misleading and provocative, and could incite people to assault doctors.

On September 3, the LF government was attacked through a large text entitled *Medical Colleger Narak* (Hell of the Medical College) on the page of the *Bartaman*, a Bengali newspaper.[141] The article stated that the Calcutta Medical College Hospital had become the residence of anti-social people. The security was very poor in the hospital, despite it being located near Writers Building (the then administrative headquarter of West Bengal) and Lalbazar (the headquarters of the Kolkata police). It was said that when Jatin Chakraborty was the Minister in-Charge of Health for a few days, there had been a massive campaign against anti-social activities in the hospital. Health Minister Prasanta Sur had also taken initiatives but failed because "in the regime of CPI (M), nobody listens to anyone. The union is bigger than the minister…the 'dada' (big political leader) is bigger than the police."[142]

On September 2, 1991 the junior doctors submitted their memorandum to the hospital superintendent of Calcutta Medical College Hospital.[143] They claimed that, in the absence of life-saving medicines, it was impossible to offer proper treatment in the hospital. According to them, the hospital had previously had around 80 life-saving medicines earlier, but this number had been reduced to just 25. Their movement was in the interests of the common people. Thus, they demanded the improvement of other services, including the supply of required medicines at the hospital. When the services of the medical college proved inaccessible, the Super of the hospital informed the Writers Building to send doctors from the health department. Health Secretary Lina Chakraborty promised to check the junior doctors' claims.[144] She said that *Health Services Doctors* would be sent to the hospital to restore normality there.[145]

The health secretary had failed to resolve the disputed issues. On September 7, junior doctors from the R.G. Kar and National Medical Colleges boycotted the outpatient departments of the hospitals. They demanded that if the government would not ensure the adequate security arrangements for doctors and health staff working at the hospitals, junior doctors would continue boycotting the pressure of outpatients. They said "junior doctors of the R.G. Kar and National Medical College would continue their movement until these demands were met."[146] ABJDF began to organize the junior doctors of different medical colleges.[147] The *Junior Doctors Council* (JDC) organized a hospital rally to solve the problems of Calcutta Medical College Hospital. They condemned the work of ABJDF and called for the withdrawal of the movement. The statement made by the JDC and government had the same message. They said that cease-work by junior doctors was contrary to the interests of the common people.[148] On the other hand, the *Medical Service Centre* held a meeting outside the gate of the R.G. Kar Medical College and Hospital on September 8, in support of the 'just demands' of the agitating doctors of Calcutta Medical College (CMC).[149]

In a bid to resolve the deadlock at the CMC, the Health Minister Prasanta Sur convened a meeting with the authorities of the hospital and the representatives of the ABJDF at Writers' Building on September 9, 1991. The demands of the agitating doctors were discussed at the meeting. Afterward, junior doctors decided to re-join the outdoor and emergency department, excluding the inpatient department. On behalf of the ABJDF, it was said that if the government did not accept the claim within seven days, they would resume the cease-work. The Health Minister promised to improve the facilities of medicines, pathology, and other services in the hospital and to provide security to doctors. He said that because of the low budget allocation of the health department it would not be possible to keep more than 32 medicines in the hospital.[150] On September 11, 1991, in a press release, ABJDF stated that the Chief Minister promised to provide X-ray, ECG, biochemistry examination facilities for 24 hours in 1987, but even then no service had been provided for a portable X-ray after 2 p.m., and no emergency blood test were available in the medical college after 3 p.m.. The reason was that no new staff appointments had been made since 1989. The government was aware, but made no attempt to resolve that problem.[151]

From the above discussion, it is clear that the movements of junior doctors of 1983 and 1987 were widespread. The movement of 1991 was also a significant event, with government hospitals made very difficult places to work. So, they struggled to bring a better treatment environment in the hospitals. The movement of junior doctors in the 1980s was a part of the overall people's health movement, attempting to speak for the people.

Following that movement, people of West Bengal have come a long way and entered the new century. There was a change in government: the administration led by Mamata Banerjee, which came to power in 2011, built super-specialty hospitals. But proper health care facilities have yet to be developed. The Left Front government had sown the seeds for the privatization of the medical system; now it grew into a tree. As result, medical care was just another consumable good. The government emphasized insurance-based health care. The PPP model has been introduced in the medical field. Now patients are required to pay for treatment even in public hospitals and often face additional charges for services such as X-rays.[152] As a result, ordinary people have been deprived of public services. Therefore, as the primary frontline soldier of the medical system, the doctors became victims of the anger of the peasants and labourers, who are constantly deprived of medical services.

According to Hiralal Koner, the leader of the student movement of the 1980s and later the secretary of the HSA, "There has been increased brightness in health. But the root cause, the problem of bed and referral, remains in the same position for four decades. As a result, junior doctors, who had nothing in their hands, have been subjected to physical assault! Surprisingly, the government's attitude towards doctors has not changed in so many years."[153] And therefore the junior doctors have chosen the path of movement repeatedly.

Drug Action Forum (1984) in the 1980s and 1990s had a great influence on junior doctors. The *Forum* used to hold seminars at Calcutta Medical College or R.G. Kar College Hospital. Those seminars were attended mainly by the medical students, along with some junior doctors, and teachers. The *Forum's* campaign served as the ideological foundation for the junior doctors' struggle for people's health. However, when the

Forum weakened, at the end of the 1990s, the speed of the people's health movement also slowed. At the same time, there was a lack of motivation for medical students.[154]

The movement of the 1990s, however, was not beyond criticism. On October 31, 1983, a leading periodical commented "It was a grim catalogue—by the end of last fortnight, six children died, 50,000 out-patients were being turned away every day from Calcutta's free government hospitals, and thousands of in-patients were sent home in various stages of uncured illness."[155] Deep Ghosh shared his experience about the junior doctors' movement of 1987. Deep, a 13-year-old student in the third grade was admitted to SSKM with an injury to his right leg. Junior doctors began to cease work next day after his admission. Lying on the bed of the hospital, he cried in agony. But no doctor treated him. He felt that his leg was starting to rot. He was eventually forced to leave the hospital and go to a private nursing home.[156]

The ABJDF was also aware of public health issues outside the hospital. In 1984, there had been an outbreak of intestinal disease in Cooch Behar, West Bengal. A team of 19 members on behalf of ABJDF, the *Medical College Students Union*, *R.G. Kar Medical College Students Union*, the *Kotnis Memorial Committee*, the *People's Health Service Association*, and the *Calcutta National Welfare Organization* went to Cooch Behar to stand by the people.[157]

The medical team had three objectives: first, to treat the people infected by the disease; second, to campaign for the prevention of intestinal diseases; and third, to determine the cause of that epidemic. Examination of the infected patient's stool revealed that a bacterium named *Shigella* was responsible for the disease. However, that bacterium alone was not responsible for the condition. The team noted the absence of proper toilets in the villages of Cooch Behar, meaning that the villagers used to defecate near ponds, rivers or tube wells or in the fields. As a result, the germs of the disease could quickly enter those sources of water. The people of the villages used that water for drinking. Most of the people in the villages were uneducated, superstitious people. They had no idea about sanitation. As a result, the disease became epidemic.[158] The team treated about 2500 patients. A simultaneous campaign in relation to proper sanitation was carried out by the team.[159]

Leaflets about the socio-economic causes of disease, as well as the prevention and treatment of stomach ailments, were also published.[160] The leaflets appealed to the people to join the health movement, urging the following:

> We know that malnutrition and the lack of adequate health care are the leading causes of intestinal disease. Sending medical teams and medicines to villages cannot prevent the disease. We want a significant improvement in the living condition of the people, as well as an organized movement to demand it. So today, all of you demand food and clean drinking water. Be united to demand a people-oriented health system.[161]

A discussion meeting was organized on May 11, 1984 at Hindi High School in Cooch Behar to expose various aspects of the disease to the common people. The topic of discussion was "In the context of the current social situation, intestinal illness and prevention."[162] The activities of ABJDF had a great impact on the future health movement in West Bengal.

People's Health Service Association (PHSA)

Along with the Alma-Ata Declaration (1978) and the movement for rational drugs in the 1980s also influenced the then medical students. Members of the DSA started to work among the labourers and peasants. Meanwhile the students of the Calcutta Medical College (CMC) and R. G. Kar Medical College joined together to form the *People's Health Service Association* (PHSA) in 1981–1982. Students of CMC began to work in the slum area of Chaul-Patti Road near Beliaghata and students of R.G. Kar Medical College chose to work in the slum area opposite to the Khanna cinema, where sex-workers lived.[163] Anup Dhar's writing tells us about the activities of the *Medical College Democratic Students' Association* (MCDSA). He wrote "In a distant village in Murshidabad district we tried to take health to the villagers. We tried to build a model of public health through people's participation; a model not sponsored by the state or by international funding agencies; a model put in place by individuals who had come together to economically and intellectually contribute to people's health. We ran free clinics in working-class colonies of jute factories along the river Ganges."[164]

The PHSA believed in serving the poor people. The organization felt that common people's health problems should be addressed properly. They felt the necessity to examine the prevalent health care system. Thus, the organization tried to expose the "anti-people" aspect of health care to the people, along with providing services. It also wanted to be a part of the struggle for the interest of the common people.[165] The PHSA wanted to organize a movement demanding pro-people health care. With that aim, they set out several programmes:

- To run clinics in urban slums and surrounding villages and create valuable and effective medical care for the poor people in those clinics.
- To conduct surveys on various issues related to health and medical care.
- To publish magazines and bulletins on medical care and health-related issues and organize seminars/discussion meetings.
- To spread health education among the people and to make health workers.
- To participate in the movement of people for health.[166]

During that period, the founding members of DSA had graduated and become doctors. Some of them entered postgraduate courses, and others joined the service. Those doctors who were associated with the DSA showed interest in working with the workers and peasants. Notable among them were Dr. Ashis Kumar Kundu and Dr. Saibal Jana of the National Medical College, Dr. Pabitra Guha, Dr. Chanchala Samajdar, Dr. Pradeep Das and Dr. Punyabrata Goon of the Calcutta Medical College, and Dr. Bhaskar Saha of R.G. Kar Medical College. All of them went to work at the Shaheed Hospital of Chhattisgarh with the idea of doing something to help the laboring poor.[167]

The Medical Service Centre

It should be added further that in the late 1970s, another organization joined the health movement: the *Medical Service Centre* (MSC), a national-level socio-medical voluntary organization supported by Socialist Unity Centre of India (SUCI), a leftist political party.[168] That organization was established in 1977 as a joint effort by doctors, nurses, medical students, and health workers. This organization believed that disease could not be cured solely by medical care. They believed it was necessary to develop a health movement which should also address people's poverty, illiteracy, and ill-health.[169]

The *Medical Service Centre* provided medical relief to the people in times of distress and disasters. Doctors, nurses, and health workers from this organization had conducted free medical camps in different districts of West Bengal (including Kolkata) and also in a few other states. The MSC organized permanent charitable medical centers, organized temporary medical camps and health-related seminars at different times. It had also provided training to non-registered rural doctors. In addition, members of this organization had campaigned against the government's negligence in health care at different times.[170] They participated in the junior doctors' movements of ABJDF.[171] The first All India conference of MSC, which was also the first international health conference in Kolkata, was held in 1986.[172] In 1992, MSC formed the *Haspatal-O-Janaswasthya Raksha Committee* in protest about user fees in government hospitals.[173]

MSC staged continuous opposed against the privatization and commercialization of health care. It has taken a stronger line against privatization in health care from its 3rd All India Conference, held at Chandigarh in 1996. Since then, it has organized many seminars, symposia and workshops on the issue of privatization and its three-pronged entry into health care, medical education, and drugs.[174] Movements were organized against hospital charge hikes at various times (1992, 1998).[175] In December 2001, members of MSC staged protest programs against the increase of service charges in government hospitals and the privatization of health care in different hospitals of Kolkata.[176] On May 31, 2005, the second state conference of the *Haspital O Janaswasthya Raksha Committee* was held at the auditorium of the Calcutta Medical College. Participants at the conference discussed a number of issues: the poor conditions of the government hospitals, privatization of healthcare, and so on. Its members marched to rule out the PPP model in health care.[177] In August 2005, the MSC organized a movement that included signature collection, badge wearing, protest demonstration and conventions throughout the state and a 'right to health' week was observed from August 25 to 31.[178] The central committee of the MSC organized a health movement at national level.[179] In 2012, after the outbreak of a fire at AMRI, a PPP model-based hospital in Kolkata, the MSC organized a movement against the use of that model in the health sector.[180]

The 6th All India Conference of the *Medical Service Centre* was held at Pandit Bhagwat Dayal Sharma Post Graduate Institute of Medical Sciences, Rohtak, Haryana on October 15 and 16, 2016. It was attended by over 500 delegates, from 19 states and 3 union territories. Fraternal delegates from Bangladesh, Nepal, and the USA also attended the conference. The exhibition on the struggles of the pioneers of science, public health challenges and role of the MSC in community service and health movements was inaugurated by Dr. Dhruba Chaudhury, head of the Department of Pulmonary and Critical Care Medicine, PGIMS Rohtak. Following the delegate session, a sit-in-demonstration was organized at Jantar Mantar, New Delhi. It was attended by more than a thousand doctors, nurses, health workers and medical-nursing-paramedical students from across the country. A memorandum was submitted to the prime minister.[181] The health activists of West Bengal belonging to the MSC played a major role in the conference. Some important demands were:

- To implement scientific, pro-people rational health policy; to oppose the pro-corporate and pro-insurance *National Health Policy* 2015 Draft.
- To stop the privatization and commercialization of the medical education system.
- To declare and implement the right to health as a fundamental right. To allocate at least 10 per cent of the annual union budget for health.
- To ensure adequate and proper government health infrastructure.[182]

The *Medical Service Centre* published two Journals: *Health Spectra* in English (first published in 1988) and *Swasthya Bikshan* in Bengali (first published in 1995). A Bengali Bulletin named *Swasthyer Sandhane* had also been published by the West Bengal State Committee of the MSC from 1990 until the launch of *Swasthya Bikshan*. MSC also published various pamphlets/booklets in English and Bengali e.g. *Janaswasthya Andoloner Ekti Raktakto Adhyay* (1983), *Sarkari Maran Phande Janaswasthya* (1992), *Swasthya Aamar Adhikar* (1993), *Medicine for Mankind—Health for the People* (1996),[183] *Sarbanasha Khasra Jatiya Swasthy-niti 2015-er Biruddhe Pratirodh Andolan Gare Tulun.*[184]

Dr. Dwarkanath Kotnis Memorial Committee

In the 1970s, another organization, the *Dr. Dwarkanath Kotnis Memorial Committee*, began to work on the people's health movement. During the Sino-Japanese War (1937–1945), the Indian National Congress sent a five-member medical team to China in 1938. Dr. Dwarkanath Shantaram Kotnis (1910–1942) was one of them.[185] He believed that communism was the only way to liberate the poorest people in the world. Dr. Kotnis had asthma, but he put his service of the people ahead of his own interests. While treating the Chinese people, he had forgotten about his health; his hard work led to him dying in 1942.[186]

After the death of Dr. Kotnis, Dr. Bijoy Kumar Basu, one of his comrades, returned to India. In 1945, inspired by Dr. Kotnis's ideology, he formed the *Kotnis Memorial Committee* (KMC). However, the committee could not play any vital role at that time. In 1973, the KMC was reconstituted under the chairmanship of Dr. Bijoy Kumar Basu. Hemanga Biswas, a Bengali singer, Dr. Anil Mukherjee, and others were associated with that reorganization. Later, many intellectuals, like Mrinal Sen and Samar Sen, were also associated with the organization.[187] The persons who tried to organize the *Cultural Revolution* in India, like that of China in the 1970s, became members of the *Kotnis Memorial Committee*. One of them was Srijan Sen.[188]

In 1978, four members of the KMC, West Bengal, Dr. Chandana Mitra, Dr. Debashis Bakshi, Dr. Mrigendra Nath Gantait went to China where they received training in acupuncture. They learned the treatment and engaged themselves in the service of the poor. Using acupuncture as an effective treatment, they formed a movement that was a part of the overall health movement. They wanted to show that medical care could be provided to the people at a meager cost through such practices. The many branches of KMC formed in different parts of West Bengal campaigned against superstition and in favour of humanism. The mouthpiece publication of this organization was *Ankure Shuru*.[189]

While discussing the days of reconstitution of the *Kotnis Memorial Committee*, Dr. Chandana Mitra, a doctor from Calcutta Medical College, highlighted both the inadequacy and inequality of the medical system of West Bengal in the 1970s. She wrote there was little more than a basic level of treatment available in health centers or village hospitals. Therefore, rural people would have to travel to Calcutta Medical College. Once there, if they did not pay a bribe, they would not have received medical services.[190] She also narrated her own experience while at medical college.

She had joined the KMC to fulfil her dream. She supported the work of the MCDSA as she had been influenced the ideals of a pro-people medical system. Despite being a service doctor, she likewise took an active part in the junior doctors' movement in 1983.[191] Dr. Bijoy Kumar Basu was another Indian doctor to be influenced by China's public health system. Therefore, he encouraged the members of the KMC to become public health workers, just like the so-called 'barefoot doctors' in China. That's why the branches of the KMC were formed in the villages or suburbs inhabited by working people.[192] In each branch, it tried to make the local boys and girls conscious with regard to health and primary health care.[193]

The KMC believed that in order to move the people's health movement forward, the obstacles must be removed. The committee tried to find out the socio-economic causes of disease and stepped in to address the problems. The KMC felt that if the people's health movement was to be successful, the necessary requirements were to gain experience through work on people's health, motivate people with that experience and then involve them in the wider movement.[194]

Norman Bethune Janaswasthya Andolan

Norman Bethune Janaswasthya Andolan, founded in 1983 with the active participation of doctors, began its journey for the proper implementation of 'health for all'. That organization was established by a group of teachers, doctors, scientists, science activists, journalists, and service personnel who were inspired by the principles of Dr. Norman Bethune (1890–1939).[195] He was a Canadian doctor, who gained international fame as a thoracic surgeon, but his workplace was global. Dr. Norman Bethune, a combatant in Spain's anti-fascist movement and a comrade in the anti-Japanese struggle, stated that "unequal economy is the mother of ill health."[196] He realized that poverty, which was increasing across the world, was the leading cause of tuberculosis and other diseases.[197] To understand his thinking we may quote some lines from his biography:

> The best form of providing health protection would be to change the economic system that produces ill health, and liquidate ignorance, poverty and unemployment. The practice of each individual purchasing his own medical care does not work. It is unjust, inefficient, wasteful and completely outmoded.[198]
>
> We go to the people! We go to the people! No more private practice; we change the whole system of medical service…That's where the doctor must go into every house, into every city, into every village, from door to door. We take medicine right down to the last individual. We don't wait until the invalid drags him down to our offices at so much per consultation; we go to him before he is ill and show him how to remain healthy. And if he is ill already, we arrest it by prompt action. From house to house, street to street, city to city…[199]

He attempted to organize a worldwide people's health movement so that people could receive free health services. Along with some doctors, Bethune set up an organization named *Montreal Group for the Security of the People's Health*. With one hundred doctors, dentists, nurses and social workers, the organization began its work in July 1936. The organization released a declaration in which it highlighted the dire state of people's health in the province of Quebec. They made various demands to the government.[200] The ideology of Norman Bethune, based on the people-centric socialist approach of medical system, was followed pretty closely by health workers in West Bengal. *Norman Bethune Janaswasthya Andolon* (NBJA) most likely attempted to pursue a program similar to that of the *Montreal Group for the Security of People's Health*. It was written in the manifesto of NBJA that "The names of Shakespeare, Rabindranath and Gorky are dear to all literature-lovers. The names of Satyendranath, Galileo and Bruno are dear to scientific workers. Similarly, to people's health workers, the name of Norman Bethune is very dear."[201]According to the pioneers of that organization, *Norman Bethune Janaswasthya Andolan* was not an isolated movement; it was part of a mainstream movement that aimed to bring about radical changes in the country's socio-economic system.[202]

Therefore, the main objective of every health movement should be the removal of social inequality. Simultaneously, health awareness would bring about benefits to the improvement of society itself. That was the main objective of *Norman Bethune Janaswasthya Andolon*. In accordance with Memorandum of Association, its aims and objectives were:

- To study the life and activities of Dr. Norman Bethune and other international people's health workers;
- To conduct and promote study and research on various aspects of sociology of health;
- To identify the factors responsible for inadequacies and ineffectiveness of the health-care delivery system in India and in other third world countries;
- To demystify medical education and healthcare delivery;
- To promote health education amongst different sections of population through compulsory curriculum in the school up to secondary level as well as non-formal methods;
- To resist unscientific and unethical practices in the health arena;
- To ban unethical use of human beings as experimental animals;

- To organise documentation centres, seminars, symposia, group discussion, mass meeting, publish journals, magazines, booklets, leaflets, posters and produce films, slides etc. for dissemination of knowledge in conformity with the objects of the society;
- To develop model health centres, hospitals and health co-operatives;
- To protect people's right in obtaining scientific healthcare and stand by the side of the people against any onslaught on them.[203]

Norman Bethune Janaswasthya Andolan was functioning to achieve those objectives. The registered office of the organisation was situated at Salt Lake, Kolkata. Founder members of the organization (as per the memorandum) were Dr. Jnanabrata Sil (President), Kalidas Samajar (Vice-President), Dr. Sukhamoy Bhattacharya (Secretary) Dr. Uma Ganguly (Treasurer), Swapan Sil, Sakuntala Bhattacharya, and Manikuntala Banerjee.[204] However, prior to joining the organization in 1983, members of NBJA had been involved in some people's health programs; many of them also wrote articles and pamphlets on people's health. They started a movement against illegal medical trials on people.[205] The main organizers of the *Norman Bethune Janaswasthya Andolan* were two doctors—Dr. Sukhamoy Bhattacharya and Dr. Jnanabrata Sil.

In 1964, Dr. Sukhamoy Bhattacharya (born in 1941) graduated from Nilratan Sircar Medical College (NRS) and worked as an Assistant Medical Officer of Railways in Palghat, Kerala. In 1969, he joined the Cholera Research Centre, Calcutta, where he became acquainted with Dr. Jnanabrata Sil. In 1980, the two of them started teaching at the University of Calcutta. Sukhamoy Bhattacharya was one of the four who formed the *Joint Action Committee of Unions & Associations of Autonomous Research Institutions* (JACARI). He had lodged a written complaint with the *Sharma Sarkar Commission* against the illegal and unethical experiments of foreign drug companies on slum dwellers and school children in Kolkata. The commission accepted that incident as their primary concern. He was a firm believer in the rationalist, defendant, and Leftist ideologies from his school days to the end of his life. On April 28, 2001, this man's struggling life came to an end.[206]

In 1961, Dr. Jnanabrata Sil, an activist of the people's movement, received his medical degree from the Calcutta Medical College. He had been drawn to rationalism and communist philosophy from his student days. He envisioned a world free of poverty and exploitation. In order to change society, he chose a revolutionary path. He had never considered medicine to be a financially rewarding profession and he entered politics not to advance his career but to serve the people.[207] Dr. Sil wrote:

> I, being a doctor with no grinding on sociology and economics, am guided by my faith in the teachings of Karl Marx within my limits of understanding. I have seen poverty from very close proximity. I personally know what is meant by "hunger pain". I understand that a socialist revolution will usher in a radical transmission when we shall get social control on all weapons of production. The State shall wither away; society will be run on the slogan "from each according to his ability and to each according to his needs".[208]

He was an activist member of *Students Health Home* from the beginning and a regular activist of *People's Relief Committee* (PRC). In 1959, he participated in the flood relief work on behalf of the PRC with Harekrishna Konar and worked for *Bangiya Pradeshik Krishak Sabha* with Binoy Chowdhury. In 1964, he joined Jamnagar Government Medical College in Gujarat as a teacher. However, he was expelled in the following year for his alleged links to the Communist Party. He then worked for some time as a doctor at Mahesh of Srirampur and Champa Road of Rishra and became an associate of the jute workers' movement. He also became the convener and first secretary of the preparatory committee of an association of scientists named JACARI.[209]

At the initiative of these two doctors, NBJA started its journey with the commitment of struggle "for a healthy life, for healthy people and for a healthy society." They wanted to work amongst the people. Dr. Sil said, "We had seen many people die in this country due to lack of health awareness or lack of treatment. So, we, two friends, tried to do something. But I will not say that we had done too much."[210]

On January 31, 1986, NBJA had arranged a seminar on the 'People's Health Movement' at the Centenary Hall of the University of Calcutta under the chairmanship of Prof. Sushil Kumar Mukherjee, Ex-Vice-Chancellor of Calcutta University. Many leading workers from different walks of social life participated in the discussion. The speakers included Prof. P.K Mukherjee, Dr. Bhaskar Roychowdhury, Bhabatosh Roy, Srijan Sen, Dr. Gouripada Dutta, Prof. Binayak Dutta Roy, and Biswajit Datta Gupta.[211] Dr. Bijoy Kumar Basu and the West Bengal Health Minister Ramnarayan Goswami sent greetings. Regarding the movement of NBJA, the Health Minister said, "People's health movement or people's science movement is the part of the mainstream struggle, which could bring fundamental change in society. However, the activists of the movement have some limitations, but they are unwavering in their determination to reach their goals."[212] On the occasion of Environment Day on June 5, 1986, the *Bangiya Bigyan Parishad* and NBJA held a seminar at Satyendra Bhavan, Bangiya Bigyan Parishad, Kolkata. The theme of the seminar was "scientific temperament in people's health movement".[213]

The NBJA recommended the *West Bengal Board of Secondary Education* (WBBSE) to make 'health education' mandatory in the secondary level syllabus. Dr. Sukhamoy Bhattacharya spoke on that subject in a workshop organized by the WBBSE. His arguments and statements were presented by the WBBSE authorities at the Eastern Conference of the *National Council of Educational Research and Training* (NCERT).[214] On August 9, 1986, a symposium on health education at the secondary level was held at Hare School in Kolkata on the initiative of NBJA and *Paschimbanga Rashtriya Shikshak Samiti*.[215] Later, on October 19, 1986, a seminar on *Public Health and Superstition* was organized by *Hajabarala* at the Pyarimohan Library in Belgharia (Kolkata).[216] On April 25, 1987, on an initiative of both *Agradut Sangha* and NBJA, a conference was held at the ground of *Agradut Sangha* (west of Ultadanga Railway Station, Kolkata) to increase the level of knowledge of common people about various aspects of medicine..[217] On March 28, 1993, at the Federation Hall in Calcutta, the NBJA and the Federation Hall Society jointly convened a conference on "Consumer Satisfaction in Medical Practice." Among the prominent people who participated in that conference, and mentioned in the leaflet of the organization, were Dr. Jyotirmoy Majumder, Dr. Bhaskar Roychowdhury, Dr. Naresh Bandopadhyay, Prof. Bela Dasgupta, and Dr. Zafrullah Chowdhury (Bangladesh).[218]

The NBJA had also worked alongside other likeminded organizations. Many social workers and science workers stood beside the NBJA. Some members of NBJA visited *Gonoshasthaya Kendra* in Bangladesh on more than one occasion and became involved in its works. On the basis of the experience gained from *Gonoshasthaya Kendra,* they wanted to build a multipurpose rural people's health project that would include a range of activities: farms, poultry, fish farming, dairy, general health care, health insurance, schools, old age homes, and so on. In this project, they also wanted to include medical and social rehabilitation systems for mentally ill adolescents.[219]

They were able to put some of their plans into action. Most notable were the establishments of two mental health centers: *Anandaniketan* in Katwa, Burdwan, and *Santisankar Monovikas Kendra* in Labpur, Birbhum, with Sukhamoy Bhattacharya as the founding working secretary of the two institutions. The *Schizophrenia Assistance Club* was also established to help the families of those affected by the condition. In addition, the mental health worker training project was initiated by NBJA.[220]

NBJA published several pamphlets on easy ways to prevent or cure common diseases. Among these were *Esab Oshudh Khaben Na* (Don't take these medicines)[221] and *Oshudh Theke Asukh* (Diseases from medicine).[222] Those pamphlets were later compiled together in three hard-bound volumes:*Sadharaner Asukh Bisukh* (A treatise on diseases of the people and their socioeconomic perspective);[223] *Maa O Sishu* (A treatise on maternal and child health);[224] and *Oshudh Bishudh* (Drugs).[225] In addition, *Deha-Mon-Samaj*, a monthly public health magazine, was published under the editorship of Sukhamoy Bhattacharya.[226] NBJA also successfully participated in the Kolkata Book Fair for a number of years. In recognition of its achievement in popularizing science, the West Bengal government honored NBJA with the Meghnad Award in 1994.[227]

After working successfully for some years, the organization was forced to stop working because of a number of problems. According to Sabyasachi Chatterjee, *Norman Bethune Janaswasthya Andolan* was not as active in the 1990s as the *Drug Action Forum*.[228] The then leading ruling party opposed the work of that organization. One of the two main pillars of the organization, Dr. Jnanabrata Sil, was accused of violating party discipline. On September 24, 1987, Dr. Gouripada Dutta, a party patriarch, had sent a letter to Sil, on behalf of the CPI (M), alleging breach of the party's discipline.[229]

In the obituary of Gouripada Datta, Dr. Kajal Krishna Banik wrote, "Professor Gouripada Datta (GPD) is a name in the socio medical movement of not only West Bengal but also the entire country."[230] One may wonder, therefore, how such a person worked primarily for the party and not for the interest of the health movement. Moreover, he knew about the works of NBJA from the very beginning since many party leaders were invited to the ceremonies of NBJA. The unpublished personal papers of Dr. Jnanabrata Sil state that pamphlets and booklets of NBJA were often sent to the leaders of the party. These also said that, on December 31, 1985, a meeting was held at the residence of Gouripada Datta on organizing people's science/health movement in West Bengal, in line with *Kerala*

Sasthra Sahithya Parishad (KSSP) of Kerala. In that meeting, it was decided to publish booklets on health problems.[231] Dr. Sil wrote that "Local Committee Secretary (Gouripada Datta) was informed of publication of first issue of *Janaswasthya Pustak Mala* (*Peter Asukh*) and seminar to be organised on January 31, 1986 entitled *Janaswasthya Andolaner Ruparekha* at Calcutta University Centenary Hall. He approved the list of speakers and agreed to give the key-note speech."[232] On August 14, 1987, in a letter to Haridas Malakar of the West Bengal Control Commission, CPI (M), -) Dr Sil wrote that:

> ...Copies of all these books have been and are being submitted to the West Bengal PC (Provincial Committee) and Cal DC (Calcutta District Committee) immediately after each publication.
>
> All these books were well appreciated by my party leaders and Com. Buddhadev Bhattacharya, comrade in charge of NBA (National Book Agency) allowed these books to be sold by NBA after personally reading the first two books and highly appreciating them. He also permitted us to mention the name of NBA amongst the list of sellers of these books.
>
> ...I had been authorised to publish such books by my leaders on December 31, 1985. I materialised their desire within a month (January 31, 86). Many leaders of the Medical LC (Local Committee) including the LCS (Local Committee Secretary) actively participated. Many of them became members on payment of subscription for one year. Other activities of NBJA were known to them. My Branch was informed of its activities.
>
> It was all appreciated till publication of the second booklet *Apusti*. Everybody encouraged us, assured us of support from the party, mass-organisation and even from the government.
>
> However, something happened in April–May in 1986. The Medical LCS verbally informed me of his determination to stop these publications, without telling me the reasons for this sudden reversal of his earlier stand as publicly committed in our Seminar on January 31, 1986. Till date I do not know these reasons...
>
> ...Our third booklet *Rog Pratirodhe Tika* was scheduled to be published at a seminar entitled the *Scientific temper in People's Health Movement*, on June 5, 1986. Cards were distributed; everything was ready. Suddenly my LCS sent me a note just a day before directing me to stop the programme of the publication of this book and threatening me of disciplinary action if the book was published. I tried to convince him of the difficulties in cancelling such a programme involving *Bangiya Bijnan Parishad* and others in vain. I understood that a trap is being laid to force me to violate party discipline. But I had no way out.[233]

At last, Dr. Sil had resigned as a member of the CPI (M). The main point was that the CPI (M) thought that the secretary of the NBJA, Sukhamoy Bhattacharya, was a Naxalite.[234] Therefore, CPI (M) was trying to stop the work of the NBJA. In Canada, Dr. Bethune could not carry out his plan because of obstacles erected by the government and the country's leading people.[235] The same thing happened with the NBJA in West Bengal. During the Left Front rule, no organization could function without the consent of the CPI (M). Sumit Sarkar has written:

> Even the leaves of the tree could not move without the consent of the CPI (M). When we went to start a small science club, we found that the CPI (M) was against it. We got an offer to work under the CPM-run *Paschim Banga Vigyan Mancha*. But we did not show interest in their proposal. As a result, CPI (M) cadres began to threat the parents of the children, among whom we wished to spread scientific awareness. Parents were told to forbid their children to join us...In the 1980s, no one dared to pronounce the name Naxalbari. No one could criticise CPI (M)'s errors.[236]

CPI (M) leader Prakash Karat argued that non-governmental organizations (NGOs)/voluntary organizations financed by foreign countries or organizations were agents of imperialism. According to him, NGOs aimed to disrupt the possibility of the largest Leftist movement in the third world.[237] Therefore, in West Bengal, the Left government viewed the non-partisan NGOs with suspicion up to the early 1980s and early 1990s. As a result, NGOs in West Bengal could not function in the same way as those of South-West India.[238] However, it's worth mentioning that the NBJA was not a foreign-funded organization.

To know some other problems which were faced by NBJA, we may quote some lines from proceedings of the meeting of the executive committee of NBJA, held on October 2, 1999.

> Society is in a very bad shape at the present moment. One of the members has died and some others have become inactive. The secretary is much incapacitated due to his visual problems and broken marriage. The financial position of the Society is also very bad; no donation is received in spite of our enlistment under section 80-G of the I.T Act. The major project of NBJA, *Santisankar Monovikas Kendra* (SMK) at Labpur, has been illegally occupied by Dr. (Mrs.) Sakuntala Bhattacharya, (she was founder member of NBJA)). She has forcibly prevented the office bearers of NBJA to enter the said project-complex and has also denied to return the official papers

> and documents of NBJA which include the deeds of gift of the lands to NBJA, records, accounts, balance-sheet, etc. of NBJA, making it difficult to run day to day function and even to submit the annual returns to the Income-Tax authorities and discharge other statutory obligations.
>
> Under the present circumstances, we have only two alternatives: 1. to dissolve the Society, or 2. to enrol new members. In view of the reputation of this Society in the state as well as at the national level for its contributions towards very relevant social causes, the general consensus was that all efforts should be made to save this state award winning NGO which is also a member of the National Council of Science & Technology Communication (NCSTC) Network, from a premature death, which can only be done through inducting new members to the Society.[239]

After the death of Dr. Sukhamoy Bhattacharya, another central pillar of NBJA, the organization became very weak. Depositing the rest of the money from the bank account of NBJA into the Chief Minister Relief Fund, the work of NBJA had been closed in 2001.[240] As Jnanabrata Sil recorded on the *Prokriti O Manush*, a feature page of *Kalantar*, "We wanted to make people aware about disease prevention techniques at low-cost by providing some necessary information about health and to stop using them as guinea pigs by foreign multinational pharmaceutical companies. But unexpectedly the order for stopping our work had come from political power. We then didn't bow our heads to the pressure but were forced to stop our activities finally. I live with grief and dissatisfaction for missing our goal."[241]

The sum-total of the movement of junior doctors, *Norman Bethune Janaswasthya Andolan* and the movement for rational drugs changed the entire scenario. The pace of the movement was accelerated by the *No More Bhopal Movement.* The movement was started to seek justice for the gas victims in the Bhopal disaster of December 1984. The doctors of West Bengal, belonging to MCDSA, had worked with that movement. The movement raised the slogan *Shahi Jankari, Shahi Ilaj*, which means 'proper information is the key to proper treatment.'[242]

Shaheed Hospital

Chhattisgarh's *Shaheed Hospital* (established on June 3, 1983) was a catalyst of the health movement. Within that setting proper medical treatment was made available to the common people. The initiative was started by a

Leftist leader Shakar Guha Niyogi (1943–1991). Niyogi had been born in Balubari village of North Dinajpur in undivided Bengal with the birth name of Dhiresh. During his student life, he became attracted to the communist ideology and the food movement of 1959 had affected him profoundly. He left home in 1961 and reached Bhilai, where he was employed as a worker in the coke oven department at the steel plant. He became a member of the undivided Communist Party. When the party split in 1964, he joined the CPI (M). Inspired by the peasant movement in Naxalbari in 1967, he left the CPI (M) and came into contact with the *All India Coordination Committee of Communist Revolutionaries.* When the CPI (ML), the Communist Party of India (Marxist–Leninist), was formed in 1969, he had been a member of that party for some time. But he was later expelled from the party for ideological reasons.[243]

Dhiresh became known as Shankar and in 1977, Shankar Guha Niyogi became the leader of the workers' movement in Dalli-Rajhara. The *Chhattisgarh Mines Shramik Sangha* (CMSS), an organization of Delhi-Rajhara miners, was formed as a result of his initiative. Shankar Guha Niyogi envisioned the CMSS as more than a trade union—it should engage with every aspect of workers' lives. With this vision, the *Chhattisgarh Mukti Morcha* (CMM) was formed in 1979, combining trade union struggles with transformative social and political activism. The workers started the movement in 1977 under the leadership of Niyogi. In an effort to suppress the movement, the police arrested him. In June 1977, when workers tried to save their leader from being detained, 11 of them were shot and killed by police. The movement, however, could not be stopped.[244]

Going beyond the three strands of the communist movement in the country, Shankar Guha Niyogi created the fourth strand, which was called the *coordination*. He wanted to establish a new alternative model built on the theory of *Sangharsh aur Nirmaan* (Struggle and construction).[245]

Niyogi said, "Construction and struggle are the two main aspects of our movement. To change the social system, the struggle and small constructions are needed, which will pave the way for the creation of an alternative system. We are experimenting with this. It should be remembered that we are talking about the politics of *Sangharsh Aur Nirmaan* (struggle and construction) in order to change the anti-people system based on exploitation."[246] To Niyogi, 'construction' was the way to create a new mentality through the cultural and social revolution. This emerged from his idea that cultural change would come when economic conditions changed. Thus, Niyogi wanted to start the cultural struggle and the class struggle, the struggle for social change. He understood that change in society was not possible without implementing the theory of 'struggle and construction'.[247] Niyogi envisioned a new world, where everyone would have access to drinking water, all cornfields would be irrigated, everyone would have jobs, the farmer would be paid fairly for his produce, all villages would have hospitals, all children would have access to schools, everyone would have land and houses, and there would be no more poverty, exploitation, or capitalism.[248] Bharat Dogra noted:

> Niyogi was first and foremost a great social thinker of the alternative development movement, but worked as a trade union leader in order to be able to implement his ideas in practical ways...Niyogi's movement provided a model to show that how poor people from an exploited backward region could be organised for real socio-economic change without any encouragement of separatist or divisive ideas or forces.[249]

The people's health movement of Dalli-Rajhara emerged from the concept of alternative development. The first initiative of CMSS was the movement against alcoholism, because of the effects of alcohol on workers, in both physical and financial terms.[250] The women of the region played a significant role in the anti-temperance movement of Dalli-Rajhara, which was to prove successful.[251] George Fernandez writes: "The campaign led by Niyogi against drinking alcohol to save the labouring poor of Chhattisgarh from ill-health was unparalleled in the history of the trade union movement in our country. After Mahatma Gandhi, there was no personality other than Niyogi who was so successful in the movement against drinking alcohol."[252]

At that time, there was a lack of government health services for workers in Dalli-Rajhara, so were often treated by the quack practitioners. Occasionally, they could get treatment from the Bhilai Steel Plant Hospital. In most cases, however, they would attend but not receive any treatment. In 1979 a tragic incident took place that affected attitudes to health services in the area. That year, Kusumbai, a union leader, died in childbirth due to doctors' negligence at the steel plant hospital. As a result, the workers took an oath to build a hospital facility for themselves, and the foundation stone of *Shaheed Prasuti Sadan* was laid the following year. The *Swasthya ke liye sangharsh karo* (Struggle for Health) movement was initiated on Independence Day 1981. Its first initiative was the cleaning campaign, when the workers forced the mine management to make arrangements to keep the workers' slums clean.[253] Ilina Sen wrote "We had run into a large crowd of people sweeping the streets with homemade khareta jhadus (hard brooms) ...Later, I learnt that this was a clean-up action as part of the '*swasthya ke liye sangharsh karo*' (struggle for health) campaign."[254]

Later, a health committee was formed, comprised of doctors and workers. On January 26, 1982, the *Shaheed Dispensary* was inaugurated. The following year, on June 3, 1983, *Shaheed Hospital* was established in the memory of those martyrs of 1977 who had been shot dead by the state police.[255] The *Mahila Mukti Morcha* also played a significant role in the health movement from the very beginning, agitating for better treatment at BSP Hospital and against unscientific medicine.[256]

Shaheed Hospital was the meeting place for activists of people's movement from different parts of India, and with a range of ideologies. Doctors like Binayak Sen, Ashish Kundu, Saibal Jana, Pabitra Guha, Punyabrata Goon, who came to CMSS, were all members of the progressive health movement. They all experienced the uniqueness of the hospital setting after joining the *Shaheed Hospital.* In 1981 Shankar Guha Niyogi was arrested under the National Security Act (NSA). At that time, Binayak and Ilina Sen went there as part of an investigating team on behalf of civil liberty groups. Before coming to Chhattisgarh, Binayak Sen had worked for some time at *Friends' Rural Centre, Rasulia Hoshangabad* (FRCH) in Madhya Pradesh (MP). However, his community-based health initiatives had proved unsuccessful there.[257]

Their goal was to make people understand the causes of illness. They tried to convince people that socio-economic causes were the root cause of all infectious and non-communicable diseases and that, therefore, to get rid of them, it was society that had to change. At the same time, they tried to make people empowered in the field of health. Simple techniques were taught to people, such as using the Oral Rehydration Solution (ORS) to combat diarrhea, and using vapor instead of syrup to cure cough. At this time, small booklets, called *Lok Shiksha Mala*, were also published in Hindi, so that people could easily understand the necessary techniques to prevent or cure disease.[258] Ilina Sen wrote:

> …a health movement was launched with a focus on health promotion and disease prevention. Its first phase was marked, as Ashish Kundu recalls, by visits to and interactions in different *mohallas*, the creation of the health exhibition, and selection of young health workers from each dafai.[259]

The workers contributed both money and labor to the construction of Shaheed Hospital. From the very beginning, the hospital decided not to receive funding from funding agencies within and outside the country in order to maintain its autonomy. As the hospital lacked the necessary funds to hire qualified medical personnel, workers were asked to work as volunteers and they responded positively. As a result, some of the workers were trained to function as health workers. Soon afterward, the book *Where There Is No Doctor* by David Werner was translated into Hindi. It was studied by both doctors and health workers. Since many of the learners lacked proper education, the use of discussion and graphical presentations was crucial. Some local girls were even given nursing training. *Shaheed Hospital*'s doctors focused on the promotion of 'rational medicine.' To make the workers aware of health issues, they held exhibitions and published several booklets on both rational medicine and infectious diseases.[260]

The experience at *Shaheed Hospital* demonstrates the close relationship between health and socio-economic conditions. Among other campaigns, people became aware of the importance of pure drinking water to prevent diarrhea. In 1989, under pressure from CMSS and the *Chhattisgarh Mukti Morcha*, the local administration and the Bhilai Steel Plant Authority installed 179 tube wells in Dalli-Rajhara and surrounding villages,. The Government Primary Health Center conducted a survey in the workers' slums of Dalli-Rajhara in 1989, six years after the opening of *Shaheed Hospital*, and found that there were no cases of polio. However, the immunization program was not the sole reason for that change. The union's movement had also raised levels of parental consciousness, which was one of the key reasons for the improvement. In addition, *Shaheed Hospital*'s establishment also compelled the Bhilai Steel Plant Hospital to upgrade its facilities. The government was forced to establish a primary health center in Dalli-Rajhara and seven in the Dondi-Lohara assembly constituency.[261]

Shaheed Hospital, founded and nurtured by workers with the support of doctors, represents an alternative model to private and corporate market-based institutions. It offers affordable and quality medical services. Following the health movement in Delhi-Rajhara, doctors and health workers adhering to Shakar Guha Niyogi's ideology shaped the health movement in West Bengal.

Legal Battle

Shakar Guha Niyogi was assassinated on September 28, 1991, but the movement's strength could not be destroyed. The *Paschimbanga Kshet Mazdoor Samity* (PBKM), an organization of agricultural laborers, organized a street rally in Kolkata on July 8, 1992 in order to launch a mass signature campaign demanding the punishment of his killers. Hakim Sheikh, a member of PBKM, came from Mathurapur block of South 24 Parganas district to attend that rally. Afterward, Hakim Sheikh and other PBKM members took the Laxmikantapur Local back to their homes in the afternoon. While getting down from the train, Hakim fell on the platform at Mathurapur station and suffered head injuries and brain hemorrhage.[262]

In that condition, he was taken to the Mathurapur Block Hospital. However, since that block hospital lacked the requisite facilities to treat such patients, the doctors referred him to any other State hospitals or medical college hospitals in Kolkata for better treatment. That night, he was taken to NRS Medical College Hospital in Kolkata. The Emergency Medical Officer in the hospital examined him and, after taking two X-ray prints of his skull, recommended that he be admitted to the hospital immediately for further treatment. He could not be admitted to the NRS, however, since neither the surgical emergency ward nor the regular surgery ward had any vacant bed. He was taken from one hospital to another overnight, but could not be admitted to any government hospital. On the morning of July 9, he was taken to SSKM Hospital and Bangur Institute of Neurology. Again, he was refused admission because neither of the hospitals had an emergency neurosurgery unit. Hakim was eventually admitted to a private medical research institute, and he survived.[263]

On the grounds of this shocking situation, in 1993, PBKM filed a petition in the Supreme Court (SC) against the indifferent and callous attitude of the medical authorities at the government hospitals of Kolkata. In an interim order issued in 1994, the SC directed the state government to form an inquiry committee to assess the situation. The state government was compelled to form an inquiry committee headed by Justice Lilamoy Ghose, a retired judge of the Calcutta High Court and the committee submitted its report to the State Health Department on March 21, 1995.[264]

The committee made some recommendations, which were accepted by the SC, to rule out such incidents in the future. The judgment of the

Supreme Court clearly stated that the main responsibility of the government of a welfare state like India is to ensure the welfare of the people. One important aspect of this public welfare is to pay special attention to the health services of the citizens. As per Article 21 of the Indian Constitution, the government has a constitutional obligation to safeguard the right to life of citizens. To fulfil this responsibility, the government has to build health centers, hospitals etc. Government hospitals, and all the medical officers working in these hospitals, have a moral responsibility to provide the necessary treatment to save the lives of the citizens. Refusing to provide medical treatment to a citizen from a government hospital is amount to a breach of Article 21.[265] The Supreme Court stated that "In the present case there was breach of the said right of Hakim Sheikh guaranteed under Article 21 when he was denied treatment at the various Government hospitals..."[266] In its judgment SC also ordered the state government that

- Adequate facilities should be maintained in the primary health centres so that immediate primary treatment can be provided to the patient to improve his/her condition.
- The quality of district level and sub-divisional level hospitals should be improved so that serious patients can be treated there.
- Specialist medical facilities should be expanded in the district and sub-divisional hospitals keeping in view the growing needs.
- A centralized communication system should be introduced to ensure that the serious patient gets a bed at the state level medical college hospital in case of emergency.
- Proper arrangements of the ambulance should be kept for transporting the patient from the primary health centre to sub-divisional and district hospitals as per requirement and similarly from sub-divisional hospital to state-level medical college hospital.
- The ambulance should be offered with the necessary medical equipment and health personnel.
- Health centres and hospitals and the doctors attached to these Centres and hospitals should be activated to treat the large number of patients who come for emergency treatment because of "higher risk of accidents on certain occasions and in certain seasons.[267]

SC directed the West Bengal government to pay Hakim Seikh a sum of Rs. 25,000 as compensation.[268] Mention may be made that the judgment of the Supreme Court in the Hakim Sheikh case considered the right to life-saving treatment of the common people as a fundamental right. As per the judgment, if a doctor or medical officer denies the admission to hospital of a critically ill patient, he or she would also be charged with violating this fundamental right. In 1996, the *Janaswasthya Adhikar Committee*, consisting of various people's organizations, women's organizations, and science organizations, publicized that verdict among the people. The committee wanted the people to use it as a weapon to fight for their rights. The first convention of the committee was held on September 27, 1996 at the Students Hall in Kolkata. The attendees of the conference were encouraged to disseminate the SC's judgment widely.[269]

Organizations like the *Association for Protection of Democratic Rights* (APDR) lend their support to the commoners fighting for their rights. In this regard, we may mention a legal battle of the APDR. Dinanath, the15-year-old son of a jute mill worker, Badri Chowdhury, a resident of Binodtala, Chandannagar, Hooghly, was bitten by a street dog on June 12, 1996; subsequently, he was given, for ten days, anti-rabies vaccines supplied by the Hopkins Biomedical Corporation Ltd. at Chandannagar Sub-Divisional Hospital. But the cold chain was not maintained to preserve the vaccine provided to Dinanath. Because of that medical negligence, after suffering from illness for a few days, Dinanath died of rabies on August 9. Badri Chowdhury then complained to the *District Consumer Dispute Redressal Forum, Hooghly*, with the support of APDR, demanding compensation. Dinnath's case reached the Supreme Court.[270] After a long legal battle, lasting 22 years, in 2018, the *District Consumer Dispute Redressal Forum, Hooghly* directed the government to pay jointly and/or severally a sum of Rs. 1,920,000 within 30 days to complainants and to issue a cheque of Rs. 10,000 in the name of the complainants for the costs of litigation.[271] Both judgements have made it clear that government hospitals are obligated to provide qualitative health care to all.

Belur Sramajibi Hospital

Inspired by the Chhattisgarh health movement, some leaders of the Indo-Japan Steel Company's labour union took an initiative to build up a hospital for the workers at Belur, a small industrial town near Kolkata. In doing so, they contacted the *People's Health Service Association* (PHSA). The *Indo-Japan Steel Limited Employees Union* was able to build a clinic with the help of the local people and some doctors belonging to the PHSA.[272]

In 1983, the *Indo-Japan Steel Limited Employees Union* and the *People's Health Service Association* combined to form *Shramajibi Swasthya Prakalpa Samiti* (Workers' Health Project Committee). Before the formal formation, those doctors and junior doctors associated with PHSA had provided health services to the workers.[273] Discussion programs on health were organized frequently by those dedicated doctors, which were regularly attended by the workers' families. Topics of discussion included the condition of government health care services, prejudice regarding health, the proper use of drugs, disease prevention and so on. As a result, the workers were able to form an anti-alcohol movement. Women in working-class families began a campaign for gaining equal status with men. The feminist magazine *Ahalya*, edited by Dr. Chandana Mitra was published from Kolkata, and was subscribed to by many of the laboring women. It contained articles on the position of girls in society, their problems, and their efforts to overcome them.[274]

On October 2, 1983, the *Shramajibi Swasthya Prakalpa Samiti* (SSPS) health project was launched at the Khamarpara Jagriti Hindi Vidya Mandir in Belur. It adopted the slogan, *Aamader Swasthya Amrai Gorbo* (We will build up our health ourselves). The outdoor facility was available in the evenings during the first phase. The cleaning operation was carried out in the mornings. There were no adequate sanitary facilities in the workers' colony. As a result, the initial emphasis was on raising the level of health consciousness among working people. The key goal of the health workers was to raise consciousness about the importance of daily hygiene among workers' families. Dr. Ranjit Ghosh, Dr. Anil Saha, Dr. Pradeep Maiti, and junior doctors were enthusiastic activists, and they were assisted by local girls.[275]

There was a lack of awareness among workers regarding hydrocele disease. They did not use the requisite precautions for hard work. Thus, there was an increase in the number of hydrocele patients among the workers. Surgery was essential for them. SSPS organized a surgical camp for hydrocele operations (a common condition involving swelling in the scrotum).[276]

Finally, in 1994, a full-fledged hospital was built in an abandoned Grand Smithy Works house. The workers were able to construct necessary objects for the hospital, such as operation tables and lamp stands for operating theaters. The hospital's outdoor specialization department was implemented gradually. A 15-bed indoor facility was built. A laboratory was also constructed. An X-ray machine was also installed. However, as a result of internal problems at the factory, workers' wages were stopped. As a result, they were unable to contribute funds to the hospital, and the hospital experienced a financial crisis. In order to meet the crisis, the workers decided to sell their blood to support the cause. They also raised money by selling coupons.[277] A leading newspaper reported:

> At a time when workers are more concerned about their wages and job security, the apolitical union of a sick unit here has set up a hospital for its members and the needy persons. The Indo-Japan Steel Employees Union members had initially set up a dispensary here a decade ago, and upgraded it to a 'full-fledged' hospital a few months ago. The trade union is not affiliated to any major political outfit. ...Operating from an abandoned building inside the Indo-Japan Steel factory's closed sister concern, the Grand Smithy Works on Grand Trunk Road, the project is the product of innovative techniques and dedication among workers and doctors. The doctors are paid a travelling allowance and provided snacks and tea for their efforts. The workers and their sympathizers collected about Rs 33,000 and invested the amount to renovate the ground floor of the three-storied building...Fees charged for operations take care of the day-to-day functioning of the hospital. Removal of cysts, gallstones, orthopaedic surgery and even skin grafts are charged between Rs 975 to Rs 3,150...A regular supply of medicine for the outdoor free clinic is maintained through the collection of unused medicines.[278]

In 1996, the factory was closed permanently. Even though the workers lost their jobs, they would still have been able to run the hospital. However, the company's owner went as far as to try to evacuate the hospital. Rajesh Goyel, a promoter, vandalized the hospital with the help of police and hooligans.[279] In an effort to save the hospital, the *Shramajibi Haspatal Bachaw Committee* was formed. Noted cultural icons such as Sankha Ghosh, Mahasweta Devi, Pratul Mukhopadhyay, Nachiketa Chakraborty, and Pijushkanti Sarkar, and mass organizations such as *Nagarik Mancha* also backed their campaign. Kirity Roy, a human rights activist, filed public interest litigation in the Calcutta High Court (WP No. 8186W of 1997 *Kirty Roy* v. *State of WB*).[280]

On January 24, 1999, Centre of Indian Trade Unions (CITU) supporters, flying a red flag, had occupied two rooms of the hospital.[281] Initially, some leaders of this health project seemed to have been influenced by Naxalite ideology. For this reason the ruling party then attacked the hospital. Sukanta Sarkar wrote in the *Anandabazar Patrika* that "initially, the initiative was spearheaded by the Naxalite Workers Union and some activists of the junior doctors' movement. As a result, their activities were marked as 'Naxalite' from the beginning. Some of those who bestowed the title later acknowledged that *Shramajibi Hospital* was kept under constant surveillance. The administration had also been utilized to do the same."[282]

Despite many obstacles, the work of the *Shramajibi Swasthya Prakalpa* has continued. The number of hospital beds has increased greatly. In 2005, they launched a project named *Hriday Chhnuye* (Touching the heart), under which bypass surgery could be done at a cost of Rs. 25,000. In 2011, they took the initiative to build a new hospital at Sriramapur in Belur. The project was named *Chai Swasthya Chai Pran,* and the aim was to have proper health care to save lives. It has a plan to build a 500-bed super-specialty hospital and provide various modern medical services. In addition, they planned to build another 120 rural hospitals. They have also taken the initiative to implement the 'KG to PG' project, which means making an arrangement of education from KG class to postgraduate, including MBBS.[283] To boost the people's health movement and to come closer to the comrades of different peoples' organizations, since 1999 *Sramajibi Hospital* has been publishing a Bengali bi-monthly magazine named *Sramajibi Swasthya.*[284]

Meanwhile, a huge building for the *Shramajibi hospital* has been constructed at Belumilki village near Srirampur (Serampore). It can be stated that this was intending to show another way. They have proved that nothing is impossible and that there is always an alternative.

Shramik Krishak Maitri Swasthya Kendra (SKMSK) and Shramajibi Swasthya Udyog

After the sudden killing of Shankar Guha Niyogi, problems arose in the Chhattisgarh movement. There were conflicts among the nine people who were associated with Niyogiji in 1991. One of them, Anup Singh, opined that, as the liberal economy had been introduced in India, it was not possible to continue the movement at the time, and workers would have to surrender. However, others, like Punyabrata Goon, opposed this idea. They wanted to sustain the movement. In that situation, doctors like Punyabrata Goon and Saibal Jana wanted to maintain the ideological class struggle. Since they were health activists, they had little experience of the workers' movement. These doctors stayed at Dalli-Rajhara, located ninety-one kilometers from Bhilai. As a result, the doctors opened a branch to communicate with the workers at Bhilai. They became popular among the workers. However, in 1994, Punyabrata Goon felt it was impossible for him to work in the docile environment because of the opposition from the Anup Singh camp.[285]

During this time, the Kanoria workers' movement in West Bengal had been developed. The labor movement of Bhilai inspired that movement. From the 1980s onward, on the one hand, various factories in West Bengal had been closed down; on the other hand, impairment was observed in the labor movements. The rights of workers in the factories were curtailed. Yet the leaders of mainstream trade unions were silent; they did not want to form any movement. They argued that if the workers had organized the movements, the factory would have been closed, which would have been detrimental to them. The workers were not prepared to accept this argument, however. So, the workers left the mainstream trade unions and started to form new unions in different factories.[286]

Similarly, in 1993, Kanoria Jute Mill's workers formed the *Kanoria Jute Sangrami Shramik Union* (KJSSU). The Kanoria workers' movement gained support from labor families, common people, and intellectuals. Although the factory was closed, they did not stop their movement. Neither did they agree with the terms imposed by the owner of the factory.[287]

The workers vowed, "We will not let any worker and their family member die due to starvation or lack of healthcare." To keep the movement moving, collective kitchens were run in 87 villages. Workers amassed money from various places in West Bengal to continue the movement and fund these collective kitchens. In addition, health camps were started by some doctors to treat the workers and their families. The children of the workers' families were trained up as health workers. In this manner, health camps also became an integral part of the Kanoria movement. Finally, the factory owner reopened the factory by accepting the demands of the workers through an agreement made on September 27, 1994. On the occasion of that victory, KJSSU organized a workers' conference on October 2, where it was announced that a hospital would be gifted to the poor people of Kanoria, as their cooperation led to the success of the labor movement. They planned to build this hospital along the lines of the

Shaheed Hospital. The hospital was named *Shramik-Krishak Maitri Swasthya Hospital* as a symbol of worker–farmer friendship.[288]

Shramik Krishak Maitri Swasthya Kendra (SKMSK) (Workers–Peasants Alliance Health Center) at Chengail in Howrah started its journey on March 21, 1995. Dr. Dhiren Ganguly inaugurated it in the presence of writer Mahasweta Devi, freedom fighter Prabir Ghosh, and others at a gathering of workers and peasants. Yet a full-time doctor was needed to continue that health center, so Dr. Punyabrata Goon arrived from the *Shaheed Hospital*. Earlier, boys and girls had been trained up, primarily in acupuncture mainly. Dr. Goon's colleague, Ajay Prasad from Chhattisgarh, came there to support the activities. The main functions of *Maitri Swasthya Kendra* were to provide rational healthcare to the people at affordable prices, to make people health-conscious, and to build a health movement. However, their path was not a smooth one. *Maitri Swasthya Kendra* had to overcome many obstacles in its journey. When the employees of the *Kanoria Jute Mill* were locked out in 2002, they lost their jobs. As a result, the meager allowance that was paid to the doctors and health workers was stopped. In this situation, they did not stop their work; rather, they remained steadfast in the goal.[289]

During the Kanoria movement, doctors from Kolkata had often paid visits there. Later, six volunteers were trained to become health workers. Those who participated in the student movement of MCDSA and the junior doctors' movement of the *All Bengal Junior Doctors Federation* (ABJDF) joined the SKMSK. It was planned to set up an organization to make the health movement more organized. As a result, in December 1999, *Shramajibi Swasthya Udyog* [SSU] (the Toilers' Health Initiative) was initiated. The intention was to bring the activists of the peoples' health movement under one umbrella.[290]

At SKMSK, patients were charged one rupee for consultation with doctors from 1995. This fee was increased to two rupees in 1996, four rupees in 1998, and five rupees in 2002. In 2013, it was raised to 10 rupees. However, there was free health service for those who could not pay this small amount.[291] *Shramajibi Swasthya Udyog* declared:

- Standing against the tide of rampant commercialization of health care services, SSU attempts to prove that scientific and modern medicine can be provided to the people at low cost.
- SSU believes that to be effective, a health program must associate with larger social movements of the people for their basic rights of

food, housing, employment, education and culture, this organization attempts to stand by the side of the just peoples' movement.
- SSU tries to educate the people on socio-economic causes of the illnesses to demystify the health sciences. It attempts to arm the people with simple technologies of disease prevention and treatment.
- SSU is against the dependence on funding agencies (foreign or Indian, governmental or non-governmental). It believes that only the health programmes initiated by people and dependent on the people's resources can be sustainable and pro-people.
- In its programmes, SSU tries to experiment with the democratic relations between doctors, health workers and the patients.[292]

The health care services were provided at a small cost in the clinics run by *Shramajibi Swasthya Udyog*. But the intention of the organization was not for it to be a substitute for government health services. Its main objective was to develop a model to show to the government that it would be possible to provide health services at low cost. At that time, the common perception was that modern medical care was so expensive that it was impossible for the government to bear its responsibility. This low-cost treatment model focused on taking detailed case histories and supplying scientific medical care. In the SSU, the trained health workers used to collect the history of the disease in a certain format and patients were then sent to the general physicians. If the general physician felt the need, the patients would be referred to a specialist physician. The patient did not have to undergo unnecessary (or additional) pathological tests. Secondly, medicines were prescribed for the patient according to the essential drugs list of either the India state or the WHO. As a result, the costs of treatment were reduced.[293] Amit Sengupta, one of the most prominent activists of people's health movement in India, noted of SKMSK that "A quiet movement in health care has been unfolding in the rural interiors of West Bengal, improving the lives of thousands of people in villages where no doctor has ever been before."[294]

In 1999, SSU opened a clinic named *Arijit Janaswasthya Kendra* at Salt Lake in Kolkata, but this proved short-lived. In 2000, *Bhaskar Rao Janaswasthya Committee*, a health organization, joined the works of SSU. In March of the same year, *Bauria Shramik Krishak Maitri Swasthya Kendra* was begun in Bauria, an industrial area near Chengail, as a joint venture of the above two organizations. Influenced by the Kanoria labour movement, the workers of Bauria the cotton mill formed their own labor union in 1995. In 2000, *Bharatiya Bijnan O Yuktibadi Samiti* (BBYS) also joined SSU. At the initiative of these SSU and BBYS, *Bainan Shramik Krishak Maitri Swasthya Kendra* was set up in 2007 at Bainan, an agricultural region.[295]

In 2007, SSU stood by the peoples in their struggles: the land struggles of Singur and Nandigram; the tribals' struggle of Lalgarh; and the anti-eviction struggle of Nonadanga. It assisted them by organizing medical relief and providing training to the activists so that they could act as health-workers. SSU tried to stand by those affected in the times of natural calamities—the super cyclone of Orissa (1999), floods in West Bengal (2001), the tsunami in the southern states of India (2004), and Aila (a cyclone) in Sundarbans (2009).[296] SSU ran a two-month residential training program to train the activists of the fraternal peoples' organizations in the management of common illnesses. The organization trained many boys and girls from the backward districts of West Bengal—South 24 Parganas, Burdwan, Bankura and Purulia—and also the neighboring states of Jharkhand, Bihar and Tripura. They provided health care in areas where there were no doctors. In doing so, they seek medical advice from SSU doctors over mobile phones.[297]

After Cyclone Aila in 2009, SSU came into contact with a small non-funded NGO *Sundarban Comprehensive Area Welfare & Environmental Research Centre*. This was a society formed by the residents of the Jamespur village of the Gosaba block of the Sundarban for the welfare of their own village. In 2009, SSU trained five girls and four boys from Jamespur as health workers. The doctors of SSU ran periodic clinics in the same area.[298]

There were a number of clinics under the common umbrella of *Shramajibi Swasthya Udyog*, such as *Shramik Krishak Maiitri Swasthya Kendra* of Chengail (1995), *Bauria Maiitri Swasthya Kendra* (2000), *Madan Mukherjee Janaswasthya Kendra* (1999) at Beliator in Bankura, *Chandipur Swasthya Kendra* (2016), and the *Barasat Citizen Forum* at Barasat.[299] These organizations wanted to open rational model clinics at low cost. Since these organizations had no doctors, however, they contacted SSU. As a result, several model clinics were set up in North Bengal in 2016.[300] It is important to note that, with the exception of Chengail, these other clinics were not primary health centers. The organizers of SSU believed that the primary health service should be provided to the poor people on a daily basis. Due to the lack of enough funds and manpower, however, health centers under SSU could not provide primary health services on a daily basis. SSU has worked without external funds. Punyabrata

Goon wrote that "We hold that 'external funding means external control'. Therefore, we are against funding of health programmes. Our health centre has been self-sufficient since 1998; we can cover the expenses through fees collected from medical consultation, tests, and sale of medicine."[301]

Apart from these model clinics, *Shramajibi Swasthya Udyog* had been working to make people aware of their right to health since 2013. The model clinics were used as a propaganda center for the health movement. In this regard, they used the report of a high-level expert group led by Srinath Reddy, published in 2011 as a weapon. They brought together 33 organizations in West Bengal and formed the *Sara Bangla Sabar Janya Swasthya Prachar Committee* (All Bengal Health for All Campaign Committee) in 2015. This combined the following organizations: *Shramajibi Swasthya Udyog*, the *All West Bengal Sales Representative Union, IFTU*, the *Association for Protection of Democratic Rights (APDR), MCDSA, Canning Juktibadi Sanskritik Sanstha, Bijnan Darbar Kanchrapara, Jansanskriti, TUCI, Tapshili Unnayan Samiti Pandaveshwar, Dishari Jansanskritik Sanstha*, the *Naihati Institute of Science & Culture, PYL, Krantikari Nawjoan Sabha, Pandaveshwar Chhatra Samiti, PDSF*, the *Foundation for Health Action, FAMA, Calcutta Ahead, Bansberia Sunday Sitting, Bijnan o Sanskritik Sanstha Chakdah, Halisahar Bijnan Parishad, Bibartan Bijnana Sanstha, Bharatiya Bijnan o Yuktibadi Samiti*, the *Dr. Bhaskar Rao Janaswasthya Committee, Madan Mukherjee Smriti Janswasthya Kendra*, the *Barasat Citizens' Forum, Bijnan Mansikata Vikash Kendra, Ragini Santipur, Sivnath Sastri Ganaswasthya Udyog, Sundarban Sramajibi Hospital, Santipur Marami*, and *Belur Sramajibi Swasthya Prakalpa*. In 2016, *Sabar Janya Swasthya Prachar Committee* invited Dr. K. Srinath Reddy to attend a people's conference at the University Institute Hall in Kolkata. Other speakers were Dr. Binayak Sen, Dr. Arun Singh, Dr. Rahul Mukherjee, Satya Sivaraman, Bankim Datta and Alakesh Mondal.[302] Later, a book of the lectures was published.[303]

During November 19–21, 2015 SSU participated in the Science March of *Bharatiya Bijnan O Yuktibadi Samiti* to convey the messages of "Health for All" in North Bengal. They also maintained their campaign in South Bengal—Siakhala, Naihati, Uttarpara, Chinsurah, Mankar, Golpark, College Street, Galsi, in the villages around Sarberia, Nonadanga, Pandaveshwar, Serampore and Behala.[304] They organized six Jathas (processions). One of those was organized in four North Bengal districts during the period January 17–20, 2016. Five other Jathas were organized in rural Howrah and the adjoining neighborhoods of Hooghly, South 24

Parganas, Bankura and Burdwan, Hooghly industrial areas and Nadia and North 24 Parganas. April 7, 2016, World Health Day, was observed as Demand Day, with organizations demanding that the government must take responsibility for the people's health.[305]

In the latter part of 2016, they campaigned in Siliguri and Tindharia tea garden, Margaret's Hope tea garden, Jalpaiguri and in along the route of a Science Expedition of *Bharatiya Bijnan O Yuktibadi Samiti* held in four districts of North Bengal. In South Bengal, they campaigned in Santipur and Kandi. To spread the campaign all over India, an All India Delegates Meet on Campaign for Universal Health Care (UHC) was held at Kolkata on World Health Day, i.e. April 7, 2017.[306] A provisional National Campaign Committee was formed. It was decided to hold its 1st public meeting at AIIMS in New Delhi. On August 26, 2017, the delegates of SSU participated in the AIIMS convention on UHC.[307]

SSU used pamphlets, booklets, magazines, Power Point Presentations (PPT), etc. as their campaign weapons. In 2002, they also published a quarterly bulletin called *Doctors' Dialogue* (Periodical Newsletter for Private Circulation), edited by Siddhartha Gupta, as a means of communication among doctors, medical students.[308] The first issue of this bulletin read:

> The movement of junior doctors in 1983 and 1986 was probably the first mass movement in West Bengal to demand health and well-being of the common man. At that time, we thought that in order to strengthen the health movement, it was necessary to publish a magazine through which the message of the health movement could be spread among the doctors. It's been two decades. We floated here and there with different needs. But slowly we are getting closer. In this situation we publish the bilingual magazine Doctor Dialogue. This is the magazine of doctors. Through which we want to protest against injustice in the health sector.[309]

Since May 2010, SSU has been associated with the bi-monthly magazine *Asukh-Bisukh* published by the *Foundation for Health Action*.[310] In 2011, they came out from the *Foundation for Health Action* and published a magazine named *Swasthyer Britte*, edited by Punyabrata Goon.[311] *Swasthyer Britte* was inaugurated on September 23, 2011 at the GLT Hall of Calcutta Medical College in the presence of activists of the people's science and people's health movements. The first issue of the magazine was presented to Dr. Jnanabrata Sil and Dr. Sanjeev Mukherjee, veteran activists of the health movement in West Bengal, who gave lectures on the health movement and the science movement. After the inauguration of the magazine, the Parthasarathi Gupta Memorial Lecture was also delivered.[312]

At the initiative of *Swasthyer Britte*, a discussion meeting was organized at the historic Indian Association Hall on November 19, 2017. The speakers were Dr. Arun Singh and Dr. Rezaul Karim. The theme of Dr. Singh's speech was the November Revolution and People's Health. He stated that it was the Bolshevik Revolution that inspired the disenfranchised people to assert their rights, which was a cause for fear of the capitalist states. The other speaker of the meeting, Dr. Karim, spoke on the doctor–patient relationship.[313]

SSU also published various booklets/pamphlets written by different writers, including such as *Banya O Prakritik Durjoge Jakhon Daktar Nei* (During Flood and Natural Calamities, When There is No Doctor),[314] *Shaheed Haspatal O Dalli-Rajharar Janaswasthya Andalon* (Shaheed Hospital and People's Health Movement of Dalli-Rajhara),[315] *Marxbader Mulsutra* (Basic Tenets of Marxism),[316] *Biswayan O Swasthya (*Globalization and Health),[317] *Chiner Swasthya-Byabasthya: Birat Biparit Jatra* (China's Health System: the Great Leap Backward),[318] *Paschimbanger Swasthyer Akashe Durjoger Ghanaghata* (The Critique of Two Acts Introduced by West Bengal Government),[319] *Bikalpa Chikitsay Homeopathy* (Homeopathy in Alternative Therapy),[320] *Sabar Janya Swasthya Marichika Nay.*[321] As a protest against the West Bengal Clinical Establishment Act 2017, the *All Bengal Health Campaign Committee* published a book named *Swasthya A-Byabastha*,[322] edited by Punyabrata Goon. In this book, articles were written by the doctors, who were associated with the health movement. This book depicted a picture of health care problems in West Bengal. A book named *Modicare: Kar Munafa Beshi, Janagan Na Corporate Company-gulor*[323] was also published to promote the formation of a movement against the insurance-centric *National Health Protection Mission* (NHPM).

On the line of *Shramik-Krishak Maitri Swasthya Kendra* (SKMSK) other small alternative initiatives were organized in West Bengal. In the 1980s, *Lokswaraj*, a Gandhian voluntary organization, started working for the development of people in Kushmashuli, a neglected tribal village in the Ramgarh region under the Binpur-I block of Jhargram subdivision. For the villagers, the organization constructed toilets and arranged for water to be available for both drinking and farming. Since there was no hospital within 20 kilometers of the village, they had no access to government health care. Usually, they depended on quack practitioners for their medical treatment. In view of the same, in around 1985, *Lokswaraj Parishad* set up a health center to provide low-cost medical care to the villagers. Yet this health center could not meet the health care needs of all the villagers. Thus, an initiative was taken to convert the health center into a hospital. Consequently, *Premseba Haspatal* was established at Kusmashuli in 1995. The *Premseba Trust* was formed to run the hospital. Ranabrata Sen, a retired officer of the Reserve Bank of India, made an important contribution to the construction of *Premseba Project.*[324] The hospital authority declared that:

> This hospital will not only treat patients but will also concentrate on disease prevention. Health workers will also take steps to raise villagers' health consciousness. Medicine alone would not be enough to cure the disease. In addition, patients should be treated with love. This is why the hospital has been named as *Premseba Haspatal.*[325]

There were two other important small alternative model clinics, named *Sundarban Sramajibi Hospital* and *Aamader Hospital*, in West Bengal. A *Krishi Chakra* was set up in 1989 with local farmers at Sarberia in the Sundarban region, 64 kilometers away from Kolkata, to oppose shrimp farming by introducing salty water into the farmland. The activities of the *Krishi Chakra* spread to nearby villages. Many people from those villages went outside the district to work in urban areas. Many returned to the village with sick health. But the people of the Sundarban had to rely on quack doctors as there were no modern medical facilities in the villages. In order to overcome that problem, in 1999, they started a fortnightly 'Health Camp' in collaboration with *Belur Sramajibi Hospital.* At the initiative of the villagers, in 2002, a four-bed hospital was initiated at Sarberia. Later, the number of beds in *Sundarbans Sramajibi Hospital* was increased from 4 to 24.[326]

In 2008, Dr. Pijush Kanti Sarkar, a former director of the *School of Tropical Medicine in Calcutta*, set up *Aamader Haspatal* at Fulberia village in Chhatna, Bankura, with the help of various well-wishers. The hospital was founded with donations from members and friends of an NGO named the *Foundation for Health Action.* According to Pijush Kanti Sarkar, "this hospital can be called an alternative model of rural healthcare." He stated that the *Drug Action Forum* continued a movement across the state for almost three decades demanding proper treatment and rational drugs; this hospital was the practical application center of that movement. The goal of the hospital was to ensure the provision of proper and rational medical care to rural people. According to the date from 2015, more than 2 lakh patients, old and new, were treated in *Aamader Haspatal.* Along with medical care, a rural health service training infrastructure was there.[327]

Janaswasthya Committee

Observing the possibilities of the *People's Health Movement*, the West Bengal state government had come forward to form the *Janaswasthya Committee* and to take part in the movement. On May 9, 1988, in a convention held at the Muslim Institute, Kolkata, *Janaswasthya Committee* was formed under the leadership of some legislators and intellectuals close to the ruling party, with state sponsorship.[328] The committee was headed by several ministers as advisers.

Basically, the health movement was strengthened in West Bengal in the 1980s and this prompted the ruling party to launch a pro-government health movement backed by the party. As with the science movement before, the health movement also attempted to bring under the control of the party.[329] As a result, the *Janaswasthya Committee* was formed by the ruling party. They started a campaign to promote health awareness among the common people in Kolkata.[330]

The *Janaswasthya Committee* focused on strengthening its organization. Therefore, regional committees were established in different regions in Kolkata. An organizational set up was established. The first annual conference of the committee was held on October 31, 1990 and the second on March 6, 1993.[331]

In October 1988, the *Janaswasthya Committee* published a bulletin for its members with the title *Janaswasthya*. Its aim of that bulletin was to publish theoretical and practical information regarding health. Later, the name was changed to *Janaswasthya Katha*. This committee highlighted the incident involving adulteration of food and cooking oil in Behala in 1988.[332] In 1990, people became terrified due to an outbreak of dengue fever in Kolkata. The *Janaswasthya Committee* took initiatives to ease the minds of the people. A campaign was launched to kill mosquitoes in order to control dengue fever. There was a comprehensive campaign, especially in Ward 49, where the fever was first discovered. It was carried out through civic conventions, leaflet distribution, street rallies, and cleaning of stagnant water. One lakh leaflet were distributed, in three languages.[333] A seminar on 'People's Health Problems' was organized at Mahajati Sadan, Kolkata on January 23, 1991. *Janaswasthya Committee* had also manned a stall on public health at the fair organized on the occasion of CITU's all India conference. There was also an arrangement for carrying out blood group testing at the stall.[334]

Citizens' Conventions were held on October 9, 1991 at the Darbhanga Building and on March 10, 1992 at the Indian Association Hall in Kolkata protesting the price hike of life-saving medicines and the intrusion of multinational companies into the pharmaceutical industry.[335] In 1992, on the occasion of World Health Day, a week-long health campaign was launched in which one lakh Bengali, 50,000 Urdu and Hindi pin badges, 5000 posters, and 50,000 leaflets were distributed.[336] On several occasions, the committee had also organized seminars, conventions, processions, and road shows to make people aware of addiction to drugs and other narcotics. Similar programs were held in Khidirpur, Garden Reach, and several other areas in Kolkata. When the intestinal disease had spread to the Hooghly Jute Mill slum, *Janaswasthya Committee*'s workers stood alongside them.[337]

They were gradually expanding their activities and strengthening the organization. Conferences were held on a regular basis. Along with the *Nagarik Committee* and the *Paschimbanga Bijnan Mancha*, the *Janaswasthya Committee* started to function as a united front. *Janaswasthya Mela* in College Square was organized by the committee on a regular basis. The committee organized seven public health fairs between 1994 and 2011. Seven souvenirs were published.[338] The first *Janaswasthya Mela* was organized in April 1994 at College Square. In that fair, Dr. Rathindra Narayan Bose, vice-chancellor of Calcutta University, was the president and the secretary was Dr. Abirlal Mukherjee. Every day, before the program of the fair, processions from Azad Hind Bag and Subodh Mallick Square had come and met at the fair premises. There were various health-related stalls, health and other book exhibitions at the fair. Seminars on health were organized and there was also an arrangement to show health-related videos.[339]

However, Dr. Gauripada Dutta wrote that the *Janaswasthya Committee* played a historic role in the beginning, but then it could not work actively because, first of all, the leading members became involved in important work in other fields; secondly, they failed to fully grasp the true significance of the public health problem.[340]

We have already discussed the history of the *People's Relief Committee* (PRC) in the first chapter. In the 1990s, an initiative was taken to construct the PRC's building in order to continue its activities. Abdullah Rasul laid the foundation stone of the new building at 26 Dilkhusa Street in 1991. Finally, the building was completed in 1997 and Jyoti Basu inaugurated *Janaswasthya Kendra*, which principally provided medical services at a low cost.[341]

CPI (M) wanted to bring the various people's health organizations under an umbrella so that it could control the people's health movement in West Bengal. The result of this was the formation of *Paschimbanga Janaswasthya Chetana Prachar Samiti* (PJCPS). The same thing happened in the case of the people's science movement.[342]

The first *National People's Health Conference* was held on 30 November and December 1, 2000 at Yuva Bharati Stadium, Kolkata. Earlier, the *Paschimbanga Janaswasthya Chetana Prachar Samiti* (PJCPS), controlled by CPI (M), had been established on March 27, 1999 at the *Bengal Academy Hall* under the leadership of the *Paschim Banga Vigyan Mancha (PBVM)* in collaboration with various mass organizations, voluntary organizations and health organizations of West Bengal. The next meeting of the committee was held on June 26 of that year in the presence of 78 people's organizations. The *National Coordinating Committee* was then formed with 18 organizations to conduct the *All India People's Health Conference*. The presidents of that association were Dr. N. H. Antia of Maharashtra and Dr. Debabar Banerji of Delhi.[343]

In June 2000, the *National Health Conference Organizing Committee* was formed in West Bengal on the initiative of PJCPS. The chairman, acting chairman, and general secretary of that committee were the then Chief Minister Jyoti Basu, Education Minister Partha De and Pradeep Bhattacharya, respectively. Initially, the office of this committee was in the state office of *Paschim Banga Vigyan Mancha* in Kolkata. On the occasion of the National Conference, a health fair was organized at the Yuva Bharati Stadium, Salt Lake from November 27 to December 3, 2000, which was inaugurated by Ashok Mitra, the former finance minister of the Government of West Bengal. The fair was attended by various organizations working in the field of health, members of UNICEF, and other organizations.[344]

The work of the national conference began at the Yuva Bharati Stadium at 9 a.m. on November 30, 2000. Dr N. H Antia, president of the National

Coordinating Committee, took up the flame. The main topics of the conference were:

- Globalization and its impact on poor people.
- Why did the Alma-Ata declaration fail?
- Minimum needs of the common people and its fulfilment.
- Reconstruction and expansion of the primary health care system.
- Commercialization of the medical system and its effect.
- Health problems of women.[345]

The noted economist Amiya Kumar Bagchi spoke on the subject of "Globalization and its impact on poor people." He was of the opinion that the economy of developing countries had been crippled by the burden of debt taken from the IMF and the rich countries. These developing countries had been forced to reduce public spending on the health sector. As a result, ordinary people were deprived of government health care.[346] Dr. Halfdan T. Mahler, former director-general of the WHO, spoke on "Health for All—A Commitment." He explained why the goal of "Health for All" could not be achieved even after the year 2000 AD. The social activist Medha Patkar discussed the impact of unplanned development activities on public health. She also spoke of forming public opinion against inequalities. Other notable participants in the conference were Dr. Mira Shiva, Dr. Amit Sengupta, M Sudha, Lakshmi Sahgal, Dr. Anant Phadke, Dr. Ravi Narayan, and Dr. Gauri Pada Dutta. All of them were prominent activists of the people's health movement and/or social movement in India. On the second day of the conference, there were various rounds of discussion on public health.[347] In the National Health Assembly, over 2000 delegates from 19 states and 18 national networks of people's movements, science movements, trade unions, health activists, and women's organizations endorsed a 20-point Indian people's health charter.[348] Indian people's health charter stated that "We declare health as a justiciable right and demand the provision of comprehensive health care as a fundamental constitutional right of every one of us."[349]

After the national health assembly, the international health assembly was held in Dhaka, Bangladesh from December 4 to 8, 2000. Along with various organizations across the world, PJCPS also participated in that conference.[350]

We know that through the *People's Health Assembly* (PHA), held in Dhaka in 2000, a worldwide people's health movement was organized. An

Indian chapter of the global *People's Health Movement* (PHM) was *Jan Swastya Abhiyan*. Since 2000 AD, 18 national networks and four resource group organizations have come together to form the People's Health Movement in India. "The National *Coordination Committee* and the *National Working Group* met subsequently in Bangalore on March 4th & 5th, in Hyderabad on April 6th and 7th, in Delhi in August and in Kolkata on November 4th and the 5th."[351]

Criticizing the health policy of India, five booklets were published. Activists across the country used those booklets to make people aware of the overall health condition in India. After a year-long health campaign, they participated in the *National People's Health Assembly 2000* held in Kolkata. Following that, *Jan Swasthya Abhiyan* (JSA) was developed.[352] Under the umbrella of JSA, a number of people's organizations belonging to the CPI (M) were present. Among those mention should be made of *Paschim Banga Vigyan Mancha* (PBVM).[353] But there was an allegation that leaders of JSA did not invite those health activists belonging to other Left groups to participate in their campaign.[354] Despite the alleged 'limitations,' a detailed study on *Jan Swasthya Abhiyan* should be made considering its huge contribution to the health movement.

Jan Swasthya Abhiyan (People's Health Movement—India)

The networks and organizations from across the country which had come together to organize the *National Health Assembly* (2000) took initiatives to continue and develop that coalition of movements in the form of the *Jan Swasthya Abhiyan* (People's Health Movement—India). It emerged from the growing health activism. *Jan Swasthya Abhiyan* (JSA) was founded in 2001 and one of the key figures was Amit Sengupta.[355] JSA was the national platform of grassroots movements, activists, and civil society organizations. Its aim was to achieve universal health care for all, irrespective of caste, creed, gender, race or sexual orientation. A document of JSA stated that "JSA is one of the most vocal voices campaigning towards achieving health as a fundamental right enshrined in the Indian constitution and making the denial of the right to good health and good healthcare a justiciable offense."[356]

The networks that constituted the *National Coordination Committee* of JSA, composed of people's science networks, national health networks, national women's organizations, networks of people's movements, and so on. State-level units of the JSA also existed in Andhra Pradesh, Assam, Bihar, Chhattisgarh, Delhi, Gujarat, Haryana, Himachal Pradesh, Jharkhand, Karnataka, Kerala, Madhya Pradesh, Maharashtra, Orissa, Rajasthan, Tamil Nadu, Tripura, Uttar Pradesh, Uttaranchal and West Bengal.[357] The National Coordination Committee members of JSA were the *All India People's Science Network* (AIPSN), the *All India Drug Action Network* (AIDAN), the *Asian Community Health Action Network* (ACHAN), the *All India Democratic Women's Association* (AIDWA), the *Association for India's Development* (AID India), *Bharat Gyan Vigyan Samiti* (BGVS), the *Breastfeeding Promotion Network of India* (BPNI), the *Catholic Health Association of India* (CHAI), the *Centre for Community Health and Social Medicine—JNU*, the *Centre for Health, Enquiry into Health and Allied Themes* (CEHAT), the *Christian Medical Association of India* (CMAI), the *Society for Community Health Awareness, Research and Action* (SOCHARA), the *Forum for Creche and Child Care Services* (FORCES), the *Federation of Medical, Representative Associations of India* (FMRAI), the *Joint Women's Programme* (JWP), *Medico Friends Circle* (MFC), the *National Alliance of People's Movements* (NAPM), the *National Federation of Indian Women* (NFIW), the *National Association of Women's Organizations* (NAWO), *Ramakrishna Mission* (RK), and the *Voluntary Health Association of India* (VHAI). According to JSA, more than 1000 organizations concerned with health care and health policy, from both within and outside the above networks, joined the campaign as participating organizations.[358]

The *Jan Swasthya Abhiyan* (JSA) took up several issues, such as abortion of female foeticide and the *National Health Policy* of 2002, to organize its campaigns. In 2001, criticizing the *draft National Health Policy*, JSA had given a letter to the health ministry. In several states, units of JSA played a significant role in the *Right to Food campaign*. Similarly, activists from JSA conducted surveys on mid-day meals and other programs in a number of states. A *JSA 'Hunger Watch' group* made up of public health and nutrition experts was set up in 2003, and it produced a draft protocol to look into cases of deaths caused by starvation. During the *Asian Social Forum* in Hyderabad in January 2003, several workshops/seminars on important health issues were conducted by JSA constituent organizations, which it supported. JSA also took part in the *World Social Forum* as a national coalition. Prior to the 2004 Lok Sabha election, JSA organized a public discussion on health issues with representatives of various political parties in Delhi on March 12. Around 300 people, including representatives from five national political parties, attended the public discussion. A prepared policy brief was presented by JSA representatives, which described the current state of health. They called for specific political initiatives in health care, which was considered as most important. JSA contributed to a people's tribunal on population policies held at Delhi in September 2004.[359]

Then the activists of JSA decided to build public opinion on the inadequacy of the government medical system. In 2003, they also commemorated the 25th anniversary of *Alma Ata 'Health for All by 2000 AD' declaration* (1978). In September 2003, JSA started the *Right to Healthcare Campaign* across the country. The initial phase of the campaign involved tracking down specific instances of health services denial and structural health care denial. The objectives of the campaign were to mobilize communities around the right to health care, to identify and highlight specific instances of health care denial, to present testimonies describing these instances of denial while also drawing attention to structural and systemic flaws.[360] Numerous representatives from 16 states attended a national public consultation that was held in Mumbai. Subsequently, JSA, in collaboration with the *National Human Rights Commission* (NHRC), arranged public hearings on the *Right to Health Care* in different parts of India such as Bhopal, Chennai, Lucknow, Guwahati, and Ranchi. At the regional hearings, selected cases of deprivation of health care in the government health systems were presented. Representatives of JSA tried to reveal a realistic picture of the government medical system. *Human Rights Commission* officials sought clarification from government officials about those cases. The hearings were widely publicized in local newspapers, and many individuals attended to offer their testimonies. "This opportunity to share was hugely empowering and the movement began to take on its own momentum." The regional hearings were followed by a national hearing in Delhi in December 2004, which was attended by the union health minister, senior health officials from 22 states across the country and the NHRC chairperson and officials. Nine sessions on topics related to health rights, such as women's and children's health rights, mental health rights, and health rights in the context of the private medical sector, were held. Over a hundred JSA delegates from more than twenty states presented numerous instances of health-rights violations. The NHRC and JSA jointly developed the national action plan to operationalize the *Right to Health*, which was announced at the end of the hearing.[361] However, there is no record of any public hearing on the health system in West Bengal, Tripura and Kerala, where CPI (M) was in power.[362]

As a result of the campaign of JSA, in 2005, the union government of UPA-I brought some pro-people modifications in some specific schemes of the *National Rural Health Mission*. In direct response to the NRHM, JSA started a program called *People's Rural Health Watch* in eight northern states. Through this program, local communities could actively monitor the standard of care and suggest ideas and alternative plans for the improvement of health. Catherine Campbell et al. stated that "JSA's most significant achievement has been its role in shaping and monitoring the Indian government's National Rural Health Mission. This included lobbying to create spaces for community monitoring of the programme, and setting up a parallel independent monitoring system called People's Rural Health Watch…the government's National Rural Health Mission has promoted many of JSA's aims, including primary health focus and community participation. Some members are willing to work with the government, while others fear that such involvement compromises JSA's critical stance."[363] Drawing from the experiences of JSA in *Right to Health Campaign*, the People's Health Movement launched an international *Right to Health and Health Care Campaign* (RTHHCC) in its second assembly in Cuenca, Ecuador, held in July 2005; and groups in other countries embarked on a similar activity that was undertaken in India.[364]

Since 2000, JSA has raised its voice against inequality and inequity in health. JSA wrote letters to various ministers and lawmakers regarding the development of health. In 2013, JSA wrote a letter to Union Health Minister Ghulam Nabi Azad on the subject of 'Saving thousands of lives by legalizing Unbanked Directed Blood Transfusion'.[365] From time to time, it published several booklets and reports on different health issues. To commemorate the occurrence of the *Second National Health Assembly* held in Bhopal in 2007, the *National Coordination Committee* of JSA published seven booklets on health issue: *Globalisation and Health* (2006), *Health System in India: Crisis & Alternatives* (2006), *Women's Health* (2006), *Campaign Issues in Child Health* (2006), *New Technologies in Public Health—Who Pays and Who Benefits?* (2007), *The Impact of the Global Trade Regime on Access to Medicines: A Case Study of HIV-AIDS Treatment Access* (2007), and *Access to Essential Medicines* (2007). Those booklets were utilized as crucial weapons in the movement for the right to health.

In 2009, before the general election, JSA published a policy brief so that people's health is given priority as a national political issue. In that brief policy JSA stated that "the current health policies and their implementation need to be seriously examined so that new policies can be implemented in the framework of quality health care for all and access to basic determinants of health as a basic right." In the first section of that document, JSA took a look at the harsh realities of people's health in India, and examined some of the maladies of current health policies. It also provided core recommendations to strengthen and reorient the health system so as to ensure quality healthcare for all. JSA hoped these recommendations would be incorporated by political parties in their election manifestos for the upcoming general election as a demonstration of their commitment to public health.[366]

It organized health-related seminars and workshops in different parts of India. The *Community Development Medicinal Unit* ([CDMU), in collaboration with *Health Action International Asia-Pacific* (HAI-AP), and JSA organized seminars on pharmaceutical policy and access to essential medicines, which were held in Kolkata, September 2, 2010, Bhubaneswar, September 3, 2010 and Siliguri on October 9, 2010.[367] In 2014, JSA published a booklet titled *Realizing the Right to Healthcare: a Policy Brief.* The main features of the then health care system were outlined in that booklet by JSA. It concluded with a list of demands made in order "to move towards a people-centric public health care system in the country." JSA urged all political parties to endorse those suggestions and put them into action when they would be elected to office. Among the major demands were:

- To act on the Social Determinants of Health.
- To enact a Right to Health Act, which assures universal access to good-quality and comprehensive health care for the entire range of primary, secondary and tertiary services, and that makes denial or non-availability for reasons of access, affordability, or quality a justiciable offence.
- To absorb, over a period, existing publicly funded health insurance schemes (RSBY and different state health insurance schemes) into an expanded public health system publicly financed through general taxation.
- To eliminate the role of multilateral and bilateral financing agencies from all areas of technical assistance or health policy formulation.

- To ensure access to treatment and care of persons with mental illness (PWMI.).[368]

The Maharashtra chapter of *Jan Swasthya Abhiyan* (JSA) undertook organized initiatives aimed at enhancing the accountability of private health care services, emphasizing both the promotion of patients' rights and the establishment of people-centric regulations within the private medical sector. In December 2012, JSA activists staged a demonstration at the Maharashtra state assembly held in Nagpur, bearing bandages (as symbolic 'patients') and masks, chanting slogans like 'Stop cheating by private hospitals', 'Adopt the Act for regulation of private hospitals in Maharashtra', and 'Protect patients' rights.' Concurrently, organized movements in various states emerged to raise awareness regarding patients' rights and the regulation of the private medical sector. Some JSA state units began documenting instances of patients' rights violations for public hearings, which were to be conducted by the National Human Rights Commission (NHRC) in partnership with JSA during the years 2015–2016. SATHI (Support for Advocacy and Training to Health Initiatives), in collaboration with JSA units and civil society groups in various states, facilitated a series of regional workshops throughout India in 2013–2014, focusing on the theme 'Promoting Patients' Rights and Ensuring Social Accountability of the Private Medical Sector.' The *Mariz Haq Abhiyan* ('Patients' Rights Campaign'), coordinated by the Healthwatch network in Uttar Pradesh, documented severe violations of patients' rights throughout the state and presented these findings at a well-attended state-level public hearing.[369]

On September 22 and 23, 2018, the third National Health Assembly (NHA) (the first was held in Kolkata in 2000 and the second was held in Bhopal in 2006) organized by JSA in Raipur, Chhattisgarh with the motto: "The time to make health and healthcare a fundamental right is Now!" It aimed to evaluate and critically analyse current policies that impact health and healthcare at national, regional and local levels. The inaugural plenary session was on *Defending Public Health System—Emerging Challenges.* Amit Sengupta stated that health is, first and foremost, a fundamental right. He said health is not just an economic, but also a political and social issue. The assembly concluded with the presentation of the *People's Health Manifesto.*[370]

Other Organizations

The *Social Action Society* was formed at Chittaranjan Avenue in Kolkata in 1983–1984 under the initiative of Shanti Roy, Dr. Dharmadas Banerjee, and others to make people aware of health of the underprivileged section of society and to protect them from drug addiction. Shanti Roy, who had long been associated with the trade union movement, understood that the so-called trade unions could not develop health awareness among working people, which is why the *Society* was formed. That organization collected medicines from different places and provided them to the poor. The poor slum dwellers were also given health cards by the *Society*. Those cardholders were entitled to receive free treatment at Hatkhola Medical Centre.[371]

People's Health Home (Vijaygarh) Samabay Samiti was founded in the 1990s by a group of residents from South Kolkata's suburbs. The organization not only attempted to reduce people's rising medical expenses, but also began a health-promoting campaign. It conducted a four-day drama festival to raise health awareness as part of that campaign.[372] Another organization in West Bengal was *Forum for People's Health*, which had the slogan "people's health by people's Health movement." A conference on primary health care on the occasion of commemoration of 30 years of Alma-Ata declarations and to celebrate 50 years of the successful public health system in Cuba and a tribute to the works of Dr. Binayak Sen, was organized by *Forum for People's Health* at Students Hall, Kolkata on May 31, 2009. Dr. Binayak Sen and Dr. Ilina Sen participated in the event immediately after their release from imprisonment after worldwide protests. Dr. Sujit Das, Dr. Haripada Das and several leaders and organizers of the people's health movement also attended.[373] At the conference, various demands were placed, such as

- People's Health demanded complete free treatment in government hospitals up to medical colleges including all necessary investigations.
- It demanded that Outpatient Departments (OPD) of all hospitals from Primary Health Centres to IPGMER and specialist clinics from sub-divisional hospitals to medical college should be remain open from 9 am to 4 pm from Monday to Friday and 9 am to 2 pm on Saturday throughout the year except eight notified holidays as per government norms.
- It demanded that emergency treatment and medicines should be available from Primary Health Centres to tertiary hospitals round

the clock and 365 days with the presence of Medical Officers and other support staff.
- It demanded for establishment of research, training and treatment centres on major public health problems.[374]

In 2017, the West Bengal government introduced the *Clinical Establishment Bill* to regulate private medical centers. However, a large portion of physicians, especially those who were associated with private practice or private hospitals, felt insecure. Some doctors of the IMA opposed the bill. Organizations such as *Doctors for Democracy* (DFD), *Doctors for Patients* (DOPA), *West Bengal Doctors Forum* (WBDF) etc. were formed to protect the professional interests of doctors. Many doctors thought that the bill would worsen the doctor–patient relationship. Thus, they started a movement.[375] The *West Bengal Doctors Forum* published a book *titled Itihaser Sankalan, Sankalaner Itihas*[376] to convey the views of doctors on current medical care to the public.

On October 30, 2017, a joint convention against violence in healthcare was held at the Moulali Youth Centre in Kolkata in the presence of members of WBDF, DOPA, the *Association of Health Service Doctors* (AHSD), DFD, the *Medical Service Centre* (MSC), the *Service Doctors Forum* (SDF), *Shramajibi Swasthya Udyog* (SSU) and several branches of IMA. The convention argued that the corporate health system had emerged at the cost of the government health system. There had been a surge of corporate activities in health care in West Bengal. It was also opined that relatives of the patient beat the doctors and medical personnel due to not receiving medical care in government hospitals. Yet no government tried to improve the infrastructure of the public hospitals. Doctors argued that the state government blamed some private hospital owners, and the entire medical community, for that unwanted situation. That's why the organizations declared that the government should be pressurized to recognize the right to health as a constitutional right. At the same time, doctors urged the people to join the health movement.[377] In a letter sent to Director of Health Services, Government of *West Bengal Joint Platform of Doctors*, WB (WBDF, SDF, AHSD, DFD, MSC and SSU) demanded that:

- Improve health infrastructure and stop harassment of ill patients. All hospitals must have 24 hours investigation and blood bank facilities

along with appropriate emergency management facilities by trained professionals and doctors from the field of modern medicine.
- Immediate arrest of all miscreants involved in assault of doctors, nurses and other hospital staff as well as damage to property as per law.
- Government must ensure *Health for All*.[378]

The organizations, the works of which have been discussed earlier, have tried to play their role with a specific priority to their field of work. On the other hand, there are others who have invested their time and energy to communicate health. Bengal has a rich heritage of both of these trends.

Junior doctors' movements constitute a significant component of the people's health movement in West Bengal. We can critically assess the extent to which these movements influenced policy reforms and compelled the government to respond to their demands. In 1983, Chief Minister Jyoti Basu ultimately conceded to the demands of the junior doctors' movement. However, the agitators soon expressed dissatisfaction over the inadequate implementation of the promises made. During the movement of 1987, the government formally accepted the demands in writing, prompting the junior doctors to withdraw their strike. This tradition of junior doctors' activism continued into the following decades, with a particularly notable episode during the nationwide protests against the National Medical Commission (NMC) Bill in 2019. The NMC Bill represented one of the most controversial legislative interventions in India's recent health policy landscape. It provoked widespread dissent among medical students and practicing doctors, who denounced it as unscientific, anti-poor, anti-professional, anti-democratic, and anti-federal. Professional associations organized mass demonstrations, including the symbolic public burning of thousands of copies of the bill. Junior doctors, in particular, emerged as the vanguard of this resistance, both nationally and in West Bengal.[379]

A significant flashpoint occurred in June 2019, when an article titled 'Nairajyer Naam NRS' ('The Name of Anarchy is NRS') appeared on the front page of *Ei Samay*, a leading Bengali daily (June 12, 2019), following an incident at Nilratan Sircar (NRS) Medical College and Hospital. On June 10, the relatives of a deceased patient allegedly assaulted junior doctors, prompting a spontaneous protest that brought hospital operations to a standstill. The agitation rapidly spread to other medical institutions in Kolkata. The crisis intensified when Chief Minister Mamata Banerjee issued a public warning: "Those who are not working should not stay in the hostel. Within four hours, I will take strict action against those who do not join the work." Rather than damping down the situation, her statement further served to galvanize the protest. In solidarity with the junior doctors, senior physicians across West Bengal submitted mass resignations. On June 14, the All India Institute of Medical Sciences (AIIMS) in Delhi staged a symbolic strike, and similar actions occurred across the country. Crucially, the movement extended beyond the medical community. Professionals from various sectors participated in rallies and demonstrations, underscoring the broader public resonance of the junior doctors' cause. Mounting public and institutional pressure eventually compelled the chief minister to meet with 31 representatives of the protesting doctors on June 17 at Nabanna, the state's administrative headquarter. Adopting a conciliatory tone, she addressed the doctors as 'Lakshmi Chhele' ('Good Boys') and assured them that their demands would be met. The meeting marked a turning point. Video clips widely circulated on social media showed jubilant junior doctors reopening hospital gates while chanting: "Jitlo kara?... Lakshmi Chhele! Amra ke?... Lakshmi Chhele!" ("Who won? Good boys! Who are we? Good boys!"). These symbolic moments captured the spirit of a youth-led mobilization that compelled the state to respond.[380]

A few years later, in 2024, West Bengal again witnessed widespread movement following the rape and death on site of a female postgraduate trainee doctor working at R.G. Kar Medical College. The tragedy sparked a powerful movement led by junior doctors across the state. What began as a strike soon escalated into a 'fast unto death.' Most of their demands were accepted following a two-phase meeting with Chief Minister Mamata Banerjee. The strike was called off after the first round of talks, and the hunger strike was withdrawn after the second.

The success of these movements can be attributed to several interrelated factors. First, junior doctors occupy the most critical position in the health care system, particularly in emergency and routine medical services, which lends their protests both urgency and broad public support. Second, although the movements were political in nature—challenging governance and institutional accountability—the participants consciously refrained from aligning with any political party or employing partisan symbols, thereby maintaining their moral legitimacy. Third, the movements were marked by a high degree of unity and coordination among the junior doctors, enhancing their collective strength. Above all, these were youth-led movements. And the youth—driven by the dream of a better world—do not easily accept defeat.

While these movements clearly showed the unity and moral strength of junior doctors, it is still unclear how much they led to lasting policy changes. After the occurrence of each and every junior doctors' movement the government took quick steps, such as promising better security in the working place. In reality, however, the problems of violence in hospitals, and poor infrastructure have not been fully addressed. So, even though the movements compelled the government to act in the short term, the long-term impact on health policy has been limited. Importantly, junior doctors have often raised their voices not just for themselves, but also for larger goals like 'Health for All' and the right to health. These movements are important moments in India's medical history because they show how young doctors can come together, and fight for a more just and accessible health system for everyone.

Notes

1. Sumit Sarkar, *Modern India, 1885–1947*, New Delhi: Macmillan India Limited, 1959, p. 4.
2. Ranajit Guha, "Bharate Gramsci: Gurur Prati Shraddhanjali", in Fakhrullah Choudhury (ed.), *Gramsci: Parichay o Tataparata*, Dhaka: Sangbed, 2012, pp. 191–201.
3. Ibid.
4. Sabyasachi Chatterjee and Nataraj Malakar, "Historicising Health Movement: A Preliminary Probe", in Suvankar Dey (ed.), *Health has a History*, Kolkata: K.P. Bagchi & Company, 2021, pp. 58–82.
5. Debabar Banerji, "The People and Health Service Development in India: a Brief Overview", *International Journal of Health Services*, Vol. 34, No. 1, p. 128.
6. Amar Jesani, "From philanthropy to human right: A perspective for activism in the field of health care", *Indian Journal of Social Work*, Vol. 59, Issue I, January 1998, pp. 291–320.
7. Abhay Shukla and Anant Phadke, "Health Movement in India", *Health Action*, Vol. 12, No. 12, December 1999, pp. 6–9.
8. Anant Phadke, "People's Health Movement in India", conference paper, available at http://www.esocialsciences.org/Download/Download.aspx?qs=Uqn/rN48N8UOPcbSXUd2VCus1JoY0J01xKbUzrxruqpklL-

WtWpt6hROJQt47wNOiSpsMHpXNFxjznExnhCRJIXh5ncdtHa2NFKjItFjPU3NwDgGvws7pMlzJ1zGBedCeH4k+KKBt4OFdayNdhZF0Rldq172Ko/ganEXD/fol6ywJO9VGHPCg4BMtn6U7aupg, retrieved on May 20, 2019.
9. Abhay Shukla and Anant Phadke, "Health Movement in India", op. cit.
10. Debabar Banerji, "The People and Health Service Development in India: A Brief Overview", op. cit.., p. 126.
11. Ibid.
12. Lawrence O. Gostin & Lindsay F. Wiley, *Public Health Law: Power, Duty, Restraint*, Oakland, CA: University of California Press, 2016, p. 7.
13. Koushik Dutta, "Swasthya Byabasthar Besarkarikaran O Amra", *4 Number Platform*, 01.03.2019, https://4numberplatform.com/?p=11036, retrieved on March 9, 2020.
14. Kumar Rana, *Health Insurance for The Poor, or Privatization by Stealth?: A Study on the Rashtriya Swasthya Bima Yojana (Rsby) in India*, A Thesis Submitted to the Faculty of The Harvard Medical School in partial fulfilment of the requirements for the Degree of Master of Medical Sciences in Global Health Delivery in the Department of Global Health and Social Medicine Harvard University Boston, Massachusetts, May 2017, p. 45.
15. Ibid., pp. 45–46.
16. Moni Nag, "Political Awareness as a Factor in Accessibility of Health Services: A Case Study of Rural Kerala and West Bengal", *Economic and Political Weekly*, Vol. 24, No. 8, February 25, 1989, pp. 417–426.
17. Sunil S. Amrith, "Health in India since Independence", BWPI Working Paper 79, Manchester: Brooks World Poverty Institute, University of Manchester, February 2009, pp. 17–18.
18. "Abhab Suchinta O Samadrishtir", Interview with Amartya Sen by Anirban Chattopadhyay and Kumar Rana published in *Anandabazar Patrika*, June 8, 2021, p. 4.
19. Moni Nag, "Political Awareness as a Factor in Accessibility of Health Services: A Case Study of Rural Kerala and West Bengal", op. cit.
20. Patralekha Chatterjee, "Seeing Health Care as a Human Right in India", *The Lancet*, Vol. 377, No. 9761, January 15, 2011, pp. 195–196.
21. Ibid.
22. Ibid.
23. Government of India: https://pmjay.gov.in/, retrieved on April 19, 2022.
24. Sabyasachi Chatterjee and Nataraj Malakar, "Shudhui Cikitsa Ebang Bima, Rog Pratirodh Jaruri Nay?", *Ei Samay*, 06.05.2019, p. 8; Sabyasachi Chatterjee and Nataraj Malakar, "Vote Boxe Janaswasthyer Kadar Nei, Tai Abahela?", *Ei Samay*, April 27, 2021, p. 8.

25. Sujit Kumar Das, "Bartaman Swasthya Byabastha O Manabik Mulyabodh", *Swasthya Siksha Unnayan*, Sharad Sankhya, 2011, pp. 30–35.
26. "Swasthyer Golakdhanda Chharun—Chikitsa Bechhe Nin" (editorial), *Asukh-Bisukh*, Vol. 1, No. 1, May–June, 2000, pp. 1–2.
27. *Health Policy Making in India*, Mumbai: CEHAT, 2002, p. 123.
28. Srijan Sen, "Kotniser Janasebar Adarshake Pathyeo Korechhe", *Prokriti O Manush, Kalantar*, September 3, 2018, Kolkata, p. 3.
29. Sabyasachi Chatterjee, *A Historical Study of the Science Movements in West Bengal 1947–1997*, PhD thesis, Department of History, Jadavpur University, 2004, pp. 310–311.
30. Anwar Jaffry and et al., "Towards a People's Science Movement", *Economic and Political Weekly*, Vol. 18, No. 11, March 12, 1983, pp. 372–376.
31. Ibid.
32. Venni venkata Krishna, "Science, Technology and Counter Hegemony—Some Reflections on the Contemporary Science Movements in India", in Terry Shinn, et al. (eds.), *Science and Technology in a Developing World, Sociology of the Science Yearbook 1995*, Netherlands: Springer, 1997, pp. 375–411.
33. Abhay Bang and Ashvin J. Patel, "Preface", in Abhay Bang & Ashvin J. Patel (eds.), *Health Care Which Way to Go?: Examination of Issues and Alternatives*, New Delhi: Medico Friend Circle, first published 1982, cited edition 1985, pp. xi–xii.
34. Prabir Gangopadhyay, "Prasangakrame", in Punyabrata Goon, *Shankar Guha Niyogir Sange Koyek Bochhor: Ek Sohojoddhar Protibedon*, Kolkata: Book Mark (Setu Prakashani), not dated, pp. 7–12.
35. Jayanta Kumar Ray, "Organising Villagers for Self-reliance: A Study of Gonoshasthya Kendra in Bangladesh", *The Calcutta Historical Journal*, Vol. V, No. 1, July–December, 1980, p. 1.
36. B.C. Ray, Presidential Speech at the All-India Medical Conference, Lahore, December 1929, *The Calcutta Review*, Third Series, Volume XXXV, April–June, 1930, p. 122.
37. Sabyasachi Chatterjee and Rakhi Chatterjee, *Banglar Mukti-Sandhani*, Kolkata: Granthamitra, 2005, pp. 186–187.
38. Samita Sen and Anirban Das, "A History of the Calcutta Medical College and Hospital, 1835–1936", in Uma Das Gupta (ed.), *Science and Modern India: An Institutional History, c.1784–1947*, Delhi: Pearson Education, 2011, p. 504.
39. Bharatjyoti Raychaudhury, *Satchallish Theke Sattor Ebong Aage Pare*, Parba 2, Kolkata: Muktaman, 2010, pp. 50–55.

40. Interview with Dr. Jnanabrata Shil (born in 1938), a medical teacher and former secretary of *Norman Bethune* Janaswasthya Andolan, Kolkata, March 2, 2019.
41. Ibid.
42. Interview with Dr. Punyabrata Goon (born in 1960), Health Activist, Kolkata, January 31, 2020.
43. Nilanjan Dutta (ed.) *Panch Prajonmer Nakshalbari*, Kolkata: Purbalok Publishers, 2018, p. 10.
44. Quoted Anil Saha, "Junior Daktar: E kon Uttarsuri", *Sramajibi Swasthya*, February 2016, pp. 25–27.
45. Abhijit Choudhury, "Medha Thaklei Valo Daktar Hoy Na", *Anandabazar Patrika*, June 16, 2015, p. 4.
46. Sthabir Dasgupta, *Swapner Sottor: Maya Rahiya Gelo*, Kolkata: Dhansere, 2018.
47. Satyaki Halder, "Amar Chhatrajiban O Ekti Chhatra Rajnitir Itikatha", *Anyakatha*, Vol. 19, January 2017, North 24 Parganas, pp. 416–423.
48. Gouri Shankar Nag, "Manabadhikar Andolan—Prasangik Vabna", in Sajal Basu (ed.), *Bharote Samajik Andolan*, Kolkata: Bookpost Publishers, 2016, pp. 198–204.
49. Jayaprakash Narayan, "Gano-andolan Lokashakti", in Sajal Basu (ed.), op. cit., pp. 249–257.
50. Rachel Carson, *Silent Spring*, USA: Houghton Mifflin Harcourt, 1962.
51. Ivan Illich, *Medical Nemesis: The Expropriation of Health*, USA: Pantheon Books, 1976.
52. Vibhuti Patel, "Human Rights Movements in India", *Social Change*, Vol. 40, No. 4, 2010, pp. 459–477.
53. Leslie J. Calman, "Women and Movement Politics in India", *Asian Survey*, Vol. 29, No. 10, October 1989, pp. 940–958.
54. *Health Policy Making in India*, op. cit.
55. *Medico Friend Circle Bulletin*, July 2013–February 2014, p. 1; Medico Friend Circle, http://www.mfcindia.org/, retrieved on March 12, 2020.
56. Asbvin J. Patel, "Ten Years with MFC: My Personal View", *Medico Friend Circle Bulletin*, April–May 1984, p. 2.
57. *Medico Friend Circle Bulletin*, January–February, 1976.
58. Ibid., p. 3.
59. The *Comprehensive Rural Health Project*, Jamkhed (CRHP) was started by doctor couple Rajanikant and Mabelle Arole in 1970. The priorities planned of CRHP were: simple symptomatic primary care available in the individual village at all times; care of pregnant and lactating mothers and deliveries; family planning and health education; control of chronic illness such as leprosy and tuberculosis; prevention of blindness.

R.S Arole, "Comprehensive Rural Health Project, Jamkhed", *Medico Friend Circle Bulletin* 49, January 1980, pp. 1–6.

60. Lok Biradari Prakalp in Gadchiroli District of Maharashtra was the project of the Maharogi Sewa Samiti, Warora. In 1973, Baba Amte set up a hut dispensary at Hemalkasa in Gadchiroli District. He stayed there for a while and got the project going. In a letter to his son, Dr. Prakash Amte accepted the responsibility of taking care of the project. The area did not have any health facilities whatsoever. The stated objectives of the project were: to provide basic health facilities; to promote education and to make people conscious of their rights; to undertake agricultural extension programmes.

    Amar Jesani, Manisha Gupte and Ravi Duggal, *NGOs in Rural Health Care* (Volume One: An Overview), Bombay: The Foundation for Research in Community Health, 1986, pp. 136–137.
61. https://chai-india.org/history_who-we-are/.
62. https://kssp.in/kssp-and-health/.
63. Neema Kudva, "Strong States, Strong NGOs", in Raka Ray and Mary Fainsod Katzenstein (eds.), *Social Movements in India: Poverty, Power, and Politics*, UK: Rowman & Littlefield Publishers, Inc., p. 243.
64. West Bengal Voluntary Health Association (WBVHA): http://www.wbvha.co.in/organization.
65. West Bengal Voluntary Health Association (WBVHA), Memorandum and Rules & Regulation, Registration No: S/14704 of 1974.
66. Manoj Sharma and Gayatri Bhatia, "The Voluntary Health Movement in India: A Strengths, Weaknesses, Opportunities, and Threats (SWOT) Analysis", *Journal of Community Health*, Vol. 21, No. 6, December 1996, p. 456.
67. Mari Marcel Thekaekara, "Where has All the Conscience gone", *New Internationalist*, Issue 200, 5 October 1989, available at: https://newint.org/features/1989/10/05/gone.
68. Sunil S. Amrith, "Health in India since Independence", op. cit., p. 19.
69. Dhruv Mankad, "Towards a Revolutionary Approach to Health", *Socialist Health Review*, Vol. 1, No. 1, June 1984, pp. 1–3.
70. Ibid., p. 2.
71. Gouri Pada Dutta, *Social Issues of Health*, Kolkata: Pratyaya, 2003, p. 97.
72. Gouri Pada Dutta, *Janaswasthya Bhabana*, Kolkata: Banglar Mukh, 2011, pp. 21–22.
73. Ibid.
74. Interview with Hiralal Konar, former secretary of Health Service Association, Kolkata, dated February 13, 2020.
75. Ibid.

76. Balai Chakraborty, "Rajyer Chikitsa O Swasthya-parishebar Bartaman O Bhabisyat", https://ritambangla.com/health/state-hospital-scenario/, retrieved on February 5, 2021.
77. Anil Saha, "Junior Doctor: E kon Uttarsuri", *Sramajibi Swasthya*, February 2016, pp. 25–27; Sujit K. Das, "Doctors in Health Care: Their Role and Class Location", *Socialist Health Review*, Vol. 2, No. 2, September 1985, p. 64.
78. *Ei Samay*, Kolkata, June 17, 2019, p. 7.
79. *Sunday Magazine*, *Amrita Bazar Patrika*, Kolkata, March 1, 1987, p. 9.
80. Punyabrata Goon, "Swasthya Andolane Sottarer Dashaker Prabhab", *Anyakatha*, 19th year, January 2017, North 24 parganas, p. 265.
81. Anil Saha, "Junior Doctor: E kon Uttarsuri", op. cit.
82. Ibid.
83. "Sara Paschimbanglar Daktar O Daktari Chhatrader Andolan", in *Bikshan*, Vol. 1, No. 9, December–January, 1973–1974, pp. 6–8; "Sara Banglar Daktar O Daktari Chhatrader Sampratik Andolan" (a report on movement of doctors and medical students), in *Bikshan*, Vol. 1, No. 10, February 1974, pp. 19–23; Debasis Bose, Sankar Kumar Nath and Jayanta K. Das (ed.), *175 Years of Medical College—Commemorative Volume*, Kolkata: Medical College Ex-Students' Association, 2009, p. 131.
84. Amaresh Banerjee, "DSA: Pragatishil Chatra Andolaner Dhara", in *Amader Katha*, a publication of Shramajibi Swasthya Udyog on account of 30th year celebration of MCDSA, Kolkata, March 21, 2007, pp. 2–3.
85. Interview with Punyabrata Goon (born in 1960), dated January 31, 2020.
86. Ibid.
87. Superintendent, N.R.S Medical College and Hospital, Calcutta, memo No. NH/E/ 351, dated April 8, 1983.
88. Punyabrata Goon, *Pa Miliye Path Chala*, Kolkata: Katha Shilpa, 2018, pp. 8–9.
89. All Bengal Junior Doctors' Federation (ABJDF), *Junior Daktarder Andolan—Ki O Keno*, Kolkata: All Bengal Junior Doctors' Federation (ABJDF), 1983, p. 2.
90. Punyabrata Goon, *Pa Miliye Path Chala*, op. cit., pp. 8–9.
91. Hiren Dasgupta and Harinaryan Adhikari, *Bhartiya Upamahadesher Chhatra Andolan*, Kolkata: Radical, 2008, pp. 463–464.
92. All Bengal Junior Doctors' Federation (ABJDF), *Junior Daktarder Andolan—Ki O Keno*, op. cit., p. 6.
93. Ibid., pp. 6–7.
94. Ibid., pp. 10–11.
95. Ibid., p. 11.
96. Ibid., p. 12.

97. Medical Service Centre, *Janaswasthya Raksha Andolaner Ekti Raktakta Adhyay*, Kolkata: Medical Service Centre, not dated, p. 13.
98. Shyamal Chakraborty, "Ar Ek Boithaker Gappo", *Rabibasariya, Anandbazar Patrika,* Kolkata, June 23, 2019, p. 4.
99. Ibid.
100. Biren Roy, "Doctors, Left Front and Health Services", *Economic and Political Weekly*, Vol. 18, No, 44, October 29, 1983, pp. 1867–1868.
101. Sumanta Sen, "Massive breakdown of medical services in Calcutta due to protest by junior doctors", in *India Today*, https://www.indiatoday.in/magazine/indiascope/story/19831031-massive-breakdown-of-medical-services-in-calcutta-due-to-protest-by-junior-doctors-771166-2013-07-15#ssologin=1#source=magazine, retrieved on February 3, 2019.
102. Ranabir Samaddar, "Chiktsa Sankater Sthayi Samadhan Adou Samvab?" *Ei Samay*, Kolkata, June 24, 2019, p. 8.
103. Sujit K Das, "Trouble on the Health Front", *Economic and Political Weekly*, Vol. 22, No. 15, April 11, 1987, pp. 629–630.
104. Biren Roy, op. cit., p. 1867.
105. *Anandabazar Patrika*, October 5, 1983, p. 1.
106. Ibid.
107. Shyamal Chakraborty, op. cit.
108. Nilanjan Dutta, *Rights and the 'Left': West Bengal 1977–2011*, Kolkata: Setu Prakashani, 2015, p. 8.
109. Biren Roy, op. cit., p. 1867.
110. Ibid.
111. Medical Service Centre, *Janaswasthya Raksha Andolaner Ekti Raktakta Adhyay*, Kolkata: Medical Service Centre, op. cit., p. 14.
112. Sujit K Das, "Trouble on the Health Front", op. cit.
113. Ibid.
114. Pradyot Sur, "Itihaser Pata Theke", in *Souvenir, 20th State Conference*, Association of Health Service Doctors, West Bengal, 2014.
115. Association of Health Service Doctors (AHSD), West Bengal, https://www.ahsdwb.org/about.html, retrieved on March 8, 2021.
116. Medical Service Centre, *Janaswasthya Raksha Andolaner Ekti Raktakta Adhyay*, op. cit., p. 4.
117. Ibid., p. 12.
118. Ibid.
119. Birendra Chattopadhyay, "Haspital Mane", in *Kabikantha: Junior Daktarder Samarthane,* published by Samir Ray on the behalf of Ganatantrik Sanskritik Samanway Committee, Kolkata, not dated.
120. Anup Maiti, "Swasthya Niye Chhelekhela Keno?" in Medical Service Centre, *Janaswasthya Raksha Andolaner Ekti Raktakta Adhyay*, op. cit., p. 25.

121. Debashish Dutta, "Ekmatra Janamati Pare Sarkarke Samasya Samadhane Badhya Karte", in Medical Service Centre, *Janaswasthya Raksha Andolaner Ekti Raktakta Adhyay*, op. cit., p. 24.
122. Ashok Samanta, "E Andalon Kebal Daktarder Nay—Amar, Apnar, Apamar Janasadharaner", in Medical Service Centre, *Janaswasthya Raksha Andolaner Ekti Raktakta Adhyay*, op. cit., p. 6.
123. In the early 1980s, Partha Chatterjee, then engineering student of Jadavpur University, along with some friends formed a group called PIX, who would screen films and also make several serious films in 8 mm.
124. Activist Canvas: https://canvaspix.wordpress.com/category/articles/, retrieved February 3, 2019.
125. *Sunday Magazine*, *Amrita Bazar Patrika*, 1 March 1987, p. 10.
126. Ibid., p. 9.
127. Ibid., p. 11.
128. Ibid., p. 11.
129. Nabarun Ghoshal, "Junior Doctors: E Kon Uttarsuri", *Shramajibi Swasthya*, August 2016, pp. 22–24.
130. Sujit K Das, "Trouble on the Health Front", op. cit., p. 629.
131. "Doctors on Strike", *Economic & Political Weekly*, Vol. 22, No. 10, March 7, 1987, pp. 401–402.
132. Ibid., p. 401.
133. Ibid.
134. *Sunday Magazine*, op. cit., p. 12.
135. Ibid.
136. Ibid., pp. 12–13.
137. Nabarun Ghoshal, "Junior Doctors: E Kon Uttarsuri", op. cit.
138. *Sandhya Aajkal*, September 2, 1991, p. 1.
139. *The Telegraph*, September 3, 1991.
140. *Sandhya Aajkal*, September 2, 1991, p. 1
141. *Bartaman*, September 3, 1991.
142. *Bartaman*, September 3, 1991.
143. *The Telegraph*, September 3, 1991.
144. *Sandhya Aajkal*, September 4, 1991, p. 7.
145. *The Statesman*, September 4, 1991.
146. *The Telegraph*, September 8, 1991.
147. *Anandabazar Patrika*, September 8, 1991.
148. *Sandhya Aajkal*, September 8, 1991.
149. *The Statesman*, September 9, 1991.
150. *Bartaman*, September 10, 1991.
151. Press release of Medical College Unit, ABJDF, September 11, 1991.
152. Sabyasachi Chatterjee and Nataraj Malakar, "Swasthya Parisheba Sarkareri Day", *Anandabazar Patrika*, December 19, 2018, p. 4.

153. *Ei Samay*, Kolkata, June 17, 2019, p. 7.
154. Speech of Subhajit Bhattacharya, a member of Bhaskar Rao Janaswasthya Committee, in a seminar on Universal Health Care organized by *Shramajibi Swasthya Udyog* and *All Bengal Health for All Campaign Committee* at West Bengal Voluntary Health Association office, Kolkata, on June 23, 2019.
155. Sumanta Sen, "Massive breakdown of medical services in Calcutta due to protest by junior doctors", op. cit.
156. *Ei Samay*, Kolkata, June 14, 2019, p. 2.
157. Punyabrata Goon, "Antrik Mahamari Ekti Samajik Rog", May 20, 1984 (unpublished).
158. Ibid.
159. Ibid.
160. Leaflet, published by *All Bengal Junior Doctor Federation*, *Health Service Association* and other organizations, date not mentioned.
161. Ibid.
162. Leaflet of *All Bengal Junior Doctor Federation*, 1984.
163. Interview with Punyabrata Goon (born in 1960), dated January 31, 2020.
164. Anup Dhar, "Genealogies of Aboriginalization Psychoanalysis and Sexuation in Cultural Crucible", in Manasi Kumar, Anup Dhar, and Anurag Mishra (eds.), *Psychoanalysis from the Indian Terroir: Emerging Themes in Culture, Family, and Childhood*, New York, London: Lexington Books, 2018, pp. 196–197.
165. Leaflet of People's Health Service Association, not dated.
166. Leaflet of People's Health Service Association, not dated.
167. *Aamader Katha*, a publication of *Shramajibi Swasthya Udyog* on account of annual conference of MCDSA, Kolkata, May 7, 2005, pp. 22–23.
168. "SUCI (C) Carries on People's Movements across the Country", *Proletarian Era*, Vol. 47, No. 23, July 15, 2014, p. 7; "Medical Service Centre running medical camps in earthquake-ravaged Nepal", May 31, 2015, http://sucicommunist.org/medical-service-centre-running-medical-camps-in-earthquake-ravaged-nepal/, retrieved on August 2, 2022.
169. Medical Service Centre, *Medical Service Centreer Abedan*, Kolkata: Medical Service Centre, 2004 (second edition), pp. 43–44.
170. Ibid., pp. 44–48.
171. *Health Spectra* (Journal of Medical Service Centre), Vol. 13, Special Bulletin, December 2000, pp. 28, 45–48.
172. Sabyasachi Chatterjee, *Bijnan Jakhan Andolan: Itihaser Path Beye, Kolkata: Setu Prakashani, 2018,* p. 110.
173. Medical Service Centre: http://www.medicalservicecentre.in/people-health.php, retrieved on September 3, 2021.

174. *Health Spectra*, Vol. 13, Special Bulletin, December 2000, pp. 28, 45–48.
175. Medical Service Centre: http://www.medicalservicecentre.in/people-health.php, retrieved on September 3, 2021.
176. *Swasthya Bikshan*, Vol. 7, Issue. 4, October–December 2001, pp. 44–45.
177. *Swasthya Bikshan*, Vol. 11, Issue. 1, October–December 2001, pp. 58–63.
178. *Health Spectra*, Vol. 15, Special Bulletin, October 2005, pp. 46–48.
179. Approach Paper for National Workshop at Lady Hardinge Medical College, New Delhi, on October 28, 2007, Central Committee of Medical Service Centre.
180. *Swasthya Bikshan*, Vol. 8, Issue. 1, January 2013, pp. 6–7.
181. *Health Spectra*, Vol. 24, February 2017, pp. 3–8.
182. Ibid., pp. 13–14.
183. *Medical Service Centre*, http://www.medicalservicecentre.in/publication.php, retrieved on August 15, 2020.
184. Medical Service Centre, *Sarbanasha Khasra Jatiya Swasthy-niti 2015-er Biruddhe Pratirodh Andolan Gare Tulun*, Kolkata: Medical Service Centre, West Bengal State Committee, 2015.
185. Amalendu Dey, "Antarjatik Rajnitir Prekshapat (1927–1938) O Chine Bharatiya Medical Mission Preran", in *Ankure Shuru* (published by *Kotnis Memorial Committee*, West Bengal), Dr. Kotins birth centenary special issue, October 2010, pp. 16–35.
186. Pamphlet published by the *Kotnis Memorial Committee* on the occasion of the 60th anniversary of the Indian Medical Mission to China (1938–1998), Kolkata, September 15, 1998.
187. Shyamal Ghosh, "Dr Kotnis Smritiraksha Committee-er Pratisthata Dr. Bijoy Kumar Basu Amader Prerana", in *Ankure Shuru* (published by Kotnis Memorial Committee, West Bengal), Dr. Bijoy Kumar Basu birth centenary special issue, October 2012, pp. 17–19.
188. Interview with Srijan Sen, Activist of Dr. Dwarkanath *Kotnis Memorial Committee*, Kolkata, dated April 3, 2019.
189. Srijan Sen, "Kotniser Janasebar Adarshake Pathyeo Korechhe", op. cit.
190. Chandana Mitra, "MCDSA Garar Aager Dingulite", in *Aamader Katha*, a publication of *Shramajibi Swasthya Udyog* on the Occasion of Annual Conference of MCDSA, 10th June, 2006, pp. 4–8.
191. Ibid.
192. Chandana Mitra, "Aamar Chokhe Dr. Bijoy Kumar Basu", *Ankure Shuru* published by *Kotnis Memorial Committee,* West Bengal, Dr. Bijoy Kumar Basu birth centenary special issue, October 2012, pp. 61–63.
193. Chandana Mitra, "MCDSA Garar Aager Dingulite", op. cit.
194. Srijan Sen, "Kotniser Janasebar Adarshake Pathyeo Korechhe", op. cit.
195. Norman Bethune Janaswastha Andolon, *Janaswasthya Andoloner Ruparekha*, Kolkata: *Norman Bethune Janaswastha Andolon*, this part

was included in different books of this organization; here the used book is: Dr. Sukhamoy Bhattacharya (ed.), *Dr. Norman Bethune*, Kolkata: NBJA, 1991, p. 73.

196. Ranatosh Chakraborty, "Dr. Norman Bethune", in Dr. Sukhamoy Bhattacharya (ed.), *Dr. Norman Bethune*, Kolkata: Norman Bethune Janaswasthya Andolan, 1991, pp. 14–34.
197. Sydney Gordon and Ted Allan, *The Scalpel, the Sword: The Story of Dr. Norman Bethune*, New York and London: Monthly Review press, revised edition 1973 (third printing), pp. 64–74.
198. Ibid., p. 95.
199. Ibid., p. 75.
200. Ibid., p. 91.
201. Norman Bethune Janaswasthya Andolan, *Peoples' Health Movement—A Manifesto,* Kolkata: *Norman Bethune Janaswasthya Andolan*, 1986, p. 10.
202. Ibid.
203. Memorandum of Association and Rules and Regulation, Norman Bethune Janaswasthaya Andolan (Registration No S/56685 of 1987–1988).
204. Ibid.
205. Norman Bethune Janaswastha Andolon, *Janaswasthya Andoloner Ruparekha*, Kolkata: *Norman Bethune Janaswastha Andolon*, op. cit.
206. Jnanabrata Sil, "Agrani Janaswasthya O Janabijnan-karmi Dr. Sukhamoy Bhattacharya-er Jibanabasan", in *Top Quark*, June-September, 2001, pp. 57–59.
207. From the Personal Papers of Dr. Jnanabrata Sil, unpublished.
208. From the Personal Papers of Dr. Jnanabrata Sil, unpublished.
209. From the Personal Papers of Dr. Jnanabrata Sil, unpublished.
210. Interview with Dr. Jnanabrata Sil, dated January 14, 2020.
211. Norman Bethune Janaswasthya Andolan, *Peoples' Health Movement—A Manifesto,* op. cit.
212. "Janaswasthya Andolan", in *Satyajug*, February 7, 1986.
213. A leaflet published by *Norman Bethune Janaswasthya Andolan* and *Bangiya Bigyan Parishad*, May 17, 1986.
214. "Janaswasthya Andolan", in *Jugantar*, February 6, 1986.
215. A leaflet published by *Norman Bethune Janaswasthya Andolan* and *Paschimbanga Rashtriya Shikkhak Samiti,* July 31, 1986.
216. A leaflet published by Hajaralaba on that seminar, Belgharia, date not mentioned.
217. A leaflet on that conference was published by Dr. Jnanabrata Sil, Kolkata, date not mentioned.
218. A leaflet of *Norman Bethune Janaswasthya Andolan* on that conference.

219. Norman Bethune Janaswastha Andolon, *Janaswasthya Andoloner Ruparekha*, Kolkata: *Norman Bethune Janaswastha Andolon*, op. cit.
220. Jnanabrata Sil, "Agrani Janaswasthya O Janabijnan-karmi Dr Sukhamoy Bhattacharya-er Jibanabasan", op. cit.
221. Sukhamoy Bhattacharya, *Esab Oshudh Khaben Na*, Kolkta: *Norman Bethune Janaswasthya Andolan*, first published in 1986 (fifth edition 1995).
222. Krishnangshu Roy, *Osudh Theke Asukh*, Kolkta: *Norman Bethune Janaswasthya Andolan*, not dated.
223. Sukhamoy Bhattacharya (ed.), *Janaswasthya Sankalan: Volume One—Sadharaner Asukh Bisukh*, Kolkata: *Norman Bethune Janaswasthya Andolan*, 1990.
224. Sukhamoy Bhattacharya (ed.), *Janaswasthya Sankalan: Volume Two—Maa O Sishu*, Kolkata: *Norman Bethune Janaswasthya Andolan*, 1990.
225. Sukhamoy Bhattacharya (ed.), *Janaswasthya Sankalan: Volume Three—Osudh Bishudh*, Kolkata: *Norman Bethune Janaswasthya Andolan*, 1993.
226. Interview with Dr. Jnanabrata Sil, age 82, Kolkata, January 14, 2020.
227. Jnanabrata Sil, "Agrani Janaswasthya O Janabijnankarmi Dr Sukhamoy Bhattacharya-er Jibanabasan", op. cit. p.
228. Sabyasachi Chatterjee, *Bijnan Jakhan Andolan Itihaser Path Beye*, op. cit., p. 105.
229. Letter of Gauripada Dutta to Comrade Dinesh Singh (Dinesh Singh was the pseudonym of Dr. Jnanabrata Sil provided by the communist party to be its member. Jnanabrata Sil was a government employee and a government employee could not join political party.), dated September 24, 1987. The letter was in Bengali, so it has been translated in English.
230. Kajal Krishna Banik "Professor Gouripada Datta: A Man of Dedication and Service", *Monthly Bulletin*, Vol. XLIX, No. 7, July 2020, Kolkata: Asiatic Society, pp. 11–13.
231. From the Personal Papers of Dr. Jnanabrata Sil, unpublished.
232. Ibid.
233. A letter of Comrade Dinesh Singh (Dr. Jnanabrata Sil) to Comrade Haridas Malakar, West Bengal State Control Committee, dated August 14, 1987.
234. A letter of Dinesh Singh (Dr. Jnanabrata Sil) to the state secretary of CPI (M), dated May 9, 1986.
235. Sydney Gordon and Ted Allan, *The Scalpel, the Sword: The Story of Dr Norman Bethune*, op. cit., p. 99.
236. Sumit Sarkar, "Biplaber Naxalbari—Pratisthaner Nakshalbari", in Nilanjan Dutta (ed.), *Panch Prajonmer Nakshalbari*, Kolkata: Purbalok Publication, 2018, pp. 260–282.

237. Prakash Karat, "Action Groups/Voluntary Organisation: A Factor in Imperialist Strategy", *The Marxist*, Volume: 2, No. 2, April–June 1984.
238. Sujit Sinha, "Bikalper Sandhane O NGO", in Subrata Kundu (ed.), *Unnayaner Khonje NGO*, Kolkata: Development Research Communication and Services Centre, 2005, p. 43.
239. Proceedings of the meeting of the executive committee of the *Norman Bethune Janaswasthya Andolan*, held on October 2, 1999, Chairman of the meeting was Dr Jnanabrata Sil.
240. Interview with Dr. Jnanabrata Sil, dated January 14, 2020.
241. Jnanabrata Sil, "Ek Daridra Bandhab Janaswasthya-Karmir Jabajjiban Karadanda", *Prokriti O Manush*, page of Kalantar, January 10, 2011, p. 3.
242. Interview with Punyabrata Goon, dated January 31, 2020.
243. Punyabrata Goon, *Shankar Guha Niyogir Sange Koyek Bachhar—Ek Saha-Joddhar Pratibedan*, Kolkata: Book Mark (Setu Prakashani), not dated, pp. 9–26.
244. *Shankar Guha Niyogi and the Chhattisgarh People's Movement* (Booklet), Delhi: People's Union for Democratic Rights, November 1991.
245. Sangharsha O Nirman—Unayan O Bikalpa (this booklet was published on the occasion of Shakar Guha Niyogi memorial lecture in 1993), published by Loksahitya Parishad, Chhattisgarh, pp. 8–9.
246. Ibid., p. 3.
247. Ibid., p. 7.
248. Punyabrata Goon, *Shankar Guha Niyogir Sange Koyek Bachhar—Ek Saha-Joddhar Pratibedan*, op. cit., p. 97.
249. *Shankar Guha Niyogi: His Work and Thinking* (Booklet), published by Jan Vikas Andolan, 1992, p. 1.
250. Frederick Engels, *The Condition of the Working Class in England in 1944* (translated by Florence Kelley Wiscunewetzky), New York: John W. Lovell Company, 1887.
251. Bharat Dogra, "Muktir Sandhane", in Punyabrata Goon and Sankar Sanyal (eds.), *Sangharsha O Nirman: Shankar Guha Niyogi O Bharater Sramik Andolaner Anya Dhara*, Kolkata: Anushtup, 2015, pp. 201–206.
252. George Fernandez, "Apaser Urrdhe", in Punyabrata Goon and Sankar Sanyal (ed.), *Sangharsha O Nirman*, op. cit., pp. 261–266.
253. Vinayak Sen, "Niyogi Ekti Natun Model Gare Tulte Cheyechilen", in Punyabrata Goon and Sankar Sanyal (ed.), *Sangharsha o Nirman*, op. cit., pp. 282–286.
254. Ilina Sen, *Inside Chhattisgarh: A Political Memoir*, India: Penguin Books Ltd, 2014, p. 55.
255. Punyabrata Goon, *Shaid Haspatal o Dalli Rajharar Janaswasthya Andolan*, op. cit., p. 6.

256. Chandana Mitra, "Chhattisgarh-er Nari Jagaran", in Punyabrata Goon and Sankar Sanyal (ed.), *Sangharsha O Nirman*, op. cit., pp. 240–250.
257. Ilina Sen, *Inside Chhattisgarh: A Political Memoir*, op. cit., pp. 52–66.
258. Punyabrata Goon, *Shaid Haspatal O Dalli Rajharar Janaswasthya Andolan*, Kolkata: Shramajibi Swasthya Udyog, 2001, pp. 1–16.
259. Ilina Sen, *Inside Chhattisgarh: A Political Memoir*, op. cit., p. 78.
260. Ibid., pp. 78–81.
261. Ibid.
262. *Jeevandayi Chikitsar Adhikar Moulik Adhikar*, a booklet of Paschim Banga Khet Mazdoor Samity, not dated.
263. Judgment of Supreme Court of India, Bench: Agrawal, S.C. (J), Paschim Banga Khet Mazdoorsamity … vs State Of West Bengal & Anr on 6 May, 1996 Equivalent citations: 1996 SCC (4) 37, JT 1996 (6) 43, available in Indian Kanoon- http://indiankanoon.org/doc/1743022/.
264. Ibid.
265. Ibid.
266. Ibid.
267. Ibid.
268. Ibid.
269. *Jeevandayi Chikitsar Adhikar Moulik Adhikar*, a booklet of Paschim Banga Khet Mazdoor Samity, not dated.
270. Bapi Dasgupta, *Sarkari Haspatale Chikitsar Gafilatite Jalatanke Mrityu: 22 Bachharer Ayini Larai*, published by Hoogly District Committee of APDR, 2018, pp. 1–8.
271. Sri Badri Chowdhury versus the Super., Chandannagar Sub Div. Hospital & Ors, Complaint Case No CC/59/1996 (Date of Filing: November 9, 1996), District Consumer Disputes Redressal Forum, Hooghly, CC of 2013 Petitioner versus Oppo; Final Order/Judgement, Dated: June 20, 2018.
272. *Bijnan o Bijnankarmi*, Vol. 17, No. 4, October–December 1995, pp. 16–17.
273. Banani Bhattacharya and Goutam Sarkar (ed.), *Shramajibi Katha* (A Short History of Shramajibi Hospital), Howrah: Belur Shramajibi Hospital, 2018 (3rd edition), pp. 4–5.
274. "Smritir Sarani Beye", in *Shramajibi Swasthya*, September 2012, pp. 4–6.
275. Ibid.
276. "Smritir Sarani Beye", *Shramajibi Swasthya*, January 2013, pp. 9–10.
277. "Smritir Sarani Beye", *Shramajibi Swasthya*, July 2013, pp. 24–28.
278. Kunal Sengupta, "Hospital Set up by Sick Unit", *The Telegraph*, November 18, 1994.
279. Akranta Gano-Udyog (A Booklet), which was published on the occasion of all India seminar on Health Rights, Workers' Rights and Human

Rights at Sarat Sadan, Howrah on August 29, 1999 organized by Sramajibi Haspatal and Manabadhikar Suraksha Mancha (MASUM), pp. 3–19.

280. Ibid.
281. "Belur Haspataler Ghar Dakhal Karlo CITU", *Bartaman*, January 25, 1994.
282. Sukanta Sarkar, "Manushke Kachhe Tanar Tirish Bachhar", Anandabazar Patrika, April 20, 2014, https://www.anandabazar.com/editorial/%E0%A6%AE-%E0%A6%A8-%E0%A6%B7%E0%A6%95-%E0%A6%95-%E0%A6%9B-%E0%A6%9F-%E0%A6%A8-%E0%A6%B0-%E0%A6%A4-%E0%A6%B0-%E0%A6%B6-%E0%A6%AC%E0%A6%9B%E0%A6%B0-1.23235, retrieved on August 18, 2020.
283. "Sustha Manush Susth Prithibi—Amader Swasthya Amarai Gorbo", *Shramajibi Swasthya*, December 2011.
284. Banani Bhattacharya and Goutam Sarkar (eds.), *Shramajibi Katha*, op. cit., p. 8.
285. Interview with Dr Punyabrata Goon (born in 1960), dated January 31, 2020.
286. Anup Mondal, "Kanoria Andolan Theke Moitri Swasthya Kendra", in *Amader Katha* (A Booklet), Kolkata: Shramajibi Swasthya Udyog, 2002, pp. 5–7.
287. Prafulla Chakraborty, *Tinti Lekhay Kanoria Jute Miler Shramik Andolan*, Kolkata: Kokata Prakashan, 2013, pp. 36–48.
288. Anup Mondal, "Kanoria Andolan Theke Moitri Swasthya Kendra", op. cit.
289. Punyabrata Goon, "Maitri Swasthya Kendra: Ekti Pratibedan", in *Akranta Gano-Udyog* (A Booklet), op. cit., pp. 24–28.
290. Interview with Dr Punyabrata Goon, dated January 31, 2020.
291. From the Personal Papers of Dr Punyabrata Goon, unpublished.
292. *Shramajibi Swasthya Udyog*, http://www.shramajibiswasthya.org, retrieved on March 12, 2020.
293. Shramajibi Swasthya Udyog, *Amader Katha*, Kolkata: Shramajibi Swasthya Udyog, 2002.
294. Amit Sengupta, "Radical Doctors: Low-cost care in rural Bengal", *Civil Society*, May 2010, http://indiaenvironmentportal.org.in/files/Radical%20Doctors.doc, retrieved on May 28, 2019.
295. Punyabrata Goon, *Pa Miliye Path Chala*, op. cit., p. 125.
296. An Unpublished write up on Shramajibi Swasthya Udyog, received by email from Punyabrata Goon.
297. Ibid.
298. Ibid.
299. Interview with Dr Punyabrata Goon, dated January 31 2020.

300. Punyabrata Goon, *Pa Miliye Path Chala*, op. cit. pp. 126–127.
301. Punyabrata Goon, *The Journey of Shramajibi Swasthya Udyog* (Working Class Health Project), http://sanhati.com/excerpted/5554/, retrieved on December 20, 2020.
302. "Introduction", in Punyabrata Goon (ed.), *Sabar Janya Swasthya—Ekti Swapna Ja Satyi Kara Jay*, Kolkata: Guruchandali, 2017.
303. Punyabrata Goon (ed.), *Sabar Janya Swasthya*, op. cit.
304. "Campaign for 'Health for All'—Presentation Booklet for PULSE 2017, AIIMS", Students Union AIIMS, Resident Doctors Association AIIMS, Society for Young Scientist AIIMS and Faculty Members, AIIMS Delhi, August 26, 2017, pp. 12–17.
305. Ibid.
306. Ibid.
307. Ibid.
308. *Doctors' Dialogue*, Volume 1, Issue 1, November 2002.
309. Ibid., p. 1 (indent lines have been translated from Bengali to English).
310. Shramajibi Swasthya Udyog, *Amader Katha*, op. cit., p. 11.
311. *Swasthyer Britte*, Vol. 1, No. 1, September 2011.
312. *Swasthyer Britte*, Vol. 1, No. 2, December 2011, p. 23.
313. Nataraj Malakar, "November Biplab Sabar Jany Swasthyer Adarshake Tule Dhoreche", *Prokriti O Manush, Kalantar*, December 25, 2017, p. 3.
314. *Banya O Prakritik Durjoge Jakhon Daktar Nei*, Kolkata: SSU, 2000.
315. Punyabrata Goon, *Shahid Haspatal O Dalli-Rajharar Janaswasthya Andalon*, Kolkata: SSU, 2001.
316. Shankar Guha Niyogi, *Marxbader Mulsutra*, Kolkata: SSU, 2006.
317. Siddhartha Gupta and Rahul Mukherjee, *Biswayan O Swasthya*, Kolkata: SSU, 2007.
318. Siddhartha Gupta, *Chiner Swasthya-Byabasthya: Birat Biparit Jatra*, Kolkata: SSU, 2007.
319. Siddhartha Gupta, *Paschimbanger Swasthyer Akashe Durjoger Ghanaghata*, Kolkata: SSU, 2010.
320. Santimay Satapati, *Bikalpa Chikitsay Homeopathy*, Kolkata: SSU, 2011.
321. Shramajibi Swasthya Udyog, *Sabar Janya Swasthya Marachika Noy*, Kolkata: SSU, 2014.
322. Punyabrata Goon (ed.), *Swasthya Abyabastha*, Kolkata: Guruchandali Publishers, 2017.
323. Punyabrata Goon and Satya Shibraman, *Modicare: Kar Munafa Beshi, Janagan Na Corporate Companygulor*, Kolkata: Guruchandali, 2018.
324. Ranabrata Sen, "Premseva Haspataler Udbodhan", *Swasthya o Paribesh*, Vol. 8, No. 2, August–September 1995, pp. 79–80.

325. A leaflet of Premseba Hospital reprinted in *Swasthya o Paribesh*, Vol. 7, No. 5, February–March 1995, p. 198. (indent lines have been translated from Bengali)
326. "Chikitsaker Avabe Dhunkchhe Sundarbaner Sramajibi Haspatal", *Ei Samay*, October 7, 2017, https://eisamay.indiatimes.com/west-bengal-news/doctors-absence-in-sunderbans-workers-hospital/articleshow/60981675.cms, retrieved on March 9, 2021.
327. "7 Bachhare 38 Hazar Rogi Dekhlo Amader Hospital", *Anandabazar Patrika*, May 11, 2015, https://www.anandabazar.com/lifestyle/unique-our-hospital-of-chhatna-have-seen-38-thousand-patients-1.144201, retrieved on March 9, 2021.
328. Gouripada Dutta, "Janaswasthya Andolaner Patabhumi O Janaswasthya Committee", in *Janaswastha Mela Souvenir*, Kolkata, 1994, p. 91.
329. Sabyasachi Chatterjee and Nataraj Malakar, "Swasthya Parisheba Sarkareri Day", *Anandabazar Patrika*, December 19, 2018, p. 4.
330. Interview with Binay Bsau Mallick, Joint Secretary of Janaswasthya Committee, dated January 31, 2020.
331. Gouripada Dutta, "Janaswasthya Andolaner Patabhumi o Janaswasthya Committee", op. cit.
332. Ibid.
333. Alok Majumder, "Janaswasthya Andolan Gore Tulun", in *Janaswastha Mela Souvenir*, Kolkata, 1994, pp. 80–82; Janaswasthya Katha, October–December, 2015, pp. 3–6.
334. Ibid.
335. Ibid.
336. Ibid.
337. Ibid.
338. "Fire Dekho Sankalan Prasange", *Janaswasthya Katha*, Special issue, January–June 2012, p. 7.
339. First Janaswasthya Mela Souvenir, Kolkata, 1994, p. 13.
340. Gauri Pada Dutta, *Amader Swasthya Samasya*, published by Ashok Kumar Pal, Kolkata, 1991, p. 37.
341. Madan Ghosh, "PRC Gathon o Naba-parjay: Agami Path Chala", in Samir Maitra (ed.), *P.R.C'R Panchattor Bochorer Ujjwal abhijan*, published by Fuhad Halim on the behalf of People's Relief Committee, Kolkata, 2018, pp. 52–55.
342. Sabyasachi Chatterjee, "Comrade, Nabajug Anle Na?", *Anandabazar Patrika*, December 1, 2018, p. 4.
343. *Jatiya Swasthya Sammelan Ebang Biswa Janaswasthya Sammelan Prasange*, published by Paschimbanga Janaswasthya Chetana Prachar Samiti, Kolkata, 2000, pp. 3–6.
344. Ibid., pp. 6–14.

345. Ibid.
346. Amiya Kumar Bagchi, "Neo-Liberal Reforms with Cosmetic Changes?", *Economic and Political Weekly*, Vol. 39, No. 32, August 7–13, 2004, pp. 3572–3574; Amiya Kumar Bagchi, "Some Public Health Issues in India", in R. Maria Saleth, S. Galab and E. Revathi (eds.), *Issues and Challenges of Inclusive Development: Essays in Honor of Prof. R. Radhakrishna*, Singapore: Springer Nature Singapore Pte Ltd., 2020, pp. 175–183.
347. *Jatiya Swasthya Sammelan Ebang Biswa Janaswasthya Sammelan Prasange*, op. cit.
348. Ravi Narayan et al., "A People's Charter for Health and Beyond", *The National Medical Journal of India*, Vol. 14, No. 2, 2001, pp. 67–70.
349. Indian people's health charter, adopted at the Indian People's Health Assembly, Kolkata, India, November 2000, available in Healthy Documents, World Alliance for Breastfeeding Action, https://healthy-documents.org/rights/healthydocuments-doc5.pdf, retrieved on May 19, 2019.
350. Gouri Pada Dutta, "Jatiya o Antarjatik Prekkhite Janaswasthya Andolan", *Janaswasthya Kotha*, Special issue, January–June 2012, pp. 19–22.
351. Amit Sengupta and T. Sundararaman, "Pre-People's Health Assembly (PHA) mobilisation in India", Building a movement for health—Case study 23, Peoples Health Movement (PHM), https://phmovement.org, retrieved on March 14, 2019.
352. "Role of Civil Society in Achieving Health for All: India Country Study", *People's Health Movement (PHM*), 2016, https://phmovement.org/wp-content/uploads/2018/06/19_IndiaReportFinal.pdf, retrieved on August 8, 2020.
353. Paschim Banga Vigyan Mancha: http://www.paschimbangavigyanmancha.org/health.php, retrieved on July 17, 2022.
354. Punyabrata Goon, "Swasthyer Jonya Sangram: Kon Patha Chalbo", in *Swasthyer* Jonya Sangram: Adhikar Banam Banijya, Kolkata: Priyatash Basu Memorial Committee, 2010, pp. 38–39.
355. Amit Sengupta (1958–2018), a leading health activist in India and the world, became involved with the *Delhi Science Forum* and the *All India People's Science Network*. He took an active role in the *All India Drug Action Network* (AIDAN). He was one of the co-founders of People's Health Movement (PHM). Sengupta had a major role in coordinating and editing Global Health Watch. (Jeetha D'Silva, "Amit Sengupta: founder and advocate of the People's Health Movement in India", *BMJ*, 7 January 2019, doi: 10.1136/bmj.k5427; Andrew Green, "Amit Sengupta", Obituary, Vol. 393, No. 10166, January 5, 2019, p. 24; Prabir Purkayastha, Indranil and Richa Chintan (eds.) *Political Journeys*

in Health: Essays by and for Amit Sengupta, New Delhi: Left World Books, 2021.)

356. Jan Swasthya Abhiyan (JSA): http://phmindia.org/, retrieved on March 20, 2019.
357. Abhay Shukla, "Jan Swasthya Abhiyan", *Yojana*, Vol. 49, July 2005, pp. 14–17.
358. Jan Swasthya Abhiyan, *Health System in India: Crisis and Alternatives*, National Coordination Committee, Jan Swasthya Abhiyan, Delhi, 2006; Jan Swasthya Abhiyan, *Universalising Health Care for All*, published by Amit Sengupta on behalf of Jan Swasthya Abhiyan, Delhi, 2012.
359. Abhay Shukla, "Jan Swasthya Abhiyan", op. cit.
360. Prem Chandran John and David G. Legge, "The People's Health Movement: health for all, now!", in Hans Lofgren et al. (eds.), *Democratizing Health: Consumer Groups in the Policy Process*, UK and USA: Edward Elgar, 2011, pp. 61–80.
361. People's Health Movement, *Global Health Watch 2: An Alternative World Health Report*, London: Zed Books, 2008, 360–363.
362. Punyabrata Goon, "Swasthyer Jonya Sangram: Kon Patha Chalbo", in *Swasthyer Jonya Sangram: Adhikar Banam Banijya,* Kolkata: Priyatash Basu Memorial Committee, 2010, pp. 38–39.
363. Catherine Campbell et al., "Heeding the Push from Below How Do Social Movements Persuade the Rich to Listen to the Poor?," *Journal of Health Psychology*, Vol. 15, No. 7, 2010, pp. 962–971.
364. Ronald Labonte, "Global right to health campaign launched", *British Medical Journal*, Vol. 331, July 30, 2005, p. 252.
365. Letter from Jan Swasthya Abhiyan to Ghulam Nabi Azad, Union Minister for Health and Family Welfare, Govt. of India, September 25, 2013. Ref. JSA/MISCV/2013.
366. *Peoples Health Manifesto—2009, Health for All Now!: A Call to all Political Parties*, published by B. Ekbal, on behalf of Jan Swasthya Abhiyan, Delhi, 2009.
367. Report on follow-up seminar 'Towards a pharmaceutical policy in India in the changed perspective', Entitled: Pharmaceutical policy and access to essential medicines, Organized by Community Development Medicinal Unit in collaboration with Health Action International Asia Pacific and Community Development Medicinal Unit Orissa, Date: Bhubaneswar, September 3, 2010, Bhubaneswar.
368. *Realizing the Right to Healthcare a Policy Brief*, published by Sarojini N and Amit Sengupta, on behalf of Jan Swasthya Abhiyan, New Delhi, March 2014.
369. Abhay Shukla, "Healthcare Corruption: Responses from People's Health Movements", in Samiran Nundy et al. (eds.), *Healer or Predators?:*

Healthcare Corruption in India, New Delhi: Oxford University Press, pp. 479–498.

370. A Document of Jan Swasthya Abhiyan, not dated. *News Click*: https://www.newsclick.in/third-national-health-assembly-concludes-demands-health-care-fundamental-right, retrieved on April 15, 2019.
371. Ashok Kumar Mukhopadhyay, "Samaj Kalyaner Kaje Anami Sangathan", *Desh*, Vol. 57, No. 21, March 24, 1990, pp. 24–25.
372. Amalratan Das, "Swasthya Panya Nay Swasthya Jatiya Sampad", *Prokriti O Manush, Kalantar*, September 11, 1995, p. 3.
373. Data received from Dr. Gourab Roy through email on December 13, 2017.
374. Programmes and Constitution of Forum for People's Health (Adopted in Third Conference of Forum for People's Health on May 31, 2009).
375. Siddhartha Gupta, "Paschimbanga Swasthya Aain 2017: Bishalyakarnir Sandhane", Punyabrata Goon (ed.), *Swasthya Abyabastha*, op. cit., pp. 11–21.
376. Koushik Lahiri et al. (eds.), *Itihaser Sankalan, Sankalaner Itihas*, Kolkata: West Bengal Doctors Forum, 2018.
377. "Chikitsakder Opar Hamla: Doctor-der Baktabya", *Swasthyer Britte*, Vol. 7, No. 2, December 2017–January 2018, pp. 55–56.
378. A letter from Joint Platform of Doctors, West Bengal to Director of Health Services, Government of West Bengal, December 27, 2017.
379. Nataraj Malakar, "A Comparative Study of the History of Different Junior Doctors' Movements during 1987–2019", *Journal of the Asiatic Society*, Vol. LXIII, No. 4, 2021, pp. 85–108.
380. Ibid.

CHAPTER 5

Probing the Movement for Essential Drugs

Nandadulal Mitra, a character in a Bengali story titled *Chikitsa Sankat*[1] written by Rajshekhar Basu (Parashuram), suffered an injury after falling from a tram. After a few days of imaginary illness, he fell into the trap of various medical treatments. On the advice of friends, he rushed to the allopathic doctor, the homeopathic doctor, the *Kabiraj*, and the *Hakim*. In a similar tale, the king, a character in *Rajar Asukh*,[2] by Sukumar Ray, also faced just such a health crisis. In the two stories, only a personal crisis was depicted. In reality, however, this has turned in to a people's crisis. The people have been confused by the range of treatments and supposed remedies on offer. Rajasekhar Basu suggested that if the conflict between *Kabiraji* (the practicing of indigenous medicine) and *Daktari* (the practicing of modern medicine) was resolved and the path of science was adopted, perhaps this crisis could be overcome.[3] Despite the improvement in medical science, however, there has been no such alleviation. The ordinary people have been deprived of modern medicines due to their lack of money. Even those who are able to purchase medicines have been victims of irrational and unnecessary drugs. At the same time, in the age of globalization, so-called 'drug imperialism' has spread rapidly. This is why the movement for essential drugs was organized. In India, "the right to health is strongly embedded in rights to essential, safe and affordable medicines."[4]

© The Author(s), under exclusive license to Springer Nature Switzerland AG 2025

N. Malakar, *Historicising the People's Health Movement in West Bengal, India*, https://doi.org/10.1007/978-3-032-02696-5_5

The main use of medicine, also known as pharmaceutical drugs, is to cure and prevent or alleviate disease or the conditions caused by disease.[5] A medicine is a chemical substance which, if applied in appropriate doses to specific bodily conditions, acts as a medicine; in other circumstances, however, it may even be poisonous.[6] Drugs have three names: a chemical name, a generic name, and a brand or trade name. For instance, *N-(4-hydroxyphenyl) ethanamide N-(4-hydroxyphenyl) acetamide* is the chemical name, *paracetamol* is the generic name and *Calpol, Crocin* etc. are the trade names. There are two other things to understand about drugs; they can come in the forms of either basic drugs or in bulk drugs and formulations. A chemical substance that is made through a process is called a basic drug. A formulation is the process of making a mixture of one or more basic drugs in different forms or shapes (pills, syrups, capsules, injections).

Medicine for All

Medicine is an important aspect of health care. In order to achieve the goal of "Health for All," free or affordable quality medicine must be made available to all, since a large proportion of medical expenses are incurred in paying for drugs.[7] In India, however, "universal access to healthcare" has not been implemented; at the same time it has also been impossible to provide free medicines for all. According to the *World Health Organization*, in 1999 an approximate number of between 499 and 649 million Indians, or 50 to 65 per cent of the population, lacked regular access to essential drugs.[8] The *National Sample Survey* [*71st Round* (2016)] showed that, in 2014, out of pocket (OOP) expenditure for medicines in terms of non-hospitalized treatment in India was 72 per cent in rural areas and 68 per cent in urban areas. If we consider West Bengal, we can see that the figures for OOP for medicine was 70 per cent in rural areas and 69 per cent in urban areas.[9] A study showed that, "*out-of-pocket* (OOP) health expenses drove 55 million Indians—more than the population of South Korea, Spain or Kenya—into poverty in 2017, and of these, 38 million (69%) were impoverished by expenditure on medicines alone."[10] In 2004, the *Consumer Unity and Trust Society, Calcutta Resource Centre* (CUTS) and the *Community Development Medicine Unit* (CDMU), two non-governmental organizations, conducted a joint survey funded by the WHO and *Health Action International* (HAI) into the prices and availability of essential drugs in West Bengal. They chose 26 public facilities (down to village hospital level) and 35 private medical outlets in Jalpaiguri,

Malda, Burdwan, Kolkata, North 24 Parganas, Midnapore, Purulia districts of West Bengal from where they attempted to collect samples of 32 essential medicines. The study found that there was a lack of availability of essential medicines at public facilities during the survey period. Of the 32 essential medicines, only 13, i.e., 40.6 per cent, were found. For example, although *albendazole* was obtainable, *aciclovir*, *fluconazole*, and *sulfadoxine pyrimethamine* were not. The lack of adequate antibiotics led to a problematic situation in terms of the treatment of bacterial and other infectious diseases in government hospitals. There was also unavailability of a number of other drugs: *isosorbide dinitrate*, a low-cost emergency treatment for severe anginal attacks; *phenytoin* or *carbamazepine* for the treatment of epilepsy (or other antiepileptics); and also of inhalers to treat asthma. In addition, there was no medicine to calm severely aggressive psychiatric patients. Medicines were available in the private sector, but in such circumstances patients had to spend more than the international reference prices for the brand name.[11]

On occasion, reports of the shortage of medicines in government hospitals has been published in newspapers. In this regard, we may give reference of two occurrences from two different times. In May 1983, a report of *India Today* stated that the Nil Ratan Sircar Medical College (NRS) and Hospital faced a shortage of medicine that provoked junior doctors to take action in protest. The report states that the NRS hospital owed Rs. 86 lakh to different medicine companies, making most of them reluctant to supply medicine to the hospital. As a result, it lacked regular supplies of *penicillin* injections, as well as of drugs like *Flagyl* and *Avil*. There was also no supply of *sorbitrates*. Patients were entitled to receive all of those drugs for free, but due to a lack of supply, they had to purchase them outside of the hospital.[12] The *World Health Organization* had announced that hydrophobia would be eradicated from the world by 2020. In order to implement that declaration, every hospital needed to have *anti-rabies vaccine* facilities. However, *Anandabazar Patrika* reported the deaths of every single one of the 36 patients admitted to Beliaghata ID Hospital in Kolkata in 2014 with hydrophobia symptoms. One of the reasons for these fatalities was the inability to obtain the *anti-rabies* vaccine at the right time. This begins fully functioning 14 days after administration. Therefore, *immunoglobulin* should be provided to the wound area during this time so that the disease does not attack. Such was the medical advice given by the WHO. However, there was a lack of *immunoglobulin* in the government hospitals as well as in the private hospitals of Kolkata and the districts. It was reported that this had occurred the private companies had reduced production of that essential medicine as they had not been able to increase their prices.[13]

The Birth of Modern Medicine in Bengal

Every ancient civilization in the world has developed its own medical system. For instance, *Ayurvedic* medicine was born in India and *Unani* medicine was introduced to India by Islamic rulers during the medieval period.[14] However, modern scientific medicine, commonly known as allopathic medicine, originated in the West, or, more specifically, Europe. European physicians arrived in India on Portuguese, French and British ships. With the spread of colonial rule, allopathic medicine shops sprang up in India. Initially, those pharmacies relied principally on imported drugs. In 1811, Bathgate, a Scottish man, first set up a drug store in Kolkata. From 1910 onwards, that institution began producing tinctures and spirits. Acharya Prafulla Chandra Roy was the pioneer who first planned to manufacture medicine in this country at the end of the nineteenth century, establishing the *Bengal Chemical and Pharmaceutical Works* in 1899. Dr. Kartik Chandra Basu, the editor of *Swasthya Samachar*, was associated with the company from its formative years.[15] The advent of antibiotics in the middle of the twentieth century brought about a revolution in the world of modern medicine.[16] Medical science has had rapid success since World War II. Effective and life-saving drugs were gradually being discovered. As there was no advanced medicine prior to this time, infant mortality due to polio, diphtheria or whooping cough was very common. There was also no medicine for tuberculosis.[17]

Due to its dependence on imports, there was a severe shortage of modern medicines in India during World War II (1939–1945). At this time bacterial infections were the leading cause of death in humans. The prevalent infectious diseases at that time were typhoid fever, tuberculosis, smallpox, malaria, measles, cholera, plague, intestinal diseases and diarrhea, respiratory diseases, pneumonia, sexually transmitted diseases, *Kala-azar*, leprosy, elephantiasis, etc. There were also non-communicable diseases, such as diabetes, mental disorders, and cancer. The provisions of modern medicine available in India at the time were insufficient to treat those diseases. At the end of the war, modern drugs began to be imported by multinational companies with Germany, England and Switzerland at the forefront of pharmaceutical production.[18] For medicine, India still had to depend on foreign industries. In the pre-independence period, the pharmaceutical industry could not be expanded in this country through domestic initiatives.[19] Accordingly, the price of medicine was very high. For this reason, it always remained largely beyond the reach of ordinary people. As a result, even if antibiotics were invented, poor people would be denied their benefits. Moreover, the government's focus was not on disease prevention but rather on cure. Financially strong people, who could afford to buy medicine, could avail themselves of the benefits of modern medicine while the poor had to rely on alternative treatment.

In the immediate post-independence period, it had been impossible to develop an indigenous pharmaceutical industry in India, which is why they were compelled to import medicine. Moreover, the government expected that in the new environment, foreign companies would help to strengthen the pharmaceutical industry within the country. Nevertheless, foreign industries did not manufacture drugs in this country; instead, they continued to import finished medicines from abroad and to sell them in India. In addition, the indigenous sector was importing fine chemical and bulk drugs from abroad for processing and formulating medicines.[20] At that time no multinational company or Indian private company was interested in developing an indigenous pharmaceutical industry.[21] As a result, even after independence, the drug market in India continued to be controlled by multinational companies. In the 1950s, "due to the higher price of imports and lack of competition, Indian drug prices were among the highest in the world."[22] However, during this period both the *Hindustan Antibiotics Limited* (1954) and *Indian Drugs and Pharmaceuticals Limited* (1961) were formed as government initiatives, with the intention of delivering medicines to the public at affordable prices. With the introduction of such government initiatives, the price of antibiotics fell by 50–70 per cent. Multinational companies were compelled to reduce the price of medicines simply to survive in the Indian market and they also began, for the first time, to manufacture drugs in the country. In the 1960s, the initiative to make bulk drugs was also observed in the private sector.[23]

Drugs and Patent Act in India

In an effort to revitalize the indigenous industry, the Government of India amended the *Patents and Designs Act, 1911*, bringing into law the *Patents Act, 1970*[24]. This act came into force on April 20, 1972, with the publication of the Patent Rules, 1972.[25] It was the most beneficial piece of legislation in respect of the development of the domestic pharmaceutical industry. The government's goal was to make medicine more accessible to the common people. Therefore, whereas in the case of other products, the patent period was of 14 years, in the case of medicine, it was set at only 5 years.[26] Thus, India transformed from a drug-importing country to an exporter of pharmaceuticals. However, the market for multinational companies did not shrink overnight. In 1970, the share of indigenous companies in the Indian market was 10–20 per cent, while the share of multinational companies was 80–90 per cent. The situation had changed little by 1980, but by 1993, the share of domestic companies stood at 61 per cent.[27] Despite the pharmaceutical success of India, the condition of the common people remained much the same. Because of poverty, "in 1973, 80 per cent of the drugs sold in India were bought by 20 per cent of the population, whereas the rest of the poor population shared amongst themselves only 20% of the drugs sold in the market."[28]

After the passage of the Patent Act of 1970, there was a degree of self-sufficiency in the pharmaceutical industry in India, but multinational pharmaceutical companies were still looking for ways to undermine this. Their opportunity came very quickly with the coming of Liberalization, Privatization and Globalization (LPG) in India. In 1991, because of its financial difficulties the Indian government was forced to borrowed a large sum from the *World Bank*.[29] As a result, Narasimha Rao's government was forced to sign the General Agreement on Tariffs and Trade (or GATT). In addition, India became a member of the *World Trade Organization* (WTO) when it formed as the institutional embodiment of the GATT.[30] Under the agreement, India was now subject to *Trade-Related Aspects of Intellectual Property Rights* (TRIPS). In 1995, sociologist Ralph Nader and Professor James Love told Michael Cantor, the US Trade Representative, "If the TRIPS agreement goes into effect, it will establish a long-term monopoly on all medicines and deprive the majority of the world's people's access to healthcare. Even the middle class has to spend a big chunk of its income on drugs."[31] Nevertheless, in 1995, the Congress government proposed to Parliament that there should be an amendment of the patent law to ratify the TRIPS agreement. However, the government's efforts failed due to opposition from both the BJP and the Left. In 1999, when the United States accused India of violating the TRIPS agreement, however, the BJP government came under pressure; this resulted in an amendment to the patent act with the support of the main opposition party, the Indian National Congress.[32] Under the new law, the patent period was extended to 20 years and Multinational companies were also given the right to import drugs from abroad. The mail-box system was also permitted. Multinational companies re-established their monopoly on the Indian pharmaceutical market.[33] As a result, the price of medicines rose.

The aggressiveness of capital monopolies in the pharmaceutical industry in the aftermath of the TRIPS agreement has been the subject of much discussion.[34] From these discussions, two clear issues have emerged: first, the steep rise in the price of medicines led to a rapid decline in the ability of people to take medicines; second, the drug production system in developing countries was disrupted. Many countries did not actually comply with all the provisions of the TRIPS, in order to protect the indigenous health system and drug industry. However, India did not follow such a route: it accepted all the provisions of the agreement and amended the *Patents Act, 1970*.[35] K. B. Saxena, a former Union health secretary in the Government of India, observed that "With the coming in of TRIPS-compliant patent regime, the patented drugs have become increasingly unaffordable for a large number of people, particularly the poor. This would be significantly more in the case of newly discovered drugs."[36] In India, the government was the largest purchaser of medicines. So, following the TRIPS agreement, many expressed concerns that the government might buy fewer drugs due to rising drug prices, causing people who relied on the government medical system to suffer.[37] To illustrate this, we may highlight the fact that, in 1980, according to a committee appointed by the West Bengal state government, medicine was purchased for 20 per cent of the patients who came to the government hospital in West Bengal. The Union government then proposed that free medicine be given to the poor patients only in government medical institutions. But the West Bengal government did not accept that proposal.[38] The *National Health Policy, 2002* read "There are some apprehensions about the possible adverse impact of economic globalisation on the health sector…the introduction of a TRIPS-consistent patent regime for drugs in a developing country results in an across-the-board increase in the cost of drugs and medical services."[39]

The *Indian Patents Act, 1970* had placed the emphasis on process patents instead of product patents, allowing Indian companies the opportunity to develop an alternative process of manufacturing patented drugs. In the wake of this development, the price of medicines in the Indian market had fallen. Companies introduced new medicine in the Indian market much earlier compared to the previous regime and they also captured some foreign markets.[40] Under the GATT, however, the people of India could no longer enjoy the benefits of the *Patents Act, 1970.* As a new member of the *World Trade Organization* (WTO), India was obliged to abide by the TRIPS agreement. Therefore, India adopted the model of product patent to provide complete security to multinational pharmaceutical companies through the amended *Patent Act, 2005.*[41] Murphy Halliburton has provided an example regarding a consequence of the act of 2005: "Pfizer, Merck, or Gilead comes out with a new AIDS medication; Indian companies can no longer produce a copy through reverse engineering without permission from the originator. Rather, they would have to obtain a license from the patent holder and pay royalties to produce the medication."[42] In the Parliament, P. Karunakaran, a Lok Sabha MP from the CPI (M), representing the Kasargod constituency of Kerala, criticized the Union government for increasing the cost of life-saving medications. According to him, while the government had introduced a drug policy, it was neither functional nor useful. The fundamental guidelines for fixing price of drugs were faulty, and it assisted the monopoly of drug companies in raising medicine prices. He urged the government to take a socially just stance to control the prices of drugs and take legal action against pharmaceutical companies that unjustly increased drug prices.[43]

Furthermore, there is evidence that the main reason why the ordinary people of India have to spend so much money on medicines is that the government of this country has reduced its expenditure on health care. The situation worsened further when the government reduced the supply of free medicines in public hospitals. The matter might be perceived more clearly by considering the table below.

Trends in access to medicines in India—1986–1987 to 2004

Period	*Free medicines*	*Partly free medicines*	*On payment medicines*	*Not received medicines*	*Total (in %) medicines*
Inpatient					
1986–1987	31.20	15.00	40.95	12.85	100
1995–1996	12.29	13.15	67.75	6.80	100
2004	8.99	16.38	71.79	2.84	100
Outpatient					
1986–1987	17.98	4.36	65.55	12.11	100
1995–1996	7.21	2.71	79.32	10.76	100
2004	5.34	3.38	65.27	26.01	100

High Level Expert Group Report on Universal Health Coverage for India submitted to Planning Commission of India, New Delhi, 2011, p. 120

Drug Colonialism

There were only a few modern pharmaceutical companies prior to the 1960s. Previous to this, doctors had compounders who used to prepare medicines (*puria* [indigenous medicine powder wrapped in a small piece of paper], mixture, ointment) for their patients. Sometimes patients would obtain their medicines made from the pharmacy according to the prescription. At that time, the most common drugs were a combination of simple chemicals such as *sodium salicylate* and *bicarbonate*, *magnesium sulphate* and *carbonate*, and plant extracts (ipca, *belladonna*). Antibiotics such as *sulpha drugs*, *penicillin*, *streptomycin*, *chloramphenicol*, and *tetracycline* were also present. There were also drugs such as *quinine* and *chloroquine* for malaria, *ametin* and *cliocunol* for dysentery, *dapsone* for leprosy, *reserpine* for high blood pressure, and so on.[44] Arunachal Datta Choudhury has written that:

> Even around 50 years ago in many places of rural Bengal the fees of the doctors were decided through a 'strange' method. Often a phial or bottle of mixture was given to the patients along with the accompanying medicines. The price of the phial was always written on the phial. And on the basis of the price of the phial the fees of the doctor were often decided. For that reason, doctors were known as 'doctors of 7.5 rupees' phial', 'doctors of 10 rupees' phial' and so on. This is very weird to imagine, but it was the fact of that time. It was only the doctors and his compounders knew what kind of substances was added in the mixtures of the phial. People of that time can remember the names of a few mixtures such as *carminative mixture* for indigestion, *alkali mixture* for fever and so on. There were other such mixtures such as *cough mixture*, *malaria mixture* and *Bromide mixture*.[45]

Pharmaceutical companies attempted to make profits by exploiting the benefits of the *Patents Act 1970*. Those companies made mixtures of multiple drugs, and sold them on the market as new drugs. The ingredients of the mixed drugs invented by each company were their own; there was no competition. Accordingly, pharmaceutical companies began to occupy the market. However, those drugs made by traders were not recognized in medical science. While the number of recognized basic drugs in medical science was less than 700, the number of drugs in the market was 60,000.[46] Later, the number rose even higher, as the result of neo-imperialism. A report of the *High Level Expert Group* stated that: "India has the dubious distinction of having its pharmaceutical market flooded with about 90,000 formulation packs and brands. The market is awash with irrational, non-essential and hazardous drugs."[47]

In 2010, the *Community Development Medicine Unit* (CDMU), in collaboration *with Health Action International* (HAI), conducted a survey on fixed-dose combinations of drugs in the Indian market. They selected Kolkata, Siliguri, and Burdwan in West Bengal to collect the samples. The report shows that a large number of irrational fixed-dose combinations (IFDCs), banned by the *Drug Control of India*, were available in the market. A large proportion of the best-selling drugs in India were found to be irrational combinations. Notable among those were cough syrups, vitamin tonics and *ayurvedic* products. The survey team also found products that had been banned all over the world, such as *Nimesulide.* Based on the *Current Index of Medical Specialties* [CIMS], April–July, 2010, the study team showed that 1356 types of irrational mixtures were being sold in the market, under a total of 4559 brand names.[48] The following table shows the number of different types of irrational fixed-dose combinations (IFDCs):

Irrational Fixed-Dose Combinations (IFDCs)

Sl. no	*Therapeutic groups*	*Number of IFDCs*	*Number of brands*
1	Gastrointestinal	169	670
2	Cardiovascular	108	526
3	Respiratory System	18	48
4	Central Nervous System	133	762
5	Musculo-Skeletal System	37	106
6	Anti-infective	80	472
7	Oncology	1	5
8	Genito-Urinary System	26	65
9	Vitamins & Minerals	2	60
10	Supplements & Adjuvant Therapy	16	38
11	Eye	79	143
12	Ear & Mouth/Throat	42	75
13	Dermatological	196	394
14	Allergy & Immune System	28	73
15	Tonics	40	101
16	Cough & Cold	167	494
17	Vitamin & Tonics	64	84
18	Hematinics	132	212
19	Oral hypoglycemics	18	231
	Total	1356	4559

Report on research project, *Fixed-dose combination in India, inception – marketing – a study*, Conducted by Community Development Medicinal Unit in collaboration with Health Action International Asia Pacific, Kolkata, 2010, p. 11

Not only West Bengal or India faced problems related to rational drugs; so also did entire developing countries. The lack of government health services alone cannot be blamed for those problems. Health planners or physicians were equally responsible for making ordinary people drug-dependent. David Werner stated:

> In Latin America, many of the new programs under the Ministry of Health, Ministry of Education, and other agencies to deliver services and promote community health in rural and marginal areas have been designed by prestigious but poorly informed and out of-date doctors and nurses. The result is that training and manuals for village health workers still tend to promote bottle feeding rather than breast feeding, restricting food to children with diarrhoea, and overuse and misuse of medication like Entero-Vioform, cough syrups, diarrhoeal plugs, etc.[49]

Diana Melrose relates a tragic incident in Bangladesh in the introduction of her book on the medicine in the third world. She wrote:

> As the boat drew into the shore we heard a strange sound from the bank. A woman was crying. We found her with a dead baby in her arms and a collection of medicine bottles beside her. She had spent all her money on these expensive drugs. She could not understand why they had not saved her baby. This Bangladeshi woman had never been told what was obvious to the doctor who found her. The baby had become severely dehydrated from diarrhoea. Her death could have been prevented with a simple home-made solution of water, salt and sugar. No amount of medicine could have kept her alive.[50]

In fact, the pharmaceutical industry, which is a part of the health care industry, became the most powerful industry in the world[51] with much higher profit margins than other industries.[52] Multinational pharmaceutical companies established a monopoly in the health sector of developing countries.[53] Dr. Halfdan Mahler, the director-general of *the World Health Organization*, who had played a key role in the Alma-Ata Conference, used the term 'drug colonialism' to describe the entire picture in the mid-1970s. He said that "some 150 essential drugs could meet the vast majority of health care needs. If you want to free yourselves from drug colonialism, let us work together to make sure that these essential drugs become available to all who need them."[54]

Medicine and the Medical Fraternity

In the context of an inundation of unnecessary and irrational drugs in the Indian market, questions about medical ethics arose repeatedly. Sanjeev Mukherjee, an activist doctor of the health movement in West Bengal, stated that the adoption of an ethical system was essential for the implementation of universal health care. He further added that privatization of medical education occurred as a result of economic liberalization. Doctors who graduated from private medical colleges also had a business mentality; they did not bother with ethical health care. Profits were given the greatest importance. In order to increase profits, it was necessary to increase the disease burden. Thus, attempts were made to cure a disease using irrational drugs, which resulted in the creation of other, new diseases. According to him, the countries where *universal health care* was introduced also had ethical health care. In such a system the doctors could not prescribe the medicine as they wished; they had to follow certain guidelines.[55] Indeed, it was impossible for multinational companies alone to capture the drug market, so they sought to establish relationships with doctors. Profit was given priority through neglect for the interests of the patient. In 2003, in a cover story for the *British Medical Journal*, doctors were compared to pigs receiving leftovers from the pharmaceutical companies.[56] In that issue, Ray Moynihan described 16 methods in which doctors were entangled with the pharmaceutical industry (so-called 'Big Pharma'). He pointed out that "entanglement between doctors and drug companies is widespread, and evidence shows that interactions with industry influence doctors' behaviour."[57] Arguing along similar lines, Anant Phadke, an activist of health movement in India, stated:

> For many years, pharma or pharmaceutical companies have been the most important corrupting influences of the medical profession. Enticing and luring doctors into prescribing unnecessary, irrational medicines has been widely prevalent in India in the last 50 years. Pharma companies have provided material incentives to doctors ranging from 'small' gifts and not so small gifts, to dinner parties, to pleasure trips inclusive of trips to foreign countries. Situation deteriorated further when doctors started buying shares of pharma companies, started investing in pharma retail stores and when hospitals invested in the pharma stores which were started in their own premises.[58]

However, not all the doctors agreed to establish a relationship with the drug companies. Thus, the drug companies stopped providing proper information to ethical doctors about their products and, therefore, doctors remained unaware of the harmful effects of drugs. Sukhamoy Bhattacharya (1941–2001), the key figure in *Norman Bethune Janaswasthya Andolan*, stated in 1987 that:

> During the initial years of our profession many multinational companies used to provide booklets on their products. Their representatives often gave literature on medicines to the doctors. Even medicine companies used to send medical journals to the doctors through postal services. Now-a-days medicine companies have almost stopped giving such medical journals or literature on their medicines. Instead, now their representatives often show off the well decorated folders with the pictures of medicines to the doctors and quickly narrate the merits of their respective medicines. It means most of the companies now don't want to inform the doctors about their medicines in detail. Even whatever information they give is full of false claims and information, and much necessary information remains hidden.[59]

The statements of Anant Phadke and Sukhamoy Bhattacharya are also supported by the writings of Dr. Swapan Jana:

> We spent our student lives in the circumstance of commercialization of the healthcare system and are still working in the same system. The incidents involving drug companies that occurred during our student years are as clear to us today as the morning light. Thirty years ago, I used to look forward to the gifts of drug companies such as medicine samples, pens, pads, etc.…After becoming a doctor, if I didn't see medical representatives, I would say to them, in a threatening tone, 'what's the matter brothers, shall I give a letter to the company?' We had no idea at that time that all of those were planned arrangements of pharmaceutical companies to expand their business and increase profits.[60]

Initiatives by the Government

The government was fully aware of these developments. In 1973, questions were raised in the Indian Parliament about the performance of public sector units in the production of drugs, the booming market of multinational companies in that field, the price of locally produced drugs, and so on. As a result, in February 1974 the Government of India formed a committee under the Ministry of Petroleum and Chemicals. The chairman of that committee was Jaisukhlal Hathi, an MP. As a result, the committee is known as the *Hathi Committee.* In 1975, the committee submitted its 275-page report to the government.[61] In that report, the committee emphasized the importance of government initiatives in drug production. The committee recommended:

- To give preference to the Indian sector without bias towards multinational companies;
- To empower the Indian pharmaceutical industry to produce bulk drugs, the government should stop the import of such items as they come to its attention;
- It opined that the focus should be placed on centrally directed research that aim to discover newer drugs for the remedies of tropical diseases such as malaria, filarial, and so on, at the same time, researches for new medicines in the treatment of ailments of the cardio-vascular system, metabolic diseases, and so on;
- Besides making the country self-sufficient in regard to drugs, medical service of a rudimentary nature in the remote villages should be introduced, where common house-hold remedies for cough, cold, fever, antacid preparations etc. should be made available in pilfer-proof packing sufficient to meet 3–4 days treatment;
- Foreign undertakings operating in this country should be directed to bring down their equity to 40 per cent forthwith and further reduce it progressively to 26 per cent.[62]

The most admirable work of the *Hathi Committee* was to compile a list of 104 essential medicines for the treatment of major diseases in India. It suggested increasing the production of these drugs so that those could be found at a fair price in all parts of the country, including rural areas. It stated that the brand names of drugs should be phased out and that generic names should be introduced instead; it was recommended that no new drugs should be marketed under a brand name. The committee spoke out against irrational fixed-dose combinations. It was stated that the drug regulatory department should take steps to eliminate those unnecessary and irrational drugs. Additionally, the committee recommended not to market any mixture not mentioned in the national pharmacopeia.[63]

At the same time, the matter of essential medicines was also being discussed at the international level. In a report presented at the 28th conference of the WHO in 1975, the director-general of WHO reviewed the drug problems in developing countries and proposed the adoption of a new drug policy. In the report, he stated that the list of essential medicines needs to be prepared according to the health needs of the people of each country and according to the structure and improvement of health services. After much discussion on the subject,[64] finally, in 1977, an expert committee of the WHO published a list of the essential medicines for the first time to offer the opportunity for developing countries to build a rational basis for the medical services. The report stated that it was not possible to provide comprehensive health care to the people through medicine. However, medicine did have an important role to play in 'protecting, maintaining and restoring' human health. Despite the increase in the production of the pharmaceutical industry, however, there was no improvement in the health of the people. The availability of essential medicines needed to improve health. Essential medicines were meant to be the medicines that most people need to maintain their health. The report gave a clear outline of the process of selection of essential drugs.[65]

Although the *Hathi Committee* recommended a pro-people drug policy, no attempt was made to apply it. Sukhamoy Bhattacharya wrote, "Despite many attempts in Delhi and elsewhere, I could not buy the report of the *Hathi Committee*. For some mysterious reason, this people-oriented report has become unavailable to the public."[66]

In 1978, the Government of India did announce a new drug policy. Its objectives were to make India self-sufficient in drugs and to make quality pharmaceuticals available to the people at a reasonable price.[67] Based on the *Drug Policy of 1978*, the *Drug Price Control Order* (DPCO) was introduced in 1979 and 347 medicines were brought under price control. Drugs formulations were divided into three categories to determine the rate of profit. The order read: "A percentage of 40 are allowed on Category I and 55 per cent on Category II and a 100 per cent on Category III has been fixed."[68] The purpose of that policy was to reduce the price of life-saving and essential medicines in order to keep them within the reach of common people. But India witnessed that the drug companies began to increase their production of the drugs which were more profitable by reducing their production of life-saving drugs. The pharmaceutical companies were not satisfied. They wanted to make higher profits. Under pressure from this lobby, the government changed the *Drug Policy of 1978*, introducing a new drug policy in 1986. A new revised price control order was enacted the following year in which the freedom of companies to make a profit in the pharmaceutical market was further enhanced.[69] Likewise, in August 1992, the government distributed a note to the members of parliament, named "Background Note on Review of Drug Policy, 1986," in which it outlined the proposed changes to the Drug Policy, 1986. Then, in 1994, the government came up with the final draft of a new drug policy.[70] Amit Sengupta wrote that "once again the government has yielded to pressure from industry and moved towards easing control mechanisms for pharmaceuticals in the new drug policy."[71] Later, *Pharmaceutical Policy 2002* stated that because of the liberalization of the Indian economy, the country's drug and pharmaceutical industry faced new challenges. Public sector units struggled to compete and were being privatized in various ways. Foreign investment was permitted up to 100 per cent.[72] The stated objective of the 2002 Pharmaceutical Policy was to reduce the "rigours of price control."[73] Thus, government control over medicine began to loosen.

Comparative Chart Summarizing Price Control Scheme under Various Drug Price Control Orders

	DPCO 1979	*DPCO 1987*	*DPCO 1995*	*Oct 2003*
No. of drugs under Price Control	347	142	76	74
No. of categories under which the above drugs were categorized	3	2	1	1
MAPE % allowed on normative/ National ex-factory costs to meet post-manufacturing expenses and to provide for margin to the mfrs.				
Category I	40%	75%	100%	100%
Category II	55%	100%	N.A.	
Category III	100%	N.A.	N.A.	
(Single ingredient Leader products)				
Total Domestic pharma sales covered under Price-Control (Approx)	90%	70%	50%	36%

S. Srinivasan and T. Srikrishna, "Chapter 1: Missing The Wood For The Trees: Drug Price Control and Pharmaceutical Policy 2002", in *Impoverishing the Poor: Pharmaceuticals and Drug Pricing in India*, Vadodara/Bilaspur: LOCOST/ Jan Swasthya Sahyog, 2004, p. 3

NA = Not Applicable

In the medical curriculum, students are taught about medicines with generic names. Although generic medicine was cost-saving for patients, doctors generally did not like to prescribe unbranded generic medicine in India until a rule was made in relation to this in 2016. This problem is exacerbated by the absence of qualified pharmacists. In 2013, a newspaper report showed that in West Bengal, there was no pharmacist in many of the private drug stores. *West Bengal State Pharmacist Council* officials stated that most of the district reserve stores under the control of the Health Department were run without pharmacists. There was also a lack of pharmacists in the government hospitals' medicine stores. According to the *Central Drug Control*, most private drug stores in West Bengal were reluctant to recruit pharmacists by providing them with reasonable salaries. They used to hire the registration number of pharmacists for between 1500 and 2000 rupees. In addition, there were 59 vacancies for drug inspectors in the state. That is why, in 2013, the *Drug Controller General of India*, Gyanendranath Singh, reprimanded the framework of state drug control, saying, "West Bengal has not been able to do what Gujarat, Maharashtra, and Karnataka have been able to do successfully."[74]

In 2002, the *Medical Council of India* (MCI) advised physicians to prescribe drugs with generic names in order to protect patients from the effects of drug companies' promotional campaigns. Then, in November 2012 and January 2013, advisories were also issued by MCI saying doctors should "prescribe generic drugs as far as possible."[75] However, these advisories were not followed fully. It was written in the *British Medical Journal* (BMJ) that "doctors across India seem unwilling to write prescriptions containing only the generic or unbranded chemical names of drugs, despite two recent advisories from the Medical Council of India urging them to do so."[76] In September 2016, the MCI amended the *Indian Medical Council Regulations* concerning the prescription of generic names of medicines by doctors, which stated that "every physician should, as far as possible, prescribe drugs with generic names legibly and preferably in capital letters and he/she shall ensure that there is a rational prescription and use of drugs."[77] In an article, Vandana Roy and Proteesh Rana argued that doctors might not prescribe unbranded generic drugs due to quality issues.[78] However, it should be noted that branded medicines might also be of low quality. Anandrao Adsul, a Lok Sabha MP of *Shiv Sena*, stated in Parliament that:

> In the year 2009–10, the number of drug samples tested was 5,877 and the number of non-standard drugs found was 378; In the year 2010–11, the number of drugs sample tested was 6,494 and the number of non-standard drugs found was 449; In the year 2011–12, the number of drug samples tested was 6,928 and the number of non-standard drugs found was 521; and in the year 2012, for the first four months, that is, from April to July, the number of drug samples tested was 2,529 and the number of non-standard drugs found was 117.[79]

According to Dr Amar Jesani, the editor of the *Indian Journal of Medical Ethics,* "the quality argument was 'a hoax' at times conveniently used to prescribe specific brands."[80] The failure of pharmaceutical companies to follow good manufacturing practices also caused concerns about the safety and effectiveness of generic drugs. Roy and Rana remarked that "a generic medicine should be bioequivalent to the innovator drug."[81] However, companies producing generic forms of drugs did not need to prove the bioequivalence with their innovator congeners prior to April 2017. This was addressed by the government of India when they brought a new amendment into law through a notification published in the *Gazette of India* on April 3, 2017 in which bioequivalence studies were made mandatory.[82] Yet it did not seem to be easy to prescribe generic drugs. Sometimes it was difficult for doctors to prescribe such medicines. In this regard, Sanjeev Kelkar relates a frightening story:

> West Bengal pharmacy owners, after a heated exchange, assaulted a group of junior doctors at College of Medicine and Jawaharlal Nehru Memorial Hospital (CMJNMH), a government hospital in Kalyani, on July 4, 2016. The doctors were prescribing generic medicines instead of branded names as per the directive. One of the attackers took out a gun and held it to a doctor's head. Before leaving, they threatened the doctors with dire consequences. This illustrates the deep and disturbing vested interest in the undue profits of selling brand drugs only.[83]

The Movement Begins

At the Fifth Conference of Heads of State or Government of Non-Aligned Countries, held in Colombo, Sri Lanka, in August 1996, a number of resolutions were adopted in relation to the global drug situation; in particular, there was a recognition of the need for affordable essential drugs and the regulation of the fast-growing pharmaceutical industry.[84] Although the Government of India could not properly follow the report of the *Hathi Committee* and the essential medicines list of the WHO, Bangladesh and Sri Lanka did follow the guidelines.[85] The government of Bangladesh constituted an eight-member committee in 1982 to evaluate the value of registered drugs and draft a national drug policy for the country. The committee stated it would not be possible to reach the goal of 'health for all by the year 2000' without providing essential medicines at an affordable price. To do this, a national drug policy must be formulated as part of the national health policy. It determined 16 criteria for the evaluation of some 4340 medicinal products. One of the criteria stated was that *cough syrups*, *throat lozenges*, *grapefruit water*, *alkalis*, etc., would not be allowed to be produced or imported as they did not have any measurable medicinal benefits. As a result of the recommendation of that committee, the government of Bangladesh banned 1666 unnecessary drugs. It was stated further that the banned drugs should be gradually removed from the market, with the process to be completed by June 1984.[86] This movement was not limited to Bangladesh, however. Mozambique stopped importing unnecessary drugs after gaining independence on June 25, 1975. In 1980, Mozambique imported a total of 355 drugs. According to an estimate in 1963, Egypt had imported 80 per cent of its essential medicines. By 1980, however, it was manufacturing 83 per cent of the medicines it needed. Lesotho, a small country in Africa, even became self-sufficient in drug production.[87] In 1989, ten groups from Africa and Asia formed the *International Network for Rational Usage of Drugs* (INRUD), a multi-institutional network dedicated to promoting the safe, effective, and cost-efficient use of drugs.[88] The HIV-positive people network also organized a worldwide movement for access to drugs.[89] Similarly, the *Treatment Action Campaign* (TAC), founded in 1998 by a small group of political activists in South Africa, launched a campaign to reduce the price of medicines for HIV-positive patients.[90] In 1999, *Médecins Sans Frontières* (MSF) launched the global 'Campaign for Access to Essential Medicines' to promote the availability of essential drugs in developing nations.[91]

It is clear from the above that the government of Bangladesh was able to ban the use of unnecessary or irrational drugs, whereas the government of India was unable to do so. In this setting, a movement to demand rational medicine sprang up across India, including West Bengal. Vimla Nadkarni et al. wrote "The essential drugs campaign gained momentum around the 1980s as a result of insufficient supply of essential drugs, an overabundance of non-essential drugs of disputable therapeutic value and the prevalence of rampant malpractices related to the manufacture and distribution of drugs. The essential drugs campaigns in India took the form of the campaign against irrational drugs and the campaign for a rational drug policy."[92] On November 7–8, 1981, a seminar on 'The Drug Industry and the Indian People' was organized in Delhi by five different groups of scientists and medicos. In that seminar, a substantial quantity of concrete material was shared regarding the growth and exploitation of the drug industry, particularly of the multinationals.[93] On January 8–10, 1982, the *Voluntary Health Association of India* (VHAI) held a workshop in Pune, Maharashtra, titled "Drug Issues—Seeking Feasible Alternatives," in which the participants were consumers, representatives of health organizations, doctors, pharmacologists, and journalists. Many activists gathered again in August 1982 in Jaipur for Drug Workshop II organized by VHAI. On this occasion, the theme was "Hazardous Drugs."[94] In March 1984, a seminar was organized by the VHAI at the Max Mueller Bhavan Kolkata on various harmful aspects of the drugs and the characteristics of the pharmaceutical industry. The speakers at that seminar were Mira Shiva of VHAI, Amitabha Guha of the *Medical Representative Association* and Zafrullah Chowdhury of *Gonoshasthya Kendra*, Bangladesh: Shiva spoke about the way in which pharmaceutical companies profit from the production of unnecessary and hazardous drugs; Guha discussed the efforts of pharmaceutical companies to entice doctors to prescribe their products; and Chowdhury detailed his own experience of organizing movement against the production of unnecessary and harmful drugs in Bangladesh.[95]

Since December 1984, a page in every issue of the *Utsa Manush* magazine had been published with the heading *Kathgaray Oshudh* (Medicine under Accusation). This page used to feature cartoons and news related to medicine.[96] Bhabani Prasad Sahu wrote a book titled *Oshudh Kheye Asukh* (*Illness from the Side-effects of Medicine*). In 1986 *Utsa Manush*[97] published a review of the book. In it, Bhabani Prasad had explained, from a Marxist perspective, how medicine became a commodity in capitalist society. Doctors, health workers, and the common people were able to learn about the anarchy and business of unnecessary drugs, as well as the banned drugs in this country at that time. However, Amit Sengupta remarked that "The powerful 'Access to Medicines' campaign was to appear only in the late 1990s and India was perhaps the only region in the world where there was an attempt to build popular resistance."[98]

History shows that the health movement attempts to build popular resistance in India. Let us present a case study in which it is made clear how the health movement has responded to the policy developments at the national level. The following case study narrates the struggle against patent monopoly.

The Case Study of Struggle Against Patent Monopoly

The movement for the people in the health sector was not in vain as it pushed the state to address the issue. We have already discussed how, in the 1970s, India had one of the most progressive patent laws in the world. *The Patents Act, 1970*, operated on a very simple principle that made it possible for the Indian domestic pharmaceutical company to produce new drugs without hindrance and at significantly lower costs. When India amended its revised *Patents Act* in 2005, this led to substantial changes in this supportive environment for Indian domestic drug companies. However, as a result of the battle against the patent monopoly conducted by the Left, progressive sections of the parliament and civil society groups brought about important amendments to the *Patent Act* 2005. We will now attempt to explore the history of this battle.

In 1986, the eighth *General Agreement on Tariffs and Trade* (GATT) round, also referred to as the Uruguay Round, was initiated. In this round, developed countries placed a number of issues on the agenda, which were related to intellectual property (IP) rights, investment, and services. IP rights demand monopoly over the production and reproduction of knowledge. At first, developing nations, led by India and Brazil, were able to delay the inclusion of these new issues. However, the opposition on the part of developing nations was defeated by the beginning of 1989. As a result of intense pressure from the US, India changed its position and agreed to negotiate the *Trade-Related Aspects of Intellectual Property Rights* (TRIPS). S.P. Shukla, India's chief negotiator at GATT, was replaced, because he was strongly active in attempting to oppose the inclusion of IP rights in the negotiating agenda.[99]

Most popular movements and civil society organizations around the world lacked clarity regarding the significance of the negotiations. In India, the *National Working Group on Patent Laws* (NWGPL) (1988), which was headed by B.K. Keayla, played a critical role in shaping opposition to the TRIPS Agreement from the late 1980s. NWGPL was formed by civil servants, lawyers, scientists, representatives of the domestic drug industry, and representatives of trade unions in the pharmaceutical industry. This laid the foundation for the global access campaign on medicines against patents and IP. It played a role as a catalyst for advocacy and mobilization. It provided studies for evidence-based debate against the proposed regime on IP in the parliament and also in the public space. The NWGPL formed the *Forum of Parliamentarians*, which included participants from virtually the entire political spectrum. In India, a number of people's organizations, non-governmental organizations, and political and social movements assembled together to oppose the GATT negotiations.[100] The first meeting of the group was held in Nehru Place, Delhi. The participants were Keayla, director, Corporate Environment in Ranbaxy; Amit Sengupta, Dinesh Abrol, and Usha Menon from the *Delhi Science Forum*; Mira Shiva from the *All India Drug Action Network*; Amitava Guha from the FMRAI; Ashok Rao of the *Confederation of Officers' Associations of Public Sector Undertakings*; B.S. Chimni from Jawaharlal Nehru University; senior journalist Balraj Mehta, several representatives from different generic drug companies, and a number of other individuals.[101] Together with civil society groups, professional bodies and student groups, the *Indian Drug Manufacturers' Association* (IDMA), an association of the Indian domestic pharmaceutical industry, pushed for public resistance, thereby generating a negative image of the TRIPS Agreement, the Dunkel Draft and the GATT in the public media.[102] NWGPL also organized several national and international seminars.

As detailed earlier, in 1994, India, along with a number of other countries, signed the GATT Agreement, which became the *World Trade Organization* (WTO) in 1995. The TRIPS Agreement set out a three-stage implementation time framework for developing countries to amend their patent laws or enact new laws within the 10-year transitional period, i.e. 1995–2005. According to that agreement, India amended its patent law in the first stage in 1999 and in the second in 2002. *The Patents (Amendment) Bill 2003*, representing the third and final amendment, was brought into parliament by the then *Bharatiya Janata Party* (BJP)-led *National Democratic Alliance* (NDA) government. It was, however, not possible for the government to pass the bill in the parliament. The bill then died a natural death due to a change in the government.[103]

Against this backdrop, four Peoples' Commissions on the TRIPS issue were set up by the NWGPL. In November 1993, the first commission was formed under the chairmanship of one of the distinguished former judges of the Supreme Court to address the constitutional issues of the Final Act of the WTO, including the TRIPS Agreement. The members of the commission were prominent scientists and economists. Another commission was set up in 1999 to address the TRIPS Agreement's obligations for the transitional period. As with the previous case, the members of that commission were eminent scientists and economists under the leadership of former judges of the Supreme Court. In 2002, the third Peoples' Commission was established to deal with the topic of a suitable patent law for India. Former Indian Prime Minister I.K. Gujral served as its chairman, and its members were distinguished senior experts. In February 2004, the Fourth Peoples' Commission came into being to evaluate the patent laws, again with the former Indian Prime Minister I.K. Gujral as chairman and a number of senior and distinguished experts as members. All of these commissions submitted reports to the government, which was also given to all political parties and lawmakers. However, these commissions were never given the opportunity to have discussions with the government.[104] *Jan Swasthya Abhiyan* (JSA) lobbied members of parliament and policymakers extensively in the run-up to the *Patents (Amendment) Act of 2005.* In 2004, the *Affordable Medicines and Treatment Campaign* (AMTC), which was launched by the *Lawyers Collective*'s HIV/AIDS Unit (established in 1998) in 2001, convened the *Global Coalition against the Indian Patent Amendmen*t (GCAIPA) in 2004. It was an informal network of NGOs from different countries. GCAIPA was composed of a number of representatives of Brazilian groups, including Alexandra Nino, Veriano Tero, and members of NWGPL, AMTC, and JSA.[105]

It is important to note that there was another stream of campaign against the policy of WTO. While recalling the campaign, Vandana Shiva said that "in 1994 we began the *neem* campaign against the patenting of *neem* by W. R. Grace. We mobilized to prevent the government from signing the GATT agreement in Marrakesh in 1994, and when the WTO still came into being, we organized to continue to question and challenge it. Internationally we organized as the *International Forum on Globalization* in 1994 and, after Seattle, as the *Our World is Not for Sale Network*. In India, 250 organizations came together in the *People's Campaign against the WTO*. The campaign was convened by S. P. Shukla, included four ex-Prime Ministers, trade unions, women's movements, farmers' unions, and environmental movements. In 2000, the movements fighting for people's natural rights to natural resources gathered. We committed ourselves to defend and reclaim our fundamental freedoms related to land, forests, biodiversity, food, and water. That is how the movements for *bijaswaraj* (biodiversity and seed democracy), *annaswaraj* (food democracy), and *jalswaraj* (water democracy) were born."[106]

The Congress-led *United Progressive Alliance* (UPA) government brought back the unchanged version of the NDA's *Third Patents (Amendment) Bill* after assuming office. The bill was strongly opposed by the Leftists, and also some regional parties. Left parties submitted a comprehensive set of amendments in December 2004. In accordance with the TRIPS Agreement, the third and final deadline was set up as 1 January 2005, for the implementation of product patents. To meet this deadline, the UPA government promulgated an ordinance on December 26, 2004.[107]

The *People Living with HIV* (PLHIV) in India network (formed in 1997) launched a protest campaign against the proposed amendments to the *Patents Act*, which, according to them, would increase the cost of treating HIV/AIDS patients. The network received technical information and analysis regarding the impact of the amendments from NWGPL and the *Jan Swasthya Abhiyan*. Numerous national and international letters of concern urged the prime minister, various ministries, and members of parliament to take the serious effects of the amendments on public health into consideration. In February 2005, the PLHIV staged protest marches against the amendments in Delhi, Mumbai, Bangalore, Kolkata, Chennai, Hyderabad, Dharwad, Panjim, Pune, and Thirupati with health organizations, trade unions, farmers' groups, environmental organizations, and many others. Colleagues and the representatives of foreign organizations who were working in India at that time joined Indian PLHIV groups in reaching out to the MPs. The activists met with several of them while sporting 'HIV-positive' t-shirts to explain the potential effects of the amendments on the medicines they had imported from India.[108]

The Leftist parties' statement claimed the government was forced to reconsider the provisions of the Bill due to persistent pressure from them, which was exerted not only through negotiations with the government but also through a nationwide campaign. The government proposed a number of amendments to the Bill on the floor of the Parliament on March 22, 2005 following a series of negotiations. Some of the key concerns which had been expressed by the Left parties were addressed by the amendments that the government tabled.[109] Amit Sengupta wrote "in the consequent negotiations between the Left and the government, the Left largely depended on advice provided by people associated with the NWGPL. These negotiations also allowed other interested parties to suggest new language. At the end, several important amendments were made to the 2004 Ordinance (ICTSD 2005)...The negotiations were held in the backdrop of protests across the country, as well as in different parts of the world—all demanding that the 'pharmacy of the South' should not be jeopardised."[110] However, if we turn our attention to the political-economic policy in West Bengal, we will get a different scenario. To depict this portrait an author alleged that "...in West Bengal the Left Front took all possible steps to make the investment environment hospitable to foreign capital. At the national level the CPM was critical of liberalization and globalization. But in the states where it was in power it created conditions for open-door capitalist development."[111]

The act introduced product patents on medicine for twenty years. However, multiple health safeguards were contained by the Indian Parliament in the amended *Patents Act*. It included a broad ground of compulsory licensing, including the unavailability and unaffordability of a medicine, state emergency, export, and government use. In the act, parallel import was introduced and the patentability criterion was made stringent. It also restored pre-grant opposition to the patent applications. The time for challenging of patent was extended from three to six months. Section 3(d) of *Patents (Amendment) Act 2005* was imposed on chemical and pharmaceutical inventions. The section reads:

> the mere discovery of a new form of a known substance which does not result in the enhancement of the known efficacy of that substance or the mere discovery of any new property or new use for a known substance or of the mere use of a known process, machine or apparatus unless such known process results in a new product or employs at least one new reactant.
>
> Explanation: For the purposes of this clause, salts, esters, ethers, polymorphs, metabolites, pure form, particle size, isomers, mixtures of isomers, complexes, combinations and other derivatives of known substance shall be

> considered to be the same substance, unless they differ significantly in properties with regard to efficacy.[112]

Section 3 (d) implies that India disallows patent monopoly on new forms or new uses of existing medicine. Section 3(d) and 'health safeguards' in the 2005 act were designed to mitigate the impact of a patent regime and to help the Indian domestic drugs industry to become the global force. Now we can testify to the ability of Section 3(d) on patents. The Swiss drugmaker Novartis applied for a patent on the anti-leukemia drug Glivec (imatinib mesylate). In 2006, the Indian Patent Office rejected the patent application for Glivec, because it was not a new drug. Novartis persisted and appealed to the *Intellectual Property Appellate Board* (IPAB). In June 2009, the IPAB upheld the decision of the patent office. Both the patent office and the IPAB invoked Section 3(d) to deny Novartis' appeal.[113] Novartis challenged IPAB's interpretation and application of Section 3(d) in the Supreme Court. In April 2013, the Supreme Court provided a historic judgment upholding the Indian Patent Office's rejection of the Novartis patent application on Glivec.[114] Furthermore, in March 2012, the Indian Patent Office granted a compulsory licence (CL) to the Indian generic drug company Natco Pharma Ltd. for Bayer's anticancer drug sorafenib. It prevented the monopoly of Bayer over the drug. Therefore, Hyderabad-based pharma company Natco was able to make and sell the drug in India. A compulsory licence (CL) was issued by the Indian Patent Office on health grounds, where patients were unable to access a life-saving medicine. As a result of CL, new drugs were manufactured at affordable costs.[115] Most countries had mandatory licence provisions in their laws, but these were rarely applied. Amit Sengupta said that "the decision was followed by reverberations across the world. A range of people working on public health and access to medicines issues welcomed the decision of the Indian patent office…The first grant of a CL in India had clear implications for the availability of new drugs at affordable costs, not just in India but in many developing countries."[116]

Drug Action Forum, West Bengal

In respect of the movement for rational medicine in West Bengal, the *Drug Action Forum,* West Bengal (DAF, WB) deserved special mention.[117] This organization was established by social workers, scientists, and doctors in 1984, and was registered on June 13, 1986. The founding members of the organization were Dr. Arun Sen (President), Dr. Pashupati Nath Chatterjee (Vice President), Dr. Sujit Kumar Das (Secretary), Dr. Pijus Kanti Sarkar (Joint Secretary), Dr. Smarjit Jana (Treasurer), Bhaskar Banerjee, Niranjan Biswas, Swapan Sil, and Dr. Ashish Thakur.[118] However, before the formal formation of the Forum, the members were active in the people's health movement. Dr. Arun Sen was the pioneering figure of *Students Health Home*.

Dr. Sujit Kumar Das was the key organizer of DAF. During his student days, he had joined the Leftist student movement. He was also one of the organizers of the *Health Services Association* (1972), an organization of doctors. Following the Bhopal gas disaster (1984), the *No More Bhopal Committee* was formed in which he played a great role in standing by the victims of the gas leak. Dr. Das also supported the junior doctors' movement of West Bengal in the 1980s.[119] The objectives of the DAF were:

- To strive for adoption and implementation of a scientific national drug policy for the country as a part of a people-oriented scientific health policy.
- To strive for the attainment of self-sufficiency and self-reliance in respect of essential drugs.
- To make all efforts to realize the goal of availability of essential drugs to all.
- To work for the elimination of all irrational drugs, chemicals, pharmaceuticals, medical devices, foods, restoratives, tonics, cosmetics and consumer goods from the country.
- To engage in all forms of democratic activity alone or in collaboration with organizations and individuals with similar aims and uphold the rights and serve the need of the consumers.
- To undertake research and survey works, data and information collection schemes on the harmful effects of different drugs and pharmaceuticals, cosmetics, pesticides, insecticides, fertilizers etc. and of various ways of environmental pollution.[120]

The DAF (WB) published several booklets/pamphlets in Bangla as a part of its movement. The subject matter of those publications were: the rational use of medicines; banned medicines; the patient–physician relationship; family planning etc. The booklet titled *Manusher Janya Oshudh, Na Oshudher Janya Manush* (1984) (Are medicines meant for the people or are people meant for medicines?) can be termed as the manifesto of the

DAF (WB). It dealt with various issues related to the treatment and medicine, the deceit of traders and rulers, the helpless condition of patients etc. It was also translated into English, Hindi, and Telugu. The booklet quickly became popular, which indicated the impact of the movement against irrational and harmful drugs on the common people. Gradually, the forum felt the need to re-publish the manifesto, resulting in the publication of *Manusher Janya Oshudh, Na Oshudher Janya Manush: Part 2* in January 1996. The forum expressed the opinion that, in the past, medicines were manufactured for the benefit of the people, but that this scenario had changed. In the new situation, first the medicine was, and then the people were prepared to take it. According to the forum, foreign pharmaceutical companies, which had been expelled from their home countries, had now taken up residence in India. As a result, numerous drugs that had been banned in other countries were still being used in the country.[121]

Several drugs were prohibited by the government, but were still available in the Indian market. In 1985, the forum published the booklet titled *Nishiddha Oshudh* (Forbidden Drugs) to make people aware of those banned drugs. Since then, as the movement of the forum gained pace, the government gradually banned harmful and unnecessary medicines. In conjunction, the forum repeatedly revised its publications. However, the revision of the booklet stopped after the 1989 edition. After this, the forum decided to publish the book in a new form. A congregation of writers was formed. After three months of their efforts, a booklet titled *Nishiddha Oshudh: Part 2* was published in December 1995 detailing 52 types of banned drugs. (The reasons behind the prohibition of those drugs was also given.) People were also informed about the adverse effects of combining *Ayurvedic* and modern medicine. In addition, the booklet also contained details of the drugs those should be prohibited for manufacture and sale.[122]

Following the popularity of these two booklets, the forum published a third one namely *Oshudh Na Velki* (Are these medicines or magic?), penned by Smarajit Jana in 1988. The booklet was published with the aim of providing scientific information about the numerous medicines available on the market. The forum used it to inform the people about the ineffectiveness of vitamin tonics, nerve/brain tonics, sex tonics, hair tonics, blood growth tonics, and health drinks as medicines. The forum stated that buying tonics and health foods was nothing but a waste of money. The forum also presented its opinions in the form of poems.[123] The book published in 1995 was well received. Its revised edition was published in

2010, under the title *Tonic Namer Velki* (The Magic of Tonics).[124] This edition also sold out quickly, necessitating a reprint.

The booklet *Darkari Oshudh*[125] (Necessary Medicine) was published in January 1996. In that booklet, the forum stated, "at numerous meetings, seminars, and through letters, many people have asked for a book to be written on essential medicines. They have said that 'it is good know about unnecessary harmful drugs, but it is the responsibility of the *DAF* to inform us about necessary medicines; the forum is not doing this.' People are still complaining." The forum published that booklet in order to address such people's opinions. There was a discussion about unnecessary drugs at the beginning of the booklet. The argument advanced by the forum was that the consumption of unscientific drugs are as harmful as the misuse of scientific drugs. Thus, a movement against unscientific drugs began. In fact, the forum did not want people to treat themselves using its booklets, as this could encourage the rise of 'quack' doctors. According to the forum, that would indulge the creation of 'quack' doctors. However, in the second part of the booklet, the practice of scientific medicine was discussed. At the end of each booklet, the forum mentioned their demands, which were:

- Adoption of a scientific people-oriented national drug policy.
- Prohibition of all unscientific medicines from being manufactured or sold.
- Prohibition of those medicines which were banned abroad.
- The DAF demanded that unethical profiteering must be stopped in the case of medicine prices.
- Doctors of *allopathy* should not prescribe *ayurvedic* medicine.
- The drug control administration should be punished for its ineptitude and corruption.
- Poor people should have access to free medicine.

The work of the forum was not beyond criticism, however. It was also accused that it of not saying anything about doctors' responsibility. It only blamed the government. It was also alleged that "health is such a matter where the so-called people's movement is not very fruitful. The presence of people at the forum's meetings and protest processions is not important…if the forum seeks its success by gathering people in meetings, it will be painful."[126] However, it would be wrong to suggest that no attempt was made to involve the doctors in the movement. As a matter of fact, the majority of the forum's members were doctors. It wanted to give the doctors the appropriate information about medicines. For that purpose, from January 1986 DAF started to publish a quarterly magazine in English called *Drug Disease Doctor* (DDD)[127].

The DDD gained international recognition, with the *International Society of Drug Bulletins* (ISDB) welcoming it as a member.[128] However, as a result of conflict within the organization, the publication of DDD was stopped in 1997.[129] The members of DAF used to write about drugs not only in the organization's own magazine, but also in other publications. For example, Dr. Pijus Kanti Sarkar, the editor of DDD, wrote a long ten-page article in the July 1986 issue of *Chaturanga* magazine under the headline *Jatiya Oshudhniti—Kar Swarthe?*[130] In this article, Dr. Sarkar attempted to address the issue of whether the national drug policy of 1986 was adopted in the interests of the people or in the interests of the pharmaceutical companies.

DAF interacted with numerous organizations involved in the medical profession, mobilized grassroots organizations associated with the people's science and health movements, inspired a number of trade unions to join the health movement, and disseminated its message among people throughout West Bengal by using posters, leaflets, street corner meetings, and other methods.[131] The activities of the DAF gained support not only in West Bengal but also in other states. Representatives of the DAF, for example, were invited from Jharkhand, Tripura to deliver a speech on 'rational medicine' in front of school or college students or teachers. Invitations also came from various branches of the *Indian Medical Association* (IMA) and the *Health Service Association* (HSA).[132] In an effort to promote the rational use of drugs (RUD) in West Bengal, a committee named *Rational Drug Campaign Committee* was formed in 1992 by some voluntary organizations and groups of medical professionals.[133]

In the other states of India, organizations similar to DAF had been present since the 1970s, including the *Medico Friend Circle*.[134] Those types of voluntary organizations from different states of India came together and took the initiative to build a platform for the movement all across India. As a result, the *All India Drug Action Network* (AIDN) was established in 1981–1982.[135] DFA, WB was just one part of that network. The DAF also established international connections with organizations working on the drug issue, particularly *Health Action International* and *Gonoshasthaya Kendra* (GK) in Bangladesh.[136]

Organizations associated with the 'Drug-Action' in India met in Wardha on 30 and 31 July 1984. The meeting received participants from

Arogya Dakshata Mandal, Pune, the *Consumer Guidance Society of India*, the *Delhi Science Forum*, the *Federation of Medical Representatives' Associations of India* (FMRAI), the *Foundation for Research in Community Health*, Bombay, *Kerala Shastra Sahitya Parishad* (KSSP*), Lok Vigyan Sangathan, Maharashtra, Low Cost Standard Therapeutics* (LOCOST), *Baroda*, the *Medico-Friend Circle*, and the *Voluntary Health Association of India* (VHAI). From West Bengal, representatives of the *Voluntary Health Association, West Bengal* and the DAF also participated in the meeting. The first day was devoted to the discussion on rational drug policy in India with notes on rational drug policy being prepared by Sujit Das (DAF, WB), Anant Phadke (MFC), and Amitab Guha (FMRAI). After thread-bare discussion a consolidated draft of a Rational Drug Policy (a kind of manifesto of the group) was finalized at the end of the meeting late in the night. On the second day, participants discussed topics such as the formation of a co-ordination committee, advancing the movement, creating slogans to build the movement across the country, etc.[137]

The DAF organized a protest march to the U.S. Consulate in Kolkata on September 3, 1984 in protest against the decision of the American Congress to allow, under certain conditions, the export of drugs which had been banned in the U.S. That protest received a very encouraging amount of public attention.[138] A convention was organized in Kolkata on January 20, being attended by 400 delegates representing various organizations working in the people's science and health movements. The convention adopted demands such as: the removal of useless, unscientific, harmful drugs; banning the banned drugs, reduce drug-prices, abolish brand names…etc. On January 30–31, 1985, at the initiative of *All India Drug Action Network* (AIDAN), a meeting was held at which the representatives of various organizations of the country participated.[139] The activities of DAF (WB) were very much appreciated at that meeting.

On May 4, 1986, at Darbhanga Hall, Calcutta University, DAF organized a meeting on national drug policy, at which political parties and trade unions were involved. Asit Ghosh (CPI), Sunil Sengupta (RSP), Swadhin Guha (AITUC), Bhaskar Gupta (SUCI), and other personalities were also in attendance. The resolution unanimously adopted at the meeting stated that "since there is a direct link between public health and drug policy, it should be discussed at all levels before it is introduced in the Parliament." The meeting also approved a proposal to prohibit the sale of harmful drugs and to compile a list of essential drugs.[140]

The second state convention of DAF on rational drug policy was held in February 1986. DAF organized a two-day workshop on February 8–9, 1986 in Kolkata, involving 72 activists and organizations working in the fields of drug, health, environment, science, and the civil rights and trade union movements. The following issues were discussed:

- Drug, health and medical care,
- Banned and bannable drugs,
- Indian drug industry,
- Drug information system,
- Drug marketing use and research,
- Useless and irrational drugs,
- Drug, government and law,
- Drug price and generic name.[141]

A panel discussion was held on the 'Role of drug in scientific and other systems of medicine.' The workshop highlighted the need to strengthen the people-oriented health movement and science movement in order to achieve a successful outcome of the drug campaign.[142]

The *International Society of Drug Bulletins* admitted *Drug Disease Doctor* (DDD) to the society's membership and the editor of DDD attended the first international conference of the society held at Stockholm, Sweden in July 1986. To meet the longstanding demand, DAF also held a two-day workshop on 'Health Care, Society and State' on November 29–30, 1986. The workshop, attended by activists from all over the state, generated tremendous interest.[143] The deliberation was conducted into four sections on the topics of:

- Health-Medicine-Physician-Society;
- State-Public Health-Medicare-India;
- Alternative Medicine-What and Why? and
- Outline of Health Movement.[144]

DAF organized its third annual convention on February 1, 1987, to which it invited the *Where There Is No Doctor* activist author David Werner. However, he was unable to attend the convention. In a letter to Dr. Sujit Kumar Das, he wrote: "I feel that this Convention is of enormous importance, and deeply regret that I will be unable to attend. However, I do wish you every success, and hope that your action will contribute to the establishment of an essential drugs policy, similar to or superior to that of Bangladesh."[145]

Local Drug Action Forum units were also established in district towns like Asansol, Bankura, and Berhampur. DAF was urged by health activists and environmentalists to join the campaign for a people-oriented health care service and safe environment. DAF also made the utmost effort to offer medical care to the victims of the Bhopal disaster (1984). DAF representatives worked in the committee appointed by the Supreme Court of India for the medical relief and rehabilitation of the gas victims following the industrial tragedy. DAF joined with several other organizations to continue *No More Bhopal Committee* in West Bengal. DAF also helped in the formation of *Bihar Drug Action Forum* which launched drug campaign in Bihar.[146] Many organizations/groups of West Bengal took up the cause of Drug Action Forum during the year 1985–1986.[147] The DAF organized a convention on February 15, 1987 at the Large Lecture Theater of Nil Ratan Sircar Medical College and Hospital to exchange views on the National Drugs Policy, 1986. Representatives of political parties and trade unions were invited to the convention.[148]

In a different domain, the new *Janata* government of India took the initiative to evaluate and alter the policies and programs of the previous Congress government. Similar initiatives were also taken in the sphere of drug policy. On May 24, 1990, the Ministry of Petroleum and Chemicals of the Government of India organized a meeting entitled 'Review of National Drug Policy' in Delhi. A number of organizations agitating for the adoption of a system of 'rational medicine' were invited to the meeting. In their contributions, representatives of the DAF, WB focused on the introduction of a scientific people-oriented drug policy.[149] On June 20, 1990, the Ministry of Petroleum and Chemicals held a joint meeting with industrialists, businessmen, and agitating organizations. *All India Drug Action Network* (AIDAN) and some of its member organizations were invited to the meeting. DAF also participated.[150]

In 1980, the *Drug Consultative Committee*, a constitutional body established under Section 7 of the *Drug and Cosmetics Act (Act 230 of 1940)*, appointed an expert subcommittee to investigate the rationality of 34 classes of *Fixed Dose Combination (FDC)* drugs. The subcommittee did its work, recommending that 23 of them should be banned. Seven of the 23 categories were advised to be weeded out over a specified period of time, while it was recommended that the remaining 16 were to be eliminated immediately. This was adopted by the Ministry of Health and Family

Welfare.[151] However, on July 23, 1983 the Government of India banned the first 12 classes of unnecessary drugs.[152] However, there were many more harmful drugs in the market. One such harmful drug was the high dose *estrogen* (E) and *progesterone* (P) combination, which was used to determine pregnancy. High dose of EP combination had been widely used around the world in the 1960s and 1970s to identify the existence of embryos. In India too, doctors, non-doctors, quack practitioners indiscriminately prescribed high doses of EP.[153] In 1967, the adverse effects of that medicine were reported. Consequently, the drug was banned in 15 countries. However, it continue to be used in India. In 1979, the research of Dr. B. Palaniappan showed that all of the women who used that drug gave birth to handicapped babies.[154] In India, "a campaign was launched on the March 8, 1982 on *International Women's Day* on the issue of drugs for women's health, the need for essential drugs and their rational use, and the need for withdrawal of unsafe potentially hazardous drugs."[155] The campaign also opposed high-dose combination of EPs. As a result, in July 1982, the *Drug Control of India* (DCI) banned that drug. However, pharmaceutical companies obtained stay order against that ban. In this scenario, Vincent Panikulanga, on behalf of the *Kerala Public Health Defence Committee*, filed a case in the Supreme Court. The apex court directed DCI to hold hearings on that drug in different cities of India.[156]

Hearings were held in Madras and Delhi at the outset, but not in Kolkata. Therefore, the *Association of Health Service Doctors, West Bengal* (AHSD, WB) organized a meeting on May 23, 1987 at Calcutta Medical College to discuss high-dose EP combinations. In order to arrange a hearing in Kolkata, AHSD, WB, *Drug Action Forum,* and the *West Bengal Medical and Sales Representatives Union* (WBMSRU) sent a letter to DCI, signed by a number of doctors. As a result, DCI held a hearing on July 10 in the auditorium of *Central Drugs Laboratory, Kolkata.*[157] Members of AHSD, DAF, WBMSRU, the *Student Federation of India* (SFI), *Nari Nirjatan Pratirodh Mancha, Norman Bethune Janaswasthya Andolan,* and other groups were all in attendance. Dr. S.K Roy, Director, Central Drugs Laboratory, Dr. Partha Dasgupta, Deputy Drugs Controller, and Dr. P.K Dutta, a former official of Drug Control, represented the government. Dr. Bhavesh Lahiri, Dr. N. Roy Chowdhury, Dr. B. Bhattacharya and others all spoke out against the banning of EP combinations. In fact, they spoke in support of the drug companies. On the other hand, Dr. Pijus Kanti Sarkar, Dr. Smarjit Jana, Dr. Sujit Kumar Das, Dr. Jnanabrata Sil, Dr. Sukhamoy Bhattacharya, Dr. Mira Shiva, and other leading physicians all presented their views against the EP combinations. At the hearing, more people were in favor of banning the drug.[158] After massive protests, in 1988 the EP Combination was actually banned.[159]

On November 3, 1988, the Government of India banned the fixed-dose combination of chloramphenicol with streptomycin (CS) and corticosteroids with any other drugs (CX) because these did not have any therapeutic justification. However, five pharmaceutical companies, Dey's Medical, Roussel, Mac Lab, Lyka Lab, and Indoco Remedies, quickly obtained stay orders from a number of high courts and continued to market it.[160] But the Congress government at the centre and the Left government in the state of West Bengal did not take any action against these actions. Therefore, DAF (WB) and AIDAN began a boycott campaign. In order to stop the sale of banned drugs, DAF (WB) sent an application to 52 drug companies, bearing the signatures of 270 doctors. The multinationals Parke Davis and Boeh-ringer-Knoll informed they would withdraw CS (Chlorostrep and Streptoparaxin, respectively) from the market. Yet Indian companies did not stop selling prohibited drugs. So, the boycott campaign continued. In fact, as consequence of the DAF's actions, doctors refused to prescribe not only harmful drugs as well as the companies' effective ones. As a result, the companies suffered huge losses. Dey's Medical attempted to persuade DAF to withdraw the boycott campaign. "Dey's Medical served a legal notice on DAF in July, 1989 stating that unless DAF immediately stops the campaign, the company shall be left with no alternative but to seek legal remedy including claim for heavy damage." However, DAF strengthened the campaign. On the other hand, Mac Lab (CS) and Indico Remedies (CX) agreed to remove harmful drugs from the market and they were exempted from the boycott by DAF. Lyka Lab simply wanted to sell its stockpile. However, the forum did not agree and continued their boycott campaign.[161]

Such a boycott movement was nothing new. In the 1970s, doctors in Scandinavian countries boycotted the products of Ciba-Geigy.[162] "As Ciba-Geigy continued to market *clioquinol* in spite of known hazards and doubtful hazards, 3000 Swedish doctors boycotted Ciba-Geigy products, causing the company to lose 25% of its market in Sweden."[163] Under intense pressure, Ciba-Geigy accepted the protestors' demands. The Indian Medical Association, a body of doctors from all over the country, expressed its moral support for the boycott campaign by DAF. In addition, the *Indian Academy of Paediatrics*, an organization of medical practitioners, played an active part in the campaign. Similarly, the *Health*

Service Association, an organization of government doctors in West Bengal, had instructed its members to observe a boycott campaign. Two unions of medical representatives also joined the movement. In West Bengal, the activists of the people's science organizations, including the *Ganabijnan Samanway Kendra*, took the initiative to make the boycott movement a success across the state.[164]

Foreign pharmaceutical corporations were concerned by the boycott campaign led by several organizations such as DAF. Accordingly, the *Organization of Pharmaceutical Producers of India* (OPPI), a joint venture of foreign drug companies in India, countered the campaigners' claims by placing advertisements in the country's most widely circulated newspapers. In opposition to this, the people's health campaigners stated that drugs were still available in the Indian market, which had been banned in other countries. However, OPPI stated that the actions of medicine in different human bodies varies due to differences in genes, dietary habits, climate, and other factors. Therefore, their argument was that drugs banned in other countries could be sold in India, and that drugs banned in India could be sold overseas. However, the pharmaceutical companies had no scientific basis for their arguments.[165] At this time DAF also began to look at prescriptions in order to prevent doctors from prescribing banned drugs.[166]

There was a major problem in that the government banned many harmful drugs, but they did not publicize this to the population. The trade names of the banned drugs were not published. Therefore, proper information about prohibited drugs remained unknown to doctors, patients, and pharmacists. The result was that voluntary organizations had to undertake the job of informing the people about the prohibited drugs. Zafrullah Chowdhury stated that one of the features of the capitalist system is that even if the government publishes a list of essential drugs or banned drugs, it is not disseminated among the people.[167] That is why the *Gonoshasthya Kendra* of Bangladesh translated the list of essential medicines of the *World Health Organization* into Bengali under the title *Prayojaniya Oshudher Byabahar*[168] (Use of Essential Medicines) and spread it among the doctors and common people. This publication crossed the borders of Bangladesh and became equally popular in West Bengal.

The Government of India banned five and ten categories of drugs on December 26, 1990, and February 11, 1991, respectively. However, it did not make the effort to have the drugs taken off the market. Although DAF attempted to inform the government of the situation, it received no reaction. Consequently, DAF collected the trade names of those banned drugs and published them in its journal *Drug Disease Doctor*. The members of DAF also tried to raise awareness about the prohibited drugs by writing articles in a variety of periodicals, including *Bijnan O Bijnankarmi, Utsa Manush*.[169] On February 10, 2011, the Union Health Ministry published "a gazette notification to ban human placental extract and its formulations along with five other drugs." The government banned the production and sale of *placentrex*, a drug made from the human placental extract, manufactured by the West Bengal-based Albert David Company. In response, the company filed a suit in the Delhi High Court. On April 6, the court ordered the government to form a committee to determine whether the ban should be lifted. On May 30, based on the recommendations of the committee, the ministry relaxed its ban on the drug, allowing it to be used for wound healing and injections for pelvic inflammatory disease.[170] It is crucial to note, however, that a group of pharmacologists had been making efforts since 1986 to impose a ban on that drug. DAF had also agitated for its removal from the market. The DDD played a significant role in raising awareness about those ineffective drugs.[171]

On July 31 and August 1, 1999, DAF organized a two-day workshop on health and medicine at the *Aikatan Cultural Centre* in Kolkata (*Eastern Zonal Cultural Centre*) as part of the *Bharat Jan Vigyan Jatha*. The workshop focused on different issues related to drugs such as a campaign against unscientific drugs, the price control of medicines, essential medicines and human rights, patent law, medicine, and health.[172] In the workshop on "Essential Medicines and Human Rights" Sujit Kumar Das stated:

> If life-saving drugs are to be delivered to all the poor, then the production of unscientific, harmful drugs must be stopped. And if the production of unnecessary drugs is stopped, the existing industrial structure can be used for the production of scientific drugs. In this case, state intervention is necessary. Moreover, the government has to bear the responsibility of providing the medicine to those who cannot afford it.[173]

According to DAF, universal health education was required to address issues such as unscientific harmful drugs, the misuse of drugs, the unfair price of drugs etc. Diseases affect the human body not just as a result of one's own activities, but also as a result of the activities of others in society. Thus, people of the society should be conscious about health. That is why DAF demanded the introduction of health education.[174]

Dr. Smarajit Jana stated that "in the absence of proper health education people often fall into ill health. Many people in this country buy drugs without prescriptions and often use harmful drugs unknowingly. Besides, many do not complete full course of antibiotics. Therefore, micro-organisms develop resistance to antibiotics and spread to the environment. Thus, antibiotics become ineffective."[175] The discovery of antibiotic *penicillin* by Alexander Fleming in 1928 was a significant breakthrough in the fight against bacteria. Later, however, it was found that the medicine was not working as before. Many bacteria produced a type of enzyme in their body to survive, which destroyed the effectiveness of the *penicillin*. This necessitated the discovery of new antibiotics, explaining the development of *methicillin*, *cephalosporin*, and so on. Their condition was similar to that of *penicillin*. In this scenario, *carbapenem*, a class of very effective antibiotic, was discovered. Yet even uncontrolled use of that developed a type of enzyme against that antibiotic. As a result, a dreadful scenario arose in the treatment of individuals suffering from serious infections. This situation had been observed in Kolkata, Mumbai, and Delhi at different times since 2000. However, no action had been taken by the government in that regard.[176] An article on the matter appeared in the September 2010 issue of *The Lancet*[177] and included the name of New Delhi. In addition, those who could come to this country from England for treatment were warned. Newspapers in this country published stories dealing with the issue. As a result, the government of India took steps to deal with the problem.[178]

According to the *Drugs and Cosmetics Rules Act*[179] of India, antibiotics cannot be dispensed without a prescription from a registered medical practitioner. Due to the poor implementation of national drugs regulations in India, however, antibiotics are easily available from drug stores. Homeopathic and *Ayurvedic* doctors can also prescribe antibiotics. The misuse of antibiotics has taken a serious turn in this country.[180] Public awareness was needed to get rid of these problems. Organizations such as DAF were working to spread awareness among the people.

Much of the objectives for which DAF was founded have now been successful, with the government cancelling many ineffective drugs. However, the activities of DAF were limited to deal with the drug-related problems. The forum was unable to build an effective movement to improve the overall health system. People were deprived of their government health services. Health care was becoming a commodity. Therefore, in the 1990s, the members of DAF felt the need for the creation of a larger health movement. They planned to turn the *Drug Action Forum* into a

Health Action Forum. Due to the lack of manpower, however, that plan was not implemented. Dr. Smarajit Jana joined the sex workers' movement. Dr. Pijus Kanti Sarkar came out of the DAF and started the *Aamader Haspatal* project at Bankura. Bhaskar Banerjee joined the mental health movement. Finally, following the death of Dr. Sujit Kumar Das (1937–2011), the work of the DAF came to an end.[181]

The Left Front government in West Bengal condemned the Union government's drug policy and demanded the nationalization of the pharmaceutical industries. 'Some organizations loyal to the CPI (M), the leading party of the Left Front' started a campaign for rational drugs and staged protests against the Union government's anti-people drug policy and the corruption of multinational drug companies.[182] The *Janaswasthya Committee* published a pamphlet entitled *Jatiya Oshudh Niti?*[183] (National drugs policy?). In that pamphlet, the *Committee* opined that there was no proper national medicine policy in operation in India. Criticizing modifications in *Drug Policy of 1986*, published in 1994 by the Ministry of Chemicals and Fertilizers, Department of Chemicals, Petrochemicals, the pamphlet stated that the government of India had changed its national drugs policy to serve the interest of multinational pharmaceutical companies.[184]

Movement Against Unethical Clinical Trials

The corruption of the pharmaceutical companies did not stop only in the sphere of unscientific drug; there was also corruption in the process of making new drugs. In order to discover a new medicine, researchers have to go through several phases. First, the effectiveness of a new drug is examined on animals in a laboratory. Then, experimentation on human beings, called a 'clinical trial,' is conducted. The conducting clinical trials in an unethical manner has a long history. During World War II, for example, the I.G. Farben Company bought women prisoned in German camps and conducted immoral experiments on them.[185]

The eighteenth *World Medical Assembly*, held in Helsinki in Finland in 1964, set out ethical principles to stop the unethical clinical trial on human beings. The Helsinki Declaration stated: "The nature, the purpose and the risk of clinical research must be explained to the subject by the doctor. Clinical research on a human being cannot be undertaken without his free consent after he has been informed; if he is legally incompetent, the consent of the legal guardian should be procured."[186] The government of

India also adopted those principles.[187] Ignoring the *Helsinki Declaration*, however, the *Cholera Research Centre, Calcutta* of the *Indian Council of Medical Research* (ICMR) in 1974, experimentally applied the sulfa drug, *phenacil*, on low-income people in the Beliaghata-Maniktala area of Kolkata. On the second occasion, in 1975–1976, a new type of cholera vaccine was administered to millions of people in that region. As a result, many people died. A few scientists from that institute mounted a protest against this unethical experiment. In response to that protest, a number of them were sacked by the management of the institution. Some of these later went on to form *Norman Bethune Janaswasthya Andolan*. Joint Action Committee of Unions and Associations of Autonomous Research Institutions (JACARI), an organization of the workers of autonomous research institutes, joined the protest movement against unethical trials. Scientists informed the Union government and the West Bengal state government about that issue, but they did not receive any response. Therefore, they complained to the *Sharma Sarkar Inquiry Commission* (1978). Among the various applications, the commission chose the issue as the first case considering the importance of the unethical medical trial on common people.[188]

There was no mention of *phenacil* in the pharmacopoeia of any country. Before it was applied in Calcutta, it had applied on the people of Morocco. According to the WHO, as a result of application of the medicine, 120 individuals per million had died. Sadly, the medicine was sent to the *Cholera Research Centre, Calcutta* by the WHO.[189] The report of the *Sharma Sarkar Commission* found in favor of the scientists. So, the *Cholera Research Centre, Calcutta* filed a case in the Calcutta High Court. The institution's management argued that they were not government employees, and that therefore the commission had no right to investigate the issue.[190] The verdict of the single bench in the Calcutta High Court was also in favor of the scientists and *Norman Bethune Janaswasthya Andolan*. Many Leftist lawyers, including Somnath Chatterjee and Bikash Bhattacharya, also supported the scientists. However, the judgment of the division bench was against the protesters. The court directed the *Sharma Sarkar Commission* to close the investigation. In addition, it became difficult for the protesters to raise money to continue the case. The scientists lodged a complaint with the West Bengal government and the West Bengal Medical Council after the *Sharma Sarkar Commission* closed its investigation. When they approached Jyoti Basu, he asked them to apply to the Commissioner of Police for investigation. While such an application was made, the Commissioner of Police delayed the report, and eventually lost. Nobody knows how it had happened.[191] Owing to the non-cooperation of the government, it was no longer possible to punish the killers. At the same time, some leaders were also accused of taking bribes from drug companies. In the quizzical words of Jnanabrata Sil in the *Prokriti O Manush*: "…the fake Leftists taking bribes from multinational drug companies…"?[192] *Norman Bethune Janaswasthya Andolan* not only spoke out against unethical drug experimentation, but also published drug-related pamphlets to improve public awareness, which had been discovered in the previous chapter.

Alternative Initiatives to Supply Affordable Generic Drugs

With the progress of the movement of the *Gonoshasthaya Kendra* (GK) in Bangladesh from1972, the need for medicines for its health centers also increased. But the medicines in Bangladesh were very expensive because its drug market was controlled by multinational companies. As a result, it became impossible for ordinary people to procure high-cost medicines. Dr. Zafrullah Chowdhury commented that "without drugs, we were like guerrillas without bullets." Thus, GK decided to set up its own pharmaceutical company, *Gonoshasthaya Pharmaceutical Limited* (GPL). In addition to covering the needs of GK, GPL was designed to supply 15–20 per cent of essential medicines (according to the list made by the WHO) to the Bangladesh market. GPL was founded in 1976 with the aim of producing essential medicines under a generic name rather than tonics and vitamins. It planned to supply medicines for 35–50 per cent less than the price of medicines supplied by multinational companies, and to still make a profit of between 10 and15 per cent.[193]

A similar initiative was also introduced in India. *Low Cost Standard Therapeutics* (LOCOST) was founded in 1983 in Vadodara (Baroda), Gujarat, with the aim of producing high-quality generics at low prices on a non-profit basis. LOCOST has been a vocal proponent of rational therapies and the adoption of a people-oriented drug policy. The *All-India Drug Action Network* (AIDAN) invited LOCOST to be a member.[194] In 1977, when a private factory in Kolkata, called *Alkaloid Research Laboratory*, closed down, 138 employees lost their jobs. Faced with uncertainty, they promised to build a pharmaceutical factory on their own initiative, setting up their own site in Behala, Kolkata. The government also supported their project. The *Federation of Medical and Sales Representatives Association of India* (FMRAI) came forward to help them and they were also supported by medical scientists. As with GPL, they started producing generic drugs and took the initiative to supply them at lower prices than other companies.[195]

The *West Bengal Voluntary Health Association* (WBVHI) also developed a similar model. WBVHI formed the *Central Drug Marketing Unit* in 1984 to supply affordable generic drugs to its member organizations. To take a more active part in providing services, however, the initiative emerged in 1986 as an independent organization called the *Community Development Medical Unit* (CDMU). This organization aimed to collect and store essential medicines from drug companies and to supply them to voluntary organizations at low cost.[196] CDMU delivered not only quality essential medicines, but also involved in the campaign for rational medicines. It published booklets in both Bengali and English.

Oshudh-Bishudh O Chikitsar Saranjam: Swasthyakarmider Nityasangi Hatiyar[197] (Drugs and Medical Equipment: A Common Tool for Healthcare Workers) was published with the help of a grant from the World Health Organization's Regional Office for Southeast Asia (Project ICP EDM 300) to assist health workers in providing information about diseases, the rational use of medicines, and other topics. With the grant from MISEREOR, the German Catholic Bishops' Organization for Development Cooperation, *Oshudher Sangata Byabahar*[198] (Rational Uses of Medicines) was published to impart knowledge about rational medicine to the people. The foreword to that book was written by the prominent Bengali writer Mahasweta Devi. In addition to these publications, CDMU also brought out both *Pharmacy Gathan O Parichalana* (Pharmacy Formation and Management) and *Drug Formulary for Community-Based Healthcare Facilities.* To make it easier for the people to understand drug labels, CDMU also issued a leaflet called *Oshudher Label Chinun O Bujhun* (Know and Understand Drug Labels). It also made some posters with titles such as *Rational Management of Storage*, *Healing Safely Serve Widely* etc. The organization was also engaged in research on both unscientific and rational medicine.[199] CDMU had also published its magazine *Rational Drug Bulletin*[200] since 1991. In 2012, the *Social Initiatives for Growth and Networking* (SIGN), Ranchi brought out the *Standard Treatment Guidelines* (STG)[201] in partnership with CDMU. The third edition of STG was published in 2019. (STG refers to a systemically developed document designed to assist practitioners and patients in making decisions about appropriate healthcare for specific clinical circumstances.) The publishing of an STG was certainly a novel approach toward strengthening the movement toward the achievement of 'right drug for right patients in right manner,'[202]

We observed earlier that the publication of the *Drug Disease Doctor*, the mouthpiece of the DAF, was discontinued in the late 1990s. However, another, similar publication, the *Bulletin on Drug and Health Information* (BODHI),[203] was launched in 1994. That bi-monthly magazine was published by the *Foundation for Health Action* (FHA), a voluntary organization. FHA was established with the following objectives:

- Adoption of scientific health policy including a rational policy for India.
- Promotion of rational use of drugs and strive to remove unscientific, irrational, harmful drugs and unscientific practices in the sphere of health.
- Launching a collective move for health for the deprived.
- Building appropriate awareness and upholding the rights of the practitioners and further the interests of the consumer.[204]

This magazine was edited by Dr. Pijus Kanti Sarkar, who had formerly been the joint secretary of DAF, WB since its inception. Dr. Sarkar was a member and editor of the *International Society of Drug Bulletins* (ISDB) and was also elected as a member of the executive committee of the ISDB. Dr. Sarkar stated that "most doctors want to do a good job but they are not getting the right information." Therefore, the aim of the magazine was to convey proper and unbiased information about rational medical procedures and medicines to the doctors, nurses or health workers.[205] From 2000, FHA began to publish another Bengali bi-monthly magazine, named *Asukh-Bisukh*.[206] Of which Dr. Sarkar was also the editor. *BODHII* was published for doctors. But the objective of the *Asukh-Bisukh* was to inform the non-doctor, i.e., the patient, the other staff involved in the medical care about diseases, medicine, and treatment. It was claimed that "if people read *Asukh-Bisukh*, they will not be misled when seeking medical treatment, will not waste money on unnecessary tests or medicines, and will be able to question doctors."[207]

After the two national seminars on Clinical Pharmacology, on May 23–24, 1996,[208] and also on November 2–3, 1998, held at North Bengal

Medical College, Darjeeling,[209] to inform the people about the concept of social pharmacology; in 2000, another organization, named the *Society for Social Pharmacology*, began its journey. In 2002, the organization's bi-monthly bulletin *Social Pharmacology*, edited by Dr. Swapan Kumar Jana, was launched. Its main objective was to spread knowledge of medicine in remote rural areas.[210] The organization also published a book titled *Prescription: Rogir Chikitsar Pratichchhabi*[211] (Prescription: Reflections of Patient's Treatment) to highlight how doctors prescribe unnecessarily harmful drugs. That book reviewed the prescriptions of several doctors, working in public hospitals or doing private practice, from 1987 to 2012. It was an attempt to make doctors, patients, and unqualified 'quack' practitioners aware of the dangers of irrational drugs.

The two organizations mentioned above showed a slight difference from the philosophy of DAF, which had advocated for legislation to prohibit unqualified quack practitioners from prescribing drugs. The *Foundation for Health Action* and the *Society for Social Pharmacology* sought to train unqualified quack practitioners so that they would not prescribe medicines unnecessarily. Perhaps because of this kind of disagreement, Dr. Pijus Kanti Sarkar left DAF and became involved in editing the BODHI and *Asukh-Bisukh* periodicals separately.

The campaign, which was started in the 1980s as a part of the people's health movement in West Bengal to demand rational medicine for all, has continued into the twenty-first century. It can be stated that the movement of the 1980s prepared the stage for this subsequent movement. Dr. Punyabrata Goon stated that the AIDAN or DAF (WB) movements inspired them when they were studying to become doctors.[212]As a result of that movement, the government had been forced to ban 344 ineffective drugs up to 2016.[213]

In Kolkata, a national seminar on *Pharmaceutical Policy and Access to Essential Medicines*, supported by WHO, was organized by *Jan Swasthya Abhiyan*, *Federation of Medical and Sales Representatives' Associations of India*, *National Campaign Committee for Drug Policy and All India Drug Action Network* on April16–17, 2005. That seminar discussed different aspects of the country's pharmaceutical policy. It noted the new situation created by the policy of LPG and the new product patent regime which threatened national self-reliance as well as the availability and affordability of essential medicines. The seminar also expressed concern about the worsening situation with regard to drug prices, with its disastrous impact on the poor. The seminar expressed the need to formulate a *National*

Pharmaceutical Policy that would address the critical issues of universal access to essential medicines and also national self-reliance.[214]

In the 1980s and 1990s, activists from the people's health movement campaigned for the implementation of the recommendations of the *Hathi Committee*. In the second decade of the twenty-first century, the health activists emphasized the recommendations of the *High Level Expert Group (HLEG) on Universal Health Coverage* for India. Here we may mention the recommendations of HLEG on drugs, which were as follows:

- Increase public spending on drug procurement to 0.5% of the GDP and provide free essential medicines to all.
- Enforce price regulation and apply price control on all formulations in the Essential Drug List.
- Ensure drug and vaccine security by strengthening the public sector and protecting the capacity of Indian private sector companies to produce low cost drugs and vaccines needed for the country.
- Strengthen institutional mechanisms for procurement and distribution of allopathic and AYUSH drugs.
- Promote rational use of drugs through prescriber, patient and public education.
- Strengthen Central and State regulatory agencies to effectively perform quality and price control functions.
- Protect the safeguards provided by the Indian patents law and the TRIPS Agreement against the country's ability to produce essential drugs.
- Transfer the Department of Pharmaceuticals to the Ministry of Health[215]

Although the HLEG recommended free medicine for all, this policy was not implemented. However, an initiative was taken to provide free medicine to patients in Tamil Nadu[216] and Rajasthan.[217] In 2012, the West Bengal government also announced the introduction of free medicines at government hospitals. A memorandum published by the Government of West Bengal on January 9, 2013 read:

> It is hereby ordered that the vital and essential medicines (drugs and consumables) & all available diagnostics services (excluding the diagnostic services under PPP) will be provided free of cost to all kinds of patients in OPD/all free beds under IPD/emergency of different Govt. Hospitals/

> health centres run by the DHFW at the level of Primary, Secondary and Tertiary level heath care facilities, as well as JSSK beneficiaries and RBSK beneficiaries.[218]

This initiative did not succeed, however, since not all medicines were available in government hospitals in West Bengal.[219] In 2012, the West Bengal government announced that fair price outlets, known as *Najyamuller Aushudher Dokan*, would be opened under PPP in 35 hospitals across the state, including all medical colleges and hospitals, all district hospitals, selected sub-divisional (SD) hospitals, and other hospitals. It was stated that 142 drugs in generic form and other medical-related items would be available at fair-price outlets at more than a 30 per cent discount on maximum retail price (MRP). The purpose of the scheme was "to ensure round the clock availability of quality medicines, consumables, surgical items, implants etc. at preapproved discounted rates over the Maximum Retail Price (MRP) to provide utmost benefits to the patients through the fair price outlets within the Medical Colleges and District Hospitals/SD Hospitals in the state of West Bengal."[220] However, that initiative was based on PPP mode, while the report of the HLEG noted the tone of opposition to the policy of PPP. In fact, PPP symbolizes the story of private capital investment and profit. Mention here can be made of the fact that the Government of India launched the *Pradhan Mantri Bhartiya Janaushadhi Pariyojna* (PMBJP) in 2008 in order to distribute generic medicines at affordable prices through exclusive outlets known as *Janaushadhi Kendra* in several districts across India.[221]

As a result of the introduction of fair-price drug outlets, people may have received more benefits than before. Dr. Jnanabrata Sil observed that for many years *Norman Bethune Janaswasthya Andolan*, along with other organizations, demanded free medicine for all from the Left Front government. But the government declined to meet this demand. He supported this initiative on the part of the TMC government, but believed that government control needed to be strengthened further in order to maintain the quality of medicines at fair-price outlets.[222] During 2013–2014, a survey was conducted by Arijita Dutta and Satarupa Bandyopadhyay to evaluate the impact of that scheme on the out-of-pocket expenditure (OOPE) of patients, selecting nine government hospitals for survey. Of 1000 hospitalized patients who were surveyed, 548 belonged to the poor category and the rest (442) were non-poor. After conducting their systematic study they concluded "…the policy is found to offer financial protection primarily to the non-poor patients by reducing OOPE…For the poorer patients visiting FPMS (Fair Price Medicine Shops), the OOPE on medicine, even bought under substantial discounts, were higher compared with those who did not. The latter group had low OOPE not because they bought the medicines from outside retail shops, but because they received them free of cost from hospital pharmacy. Hence, the program failed to provide financial protection, although they increased the access to medicines significantly."[223] Truly, the achievement of "health for all" is not possible simply through the taking such of initiatives. How do people who do not have enough money to feed themselves buy medicine? Thus, the people's health movement opposes this limited initiative. It demanded that the government should provide free medicines to the people, stop the production of medicines under brand names, and produce them in generic form. In addition, it was demanded that the main medicine, i.e. food, should also be provided in sufficient amounts.

Notes

1. Parashuram, "Chikitsa Sankat", in Parashuram, *Gaddalika*, published by Brajendranath Bandopadhyay, Kolkata, BS 1331 (1924), pp. 40–68.
2. Sukumar Ray, "Rajar Asukh", in Prafulla Kumar Patra (ed.), *Sukumar Rachanabali*, Kolkata: Patra's Publication, not dated, pp. 313–317.
3. Rajshekhar Basu, "Daktari O Kabiraji", in *Laghuguru Prabandhabali*, Kolkata: Ranjan Publishing House, BS 1346 (1939), pp. 8–27.
4. Phares G.M. Mujinja et al., NGOs, Consumer Rights and Access to Essential Medicines: Non-Governmental Public Action in a Low-Income Market Context", in Jude Howell (ed.), *Non-Governmental Public Action and Social Justice*, Basingstoke: Palgrave Macmillan, 2013, p. 130.
5. David L. Rabin and Patricia J. Bush, "The Use of Medicines: Historical Trends and International Comparisons", *International Journal of Health Services*, Vol. 4, No. 1, Winter 1974, pp. 61–87.
6. David I. Macht, "A Drug or Poison?", *The Scientific Monthly*, Vol. 47, No. 1, July 1938, pp. 34–40.
7. S. Srinivasan, "'Medicines for All', the Pharma Industry and the Indian State", *Economic and Political Weekly*, Vol. 46, No. 24, June 11–17, 2011, pp. 43–50.
8. World Health Organization, *The World Medicines Situation*, Geneva: World Health Organization, 2004, pp. 62–63.

9. Health in India: NSS 71st Round, January–June 2014, National Sample Survey Office, Ministry of Statistics and Programme Implementation, Government of India, 2016, p. 42.
10. "Out-of-pocket health expenses plunge 55 mn Indians into poverty in 2017", *Business Standard*, Mumbai, 19/07/2018, https://www.business-standard.com/article/current-affairs/out-of-pocket-health-expenses-plunge-55-mn-indians-into-poverty-in-2017-118071900115_1.html, retrieved on April 2, 2019.
11. Santanu Kumar Tripathi, Dalia Dey and Avijit Hazra, *Medicine Prices and Affordability in the State of West Bengal, India*, Report of a survey supported by World Health Organization and Health Action International, not dated, pp. 7–43, Available at: https://haiweb.org/wp-content/uploads/2015/07/India-West-Bengal-Report-Pricing-Surveys.pdf.
12. Sumanta Sen, "Calcutta's Nilratan Sircar Hospital Faces Medicine Shortage, Doctors Threaten Agitation", *India Today*, May 15, 1983, https://www.indiatoday.in/magazine/living/story/19830515-calcuttas-nilratan-sircar-hospital-faces-medicine-shortage-doctors-threaten-agitation-770643-2013-07-22, retrieved on April 6, 2022.
13. Soma Mukhopadhyay, "Jalatanker Osudh Amil", *Anandabazar Patrika*, Kolkata January 25, 2015.
14. P.K. Sanyal, *A Story of Medicine and Pharmacy in India*, Kolkata: B. Pharm, 1960, pp. 47–130.
15. Ibid., pp. 133–135.
16. K. Park, *Park's Text Book of Preventive and Social Medicine*, India: Bhanot Publishers, 23rd edition 2015, p. 6.
17. James Le Fanu, *The Rise and Fall of Modern Medicine*, UK: Hachette, 2011, Introduction page.
18. Prasanta Kumar Ghosh, *Government's Policies and Growth of Pharmaceutical Industry in India 1947–2018: A Review*, Discussion Paper 236, Research and Information System of Developing Countries (RIS), New Delhi, 2019, pp. 1–3.
19. Anil Kumar, "The Indian Drug Industry under the Raj, 1860–1920", in Biswamoy Pati and Mark Harrison (ed.), *Health, Medicine and Empire: Perspective of Colonial India*, India: Orient Longman, 2001, reprint 2006, p. 356.
20. Biswajit Dhar and Reji Joseph, "Developments in India's Domestic Pharmaceutical Sector and Implications for Universal Health Care in India", in Imrana Qadeer (ed.), *India Social Development Report 2014: Challenges of Public Health*, New Delhi: Oxford University Press, 2015, pp. 138–139.
21. Prasanta Kumar Ghosh, op. cit., p. 5.

22. Labanya Pal, "Foreign Direct Investment and Productivity Spill-overs: Evidence from the Indian Pharmaceutical Industry", in Byasdeb Dasgupta, Archita Ghosh, and Bishakha Ghosh (eds.), *Neoliberalism in the Emerging Economy of India: The Political Economy of International Trade, Investment and Finance*, London, New York: Routledge, 2021, p. 174.
23. Amit Sengupta et al., *Economic Constraints to Access to Essential Medicines in India*, New Delhi: Society for Economic and Social Studies & Centre for Trade and Development, 2009, p. 13.
24. Government of India, *The Patents Act, 1970* (No. 39 of 1970), which received the assent of the President on September 19, 1970 and was published in the Gazette of India, Extraordinary, Part II—Section i dated the September 21, 1970.
25. Government of India, Patents Rules, 1972, published in the Gazette of India, vide S.O. 301(E) dated April 20, 1972 in Part II, Section 3, sub-section (ii).
26. Anindya Bhukta, *Patent Katha*, Kolkata: Nagarik Mancha, 2006, pp. 27–31.
27. Amit Sengupta et al, *Economic Constraints to Access to Essential Medicines in India*, op. cit., p. 14.
28. A. R. Phadke, "The Drug Industry—An Analysis", in Ashvin J. Patel (ed.), *In Search of Diagnosis: Analysis of Present System of Health Care*, New Delhi: Medico Friend Circle, first edition 1977, cited edition 1985, p. 82.
29. *The IMF Loan: an Exercise in Mortgage*, New Delhi: All India Revolutionary Student Federation (AIRSF), 1991, p. 1.
30. Jyoti Basu (ed.), *Documents of the Communist Movement in India 1994–96*, Vol. 25, Kolkata: National Book Agency, 1998, p. 104.
31. Gopinath Chattopadhyay, *Patent O Janaswasthya*, Kolkata: Forum for Scientist, Engineers and Technologists (FOSET), 1999, p. 19.
32. Ibid., pp. 3–7.
33. Anindya Bhukta, *Patent Katha*, op. cit., pp. 15–17.
34. Amitava Guha, "TRIPS Chukti o Prayojaniya Oshudh", in Amiya Kumar Bagchi (ed.), *Viswayan: Bhabna-Durbhabna* (Vol. II), Kolkata: National Book Agency, 2008 (first published 2002), pp. 386–398.
35. Ibid.
36. K. B. Saxena, "Trade in Health Services Implications for People's Health", in P. M. Arathi (ed.), *Public Health in India: Policy Shifts and Trends* (Series Editor: Manoranjan Mohanty, Social Change in Contemporary India, Volume VI), New Delhi: SAGE Publications India Pvt Ltd, 2022, p. 69.

37. Shuvendu Dasgupta, *GATT Chuktir Edik Sedik*, North 24 Parganas: Janasanghati Kendra, 1995, p. 26.
38. Sujit Kumar Das, "Janamukhi Boigyanik Oshudhnitir Mulkatha", *Utsa Manush*, Vol. 10, No. 2, February 1989, pp. 33–35.
39. Government of India, *National Health Policy 2002*, New Delhi: Ministry of Health and Family Welfare, Department of Health, 2002, p. 17.
40. C. Niranjan Rao, "Patents and Pharmaceuticals in India", *Economic and Political Weekly*, Vol. 41, No. 20 May 20–26, 2006, pp. 1975–1977.
41. The Patents (Amendment) Act, 2005 No. 15 of 2005, the Gazette of India, New Delhi, April 5, 2005.
42. Murphy Halliburton, *India and the Patent Wars: Pharmaceuticals in the New Intellectual Property Regime*, USA: Cornell University Press, 2017, p. 38.
43. Speech of P Karunakaran on Need to Control the Increase in Prices of Life-saving Medicines, in Lok Sabha Debates, Fifteenth Series, Vol. XXXIII, Thirteenth Session, 2013/1935 (Saka), No. 23, Tuesday, April 23, 2013/Vaisakha 03, 1935 (Saka), p. 34.
44. "Nishiddha Osudher Panchali", *Asukh-Bisukh 65*, January–February, 2011, p. 7.
45. Arunachal Datta Choudhury, "Hariye Jawa Osudh, Fire Asbe Na Aar", *The Doctors Dialogue*, January 6, 2020, https://thedoctorsdialogue.com/medicines-of-the-yester-years/, retrieved on January 16, 2020.
46. Sujit Kumar Das, *Darkari Osudh*, Kolkata: Drug Action Forum, West Bengal, 1996, p. 6.
47. High Level Expert Group Report on Universal Health Coverage for India, op. cit., p. 127.
48. Report on research project, *Fixed-dose combination in India, inception – marketing – a study*, Conducted by Community Development Medicinal Unit in collaboration with Health Action International Asia Pacific, Kolkata, 2010, pp. 3–15.
49. Dianna Melrose, *Bitter Pills: Medicines and the Third World poor*, England: OXFAM, reprinted version 1987 (first published 1982), p. 92.
50. Ibid., p. 1.
51. Vincent Tucker, "Health, Medicine and Development: A Field of Cultural Struggle", in Vincent Tucker (ed.), *Cultural Perspective on Development*, London: Frank Class, reprinted version 2002 (first published 1997), p. 111.
52. Paul Farmer, *Pathologies of Power: Health, Human Rights, and the New War on the Poor*, Berkeley, Los Angeles and London: University of California Press, 2002, p. 303.

53. Subrata Pahari, "Oshudher Upanibeshbad O Adhunik Bangla", in Goutam Chattopadhyay (ed.), *Itihas Anusandhan 15*, Kolkata: Paschimbanga Itihas Samsad, 2001, pp. 722–731.
54. "A Blueprint for Health for All" (Text of Address by Dr H. Mahler in the First Meeting, August 2, 1977; Originally issued as document SEA/RC30/Min. 1, on 3 August 1977), in *Report and Minutes of the Thirtieth Session of the WHO Regional Committee for South-East Asia*, Bangkok, Thailand, 2–8 August 1977, New Delhi: September, 1977, p. 83.
55. Speech by Dr. Sanjeev Mukherjee in the discussion meeting on universal health care organized by the *Shramajibi Swasthya Udyog* and *All Bengal Health for All Campaign Committee* at the office of *West Bengal Voluntary Health Association*, Kolkata on 23.06.2019.
56. *British Medical Journal*, Vol. 326, No. 7400, 31 May 2003.
57. Ray Moynihan, "Who Pays for the Pizza?: Redefining the Relationship between Doctors and Drug Companies. 1: Entanglement", *British Medical Journal*, Vol. 326, No. 7400, 31 May 2003, pp. 1189–1192.
58. Anant Phadke, "Regulation of Doctors and Private Hospitals in India", *Economic and Political Weekly* (EPW), Vol. 51, No. 6, February 6, 2016, p. 49.
59. Sukhamoy Bhattacharya, *Prasanga Oshudh*, Kolkata: Norman Bethune Janaswasthya Andolan, 1987, p. 17.
60. Swapan Jana, "Oshudh Company O Chikitsak Samaj", *Social Pharmacology*, Hoogly: Society for Social Pharmacology, 2007, p. 75.
61. Government of India, *Report of the Committee on Drugs and Pharmaceutical Industries*, (Hathi Committee Report), Ministry of Petroleum & Chemicals, April 1975, pp. 1–3 (available online now).
62. Ibid., p. 104.
63. Ibid., pp. 257–264.
64. World Health Organization, The Selection of Essential Drugs: Report of a WHO Expert Committee, World Health Organization Technical Report Series 615, Geneva: World Health Organization, 1977, pp. 7–8.
65. Ibid., pp. 9–13.
66. Sukhamoy Bhattacharya, *Prasanga Oshudh*, op. cit., p. 7.
67. "New Drug Policy (Contributed)", *Economic and Political Weekly*, Vol. 13, No. 21, May 27, 1978, pp. 875–879.
68. Government of India, Drugs (Prices Control) Order, 1979, Government of India: Department of Pharmaceuticals http://pharmaceuticals.gov.in/sites/default/files/DPCO1979.pdf, retrieved on July 16, 2019.
69. Report: Task Force to Explore Options other than Price Control for Achieving the Objective of Making Available Life-saving Drugs at Reasonable Prices, Submitted to the Department of Chemicals & Petrochemicals, Government of India, 2005, pp. 12–13.

70. Amit Sengupta, "New Drug Policy: Prescription for Mortgaging Drug Industry", *Economic and Political Weekly*, Vol. 29, No. 39, September 24, 1994, p. 2526.
71. Ibid.
72. Government of India, Pharmaceutical Policy 2002, February 15, 2002, available from: https://www.nppaindia.nic.in/wp-content/uploads/2020/07/PHARAMACEUTICAL-POLICY-2002.pdf, retrieved on February 20, 2022.
73. Ibid.
74. Parijat Bandyopadhyay, "Pharmacist Niye Dhalaw Durniti, Bartsana Rajyake", *Anandabazar Patrika*, Kolkata, January 11, 2013.
75. Ganapati Mudur, "Doctors in India defy guidelines on generic drugs", *British Medical Journal*, 1 July 2013, Vol. 347, doi: https://doi.org/10.1136/bmj.f4244.
76. Ibid.
77. Government of India, Memorandum No Z15025/83/2017/DIR/CGHS, Dated September 8, 2017, New Delhi: Ministry of Health and Family Welfare.
78. Vandana Roy and Proteesh Rana, "Prescribing generics: All in a name", *Indian Journal of Medical Research*, vol. 147, No. 5, May 2018, pp. 442–444.
79. Speech of Anandrao Adsul, in Lok Sabha Debates, Fifteenth Series, Vol. XXX, Twelfth Session, 2012/1934 (Saka), No.11, Friday, December 7, 2012/Agrahayana 16, 1934 (Saka), p. 18.
80. Ibid.
81. Vandana Roy and Proteesh Rana, "Prescribing generics: All in a name", op. cit.
82. Government of India, Notification (Drug and Cosmetic (Ninth Amendment) Rules), New Delhi: Ministry of Health & Family Welfare, in the Gazette of India, April 3, 2017.
83. Sanjeev Kelkar, *India's Private Health Care Delivery: Critique and Remedies*, Singapore: Palgrave Macmillan, 2021, pp. 153–154.
84. Zafrullah Chowdhury, *The Politics of Essential Drugs—the Makings of a Successful Health Strategy: Lessons from Bangladesh*, Dhaka, Bangladesh: The University Press Limited, 1996, p. 39.
85. Amit Sengupta et al., *Economic Constraints to Access to Essential Medicines in India*, op. cit., p. 14.
86. Government of the People's Republic of Bangladesh, *Report of the Expert Committee for Drugs on the National Drug Policy of Bangladesh 1982*, Ministry of Health & Population Control, Government of the People's Republic of Bangladesh, Dhaka, 1986, pp. 1–14.
87. *Utsa Manush*, Vol. 5, No. 4, April 1984, pp. 112–113.

88. John Chalker, "The International Network for Rational Use of Drugs (INRUD)", in *The Politics of Medicines* (e-Encyclopaedia), 2012, Available from: https://haiweb.org/encyclopaedia/theinternational-network-for-rational-use-of-drugs/, retrieved on June 16, 2022.
89. Smarajit Jana, *Swasthyer Utsa Sandhane*, Kolkata: Durbar Prakashani, 2016, pp. 141–143.
90. Mark Heywood, "South Africa's Treatment Action Campaign: Combining Law and Social Mobilization to Realize the Right to Health", *Journal of Human Rights Practice*, Vol.1, No. 1, March 2009, pp. 14–36.
91. Médecins Sans Frontières (MSF): https://www.msf.org/access-medicines, retrieved on July 24, 2022.
92. Vimla Nadkarni, Shubhada Maitra, Gurmeet Hans and Anil Kumar, "Health Advocacy: Implications for the Social Work Profession", *The Indian Journal of Social Work*, Vol. 59, No. 1, 1998, p. 324.
93. Anant Phadke, "Multinationals in Indian Drug Industry", in Kamala S. Jayarao and Ashvin J. Patel (eds.), *Under the Lens: Health and Medicine*, New Delhi: Medico Friend Circle, 1986, pp.105–120.
94. Mira Shiva, "Towards a Healthy Use of Pharmaceuticals: An Indian Perspective", in *Development Dialogue* (published in two issues per year by Dag Hammarskjöld Foundation), issue on Another Development in Pharmaceuticals, Vol. 2, 1985, pp. 90–91.
95. Smarajit Jana, "Oshudh Banam Swasthya", *Utsa Manush*, Vol. 5, No. 4, April 1984, p. 112.
96. *Utsa Manush*, Vol. 6, No. 3, March 1985, p. 69.
97. *Utsa Manush*, Vol. 7, No. 12, December 1986, p. 338.
98. Amit Sengupta, "Globalization, Intellectual Property Rights, and Pharmaceuticals", in Purendra Prasad and Amar Jesani (eds.), *Equity and Access: Health Care Studies in India*, New Delhi: Oxford University Press, 2018, p. 132.
99. Amit Sengupta, "Two Decades of Struggle", *Economic & Political Weekly*, Vol. 48, No. 32, August 10, 2013, pp. 43–45. (The article has also been incorporated in Prabir Purkayastha, Indranil and Richa Chintan edited *Political Journeys in Health: Essays by and for Amit Sengupta*, New Delhi: Left World Books, 2021, pp. 73–82.)
100. Ibid.
101. Amit Sengupta, "B.K. Keayla: A Personal Reminiscence", *Economic & Political Weekly*, Vol. 45, No. 51, December 18–24, 2010, pp. 25–26. (The article has also been incorporated in Prabir Purkayastha, Indranil and Richa Chintan (eds.) *Political Journeys in Health: Essays by and for Amit Sengupta*, op. cit., pp. 83–87.)

102. Amaka Vanni, *Patent Games in the Global South: Pharmaceutical Patent Law Making in Brazil, India and Nigeria*, UK & US: Hart Publishing, Bloomsbury Publishing Plc, 2019, p. 127.
103. Amit Sengupta, "Globalization, Intellectual Property Rights and Pharmaceuticals", in Purnendu Prasad and Amar Jesani (eds.), *Equity and Access: Health Care studies in India*, New Delhi: Oxford University Press, 2018, pp. 127–153.
104. B.K. Kealya, "Amended Patents Act 1970: A Critique", in Harsh Dobhal (ed.), *Writing on Human Rights, Law, and Society in India: A Combat Law Anthology*, New Delhi: Human Rights Law Network, 2011, pp. 317–318.
105. Duncan Matthews, *Intellectual Property, Human Rights and Development: The Role of NGOs and Social Movements*, UK & USA: Edward Elgar, 2011, pp. 176–185.
106. Vandana Shiva, *Earth Democracy: Justice, Sustainability and Peace*, London: Zed Books, 2006, p. 93.
107. Left Parties on Patents Amendment—Left Parties Statement: Amendment to the Indian Patents Act, The Battle is Joined, The War is Not Over, March 23, 2005, https://www.cpim.org/content/left-parties-patents-amendment, retrieved in 01.04.2023.
108. People's Health Movement, *Global Health Watch 5: An Alternative World Health Report*, UK: Zed Books, 2017, pp. 394–404.
109. Left Parties on Patents Amendment—Left Parties Statement: Amendment to the Indian Patents Act, The Battle is Joined, The War is Not Over, March 23, 2005, https://www.cpim.org/content/left-parties-patents-amendment, retrieved in April 1, 2023.
110. Amit Sengupta, "Two Decades of Struggle", op. cit.
111. Manoranjan Mohanty, "Dimensions of Power and Social Transformation", in Bijayalaxmi Nanda and Nupur Ray (eds.), *Discourse on Rights in India: Debates and Dilemmas*, London & New York: Routledge, 2019, p. 35.
112. The Patents (Amendment) Act, 2005, No. 15 of 2005 (The Act of Parliament received the assent of the President on April 4, 2005), The Gazette of India, New Delhi, April 5, 2005/Chaitra 15, 1927 (Saka).
113. Amit Sengupta, "Patent to plunder", *Frontline*, May 4, 2012. (The article has also been incorporated in Prabir Purkayastha, Indranil and Richa Chintan (eds.) *Political Journeys in Health: Essays by and for Amit Sengupta*, op. cit., pp. 64–74.)
114. *Novartis Ag* v *Union Of India & Ors* on April 1, 2013, In The Supreme Court of India Civil Appellate Jurisdiction, full text of final judgment is available at: https://indiankanoon.org/doc/165776436/, retrieved on April 1, 2023.

115. Ankur Paliwal, "Indian company gets licence to manufacture and sell patented cancer drug", Down To Earth, March 12, 2012, https://www.downtoearth.org.in/news/indian-company-gets-licence-to-manufacture-and-sell-patented-cancer-drug-37393.
116. Amit Sengupta, "Patent to plunder", op. cit.
117. Sabyasachi Chattopadhyay, "Paschimbange Ashir Dashake Janaswasthya Andolan", in Goutam Chattopadhyay (ed.), *Itihas Anusandhan 15*, Kolkata: Paschimbanga Itihas Samsad, 2001, pp. 741–747.
118. Memorandum & Rules (1/S/52867), Drug Action Forum, West Bengal, 1987.
119. Swapan Kumar Jana, "Ajiban Joddha Chhilen Dr Sujit Das", *Prokriti O Manush, Kalantar*, May 16, 2011, p. 3; Calcutta Notebook, in *Frontier*, Vol. 43, No. 45, May 22–28, 2011; Punyabrata Goon, "Smarane: Dr Sujit Kumar Das", in *Swasthyer Britte*, Vol. 1, No. 1, September 2011, Kolkata, p. 24.
120. Memorandum & Rules, op. cit., Item No. 1.
121. Sujit Kumar Das, *Manusher Janya Oshudh, Na Oshudher Janya Manush (Parba 2)*, Kolkata: Drug Action Forum, West Bengal, 1996.
122. Sujit Kumar Das (ed.), *Nishiddha Oshudh (Parba 2)*, Kolkata: Drug Action Forum, West Bengal, 1995.
123. Smarajit Jana, *Oshudh Na Velki*, Kolkata: Drug Action Forum, West Bengal, second edition 1995.
124. Smarjit Jana, *Tonic Namer Velki*, Kolkata: Durbar Publishers, 2010, second edition 2013.
125. Sujit Kumar Das, *Darkari Oshudh*, Kolkata: Drug Action Forum, West Bengal, 1996.
126. Ranjan Bhadra, "Chikitsaker Bhumikar Upar Jor Paruk", in *Bijnan O Bijnankarmi*, Vol. 9, No. 3, November–December, 1985, pp. 20–22.
127. *Drug Disease Doctor*: R.N. 48196/87; *Drug Disease Doctor*, Vol. 1, No. 1, January 1986.
128. "Nishiddha Oshudher Panchali", in *Asukh-Bisukh* 65, January–February 2011, p. 10.
129. Punyabrata Goon, "Smarane: Dr Sujit Kumar Das", op. cit.
130. Pijus Kanti Sarkar, "Jatiya Oshudhniti—Kar Swarthe?" *Chaturanga*, Vol. 47, No. 3, July 1986, pp. 191–200.
131. Sujit K Das, "Humbling the Mighty: A Small Beginning", *Economic and Political Weekly*, Vol. 24, No. 37, September 16, 1989, p. 2057.
132. "Nishiddha Oshudher Panchali", *Asukh-Bisukh 65*, op. cit., p. 9.
133. SK Jana et al., "A Historical Perspective on the Rational Use of Drugs (RUD) in India", *Indian Journal of Pharmacology*, Vol. 38, No. 5, October 2006, pp. 374–375.

134. Medico Friend Circle: http://www.mfcindia.org/main/history.html.
135. S. Srinivasan, "A Network for the Rational and Ethical Use of Drugs", *Indian Journal of Medical Ethics*, Vol. 1, January–March 2004, p. 13.
136. Souvenir of second state convention of *Drug Action Forum* on the Rational Drug Policy, WB, Kolkata, February 1986, p. 5.
137. Anant Phadke, "All India Drug Action Network", *Medico Friend Circle Bulletin 105*, September 1984, pp. 10–13.
138. Souvenir of Second State Convention of Drug Action Forum on the Rational Drug Policy, WB, Kolkata, February 1986, p. 4.
139. Anant Phadke, "All India Drug Action Network: Report of The All-India Meeting on 30th & 31st January, 1985", *Medico Friend Circle Bulletin 111*, March 1985, pp. 12–13.
140. Ajkal, May 5, 1986, p. 2.
141. Souvenir of Second State Convention of Drug Action Forum on the Rational Drug Policy, WB, Kolkata, February 1986, pp. 7–8.
142. Ibid., p. 8.
143. Souvenir of the Third Annual Convention of *Drug Action Forum* on the National Drug Policy, WB, Kolkata, February 1987, p. 6.
144. Ibid.
145. A letter from David Werner to Dr Sujit Kumar Das dated November 28, 1986, reprinted in the Souvenir of the third annual convention of *Drug Action Forum* on the National Drug Policy, WB, Kolkata, February 1987, p. 3.
146. Souvenir of the Third annual Convention of *Drug Action Forum* on the National Drug Policy, WB, Kolkata, February 1987, pp. 5–6.
147. Souvenir of the Second State Convention of *Drug Action Forum* on the Rational Drug Policy, WB, Kolkata, February 1986, pp. 10–11.
148. *Utsa Manush*, Vol. 8, No. 2, February 1987, p. 55.
149. Sujit Kumar Das, "Samasta Aboigyanik Oshudh Batil Karte Hobe", *Utsa Manush*, Vol. 11, No. 6, June 1990, pp. 146–147.
150. Sujit Kumar Das, "Boigyanik Ganamukhi Oshudhnitir Dabite Janamat Gare Tulun", *Utsa Manush*, Vol. 11, No. 8, August 1990, pp. 203–204.
151. Arun Bal, "Distortions in Drug Policy: Who is to be Blamed?", *Economic and Political Weekly*, Vol. 21, No 23, June 7 1986, p. 1029.
152. Drugs Control Media Services: https://www.drugscontrol.org/banned-drugs.php, retrieved on March 20, 2019.
153. Anik Sen, "Central Drugse Tulkalam—Drug Control Ki Sarkari Nitir Biruddhe?", *Bijnan O Prajukti, Ajkal*, July 13, 1987, p. 6.
154. Sudipta Saraswati, "Aar Bikalanga Shishu Athaba Aar High-dose E.P. Noy", *Bijnan O Bijnankarmi*, September–December, 1987, p. 19.
155. Anjali Shenoi, Jacob Puliyel and Mira Shiva, "Unethical Testing and Promotion of Vaccines", in Gabriella Wass (ed.), *Corporate Activity and*

Human Rights in India, New Delhi: Human Rights Law Network, 2011, pp. 51–52.
156. Sudipta Saraswati, "Aaro Bikalanga Shishu Athaba Aar High-dose E.P. Noy", op. cit., p. 19.
157. Ibid., pp. 19–20.
158. Ibid., pp. 20–21.
159. Mihir Desai, Kamayani Bali Mahabal (ed.), *Health Care Case Law in India*, Mumbai: Centre for Enquiry into Health and Allied Themes (CEHAT) and India Centre for Human Rights & Law (ICHRL), 2007, p. 94.
160. Sujit K. Das, "Humbling the Mighty: A Small Beginning", op. cit. p. 2057.
161. Ibid., p. 2058.
162. Sujit Kumar Das, "Boycott-er Dak—Ebong Tarpor", *Utsa Manush*, Vol. 10, No. 9, September, 1989, pp. 246–249.
163. Philippa Saunders and Andrew Herxheimer, "Networking: Some Reflections on 25 Years of HAI", in Radha Holla (ed.), *Fast Furious and Flexible: The Story of Health Action International (HAI) 1981–2006*, Colombo: Health Action International Asia Pacific, 2006, pp. 18–19.
164. Sujit Kumar Das, "Boycott-er Dak—Ebong Tarpor", op. cit.
165. Sujit Kumar Das, "Oshudh Andolan o Byabsayider Apaprchar", *Utsa Manush*, Vol. 8, No. 1, January 1987, pp. 13–14.
166. "Kichhu Daktarer Sahajyei Bajare Nishiddha Oshudh", *Anandabazar Patrika*, May 12, 2012, http://archives.anandabazar.com/archive/1120512/12swasth4.html, retrieved on April 19, 2019.
167. Interview with Zafrullah Chowdhury (born in 1941) by Farhad Mazhar, Bangladesh,2018,https://www.youtube.com/watch?v=BQLjPkMQte8, retrieved on October 20, 2021.
168. *Prayojaniya Oshudher Byabahar* published by Gonoprakashani, Dhaka, Bangladesh, 1992.
169. Sujit Kumar Das (ed.), *Nishiddha Oshudh (Parba-2)*, op. cit., p. 15.
170. "Drug Made from Human Placenta Back in the Market", *The Times of India*, June 20 2011, https://timesofindia.indiatimes.com/city/chennai/Drug-made-from-human-placenta-back-in-the-market/articleshow/8930661.cms, retrieved on July 12, 2019.
171. Swapan Kumar Jana, "Panchmisheli (thirteenth bout)", *Asukh-Bisukh 65*, January–February, 2011, p. 21.
172. Drug Action Forum, *Swasthya O Chikitsa: Parisheba, Krishti O Shiksha Bishoye Karmashalar Alochya Bishay*, Kolkata: Drug Action Forum, 1999, pp. 1–21.
173. Ibid., pp. 10–11.
174. Ibid., pp. 17–18.

175. Smarajit Jana, "Hatbaralei Oshudh", *Bijnan O Bijnankarmi*, Vol. 9, No. 3, November–December, 1985, pp. 19–20.
176. "Antibioticer Apabyabahar: Sarkari Padakkhep" (Editorial), *Asukh-Bisukh 67*, May–June, 2011, pp. 2–4.
177. Karthikeyan K. Kumarasamy et al., "Emergence of a new antibiotic resistance mechanism in India, Pakistan, and the UK: a molecular, biological, and epidemiological study", *The Lancet*, Vol. 10, No. 9, September, 2010, pp. 597–602.
178. "Antibioticer Apabyabahar: Sarkari Padakkhep" (Editorial), op. cit.
179. Government of India, *The Drugs and Cosmetics Rules, 1945* [As amended up to August 15, 2013], New Delhi: Ministry of Health and Family Welfare.
180. Gerard Porter et al, "Over-the-counter sales of antibiotics for human use in India: The challenges and opportunities for regulation", *Medical Law International*, Vol. 21, No. 2, 2021, pp. 149–150.
181. Interview with Dr. Smarajit Jana (1952–2021), Kolkata, February 14, 2020.
182. Sujit Kumar Das, "Janamukhi Boigyanik Oshudhnitir Mulkatha", *Utsa Manush*, Vol. 10, No. 2, February 1989, pp. 33–35.
183. *Jatiya Oshudhniti?*, Kolkata: Janaswasthya Committee, 1994.
184. Ibid., p. 3.
185. Jonathan Glover, *Causing Death and Saving Lives*, England: Penguin, 1977, p. 58.
186. Declaration of Helsinki, Recommendations guiding doctors in clinical research adopted by the 18th World Medical Assembly, Helsinki, Finland, June 1964.
187. Sukhamoy Bhattacharya, "Janaganer Opar Oshudh Pariksha", in Sukhamoy Bhattacharya (ed.), *Oshudh-Bishudh: Janaswasthya Sankalan* (part 3), Kolkata: Norman Bethune Janaswasthya Andolan, 1993, pp. 102–103.
188. Sukhamoy Bhattacharya, *Bishay Janaswasthya*, Kolkata: Dasgupta and Company Private Limited, 1983, pp. 74–81.
189. Siddhartha Ghosh, "Chikitsar Name E Kon Apakirti", *Utsa Manush*, Vol. 2, No. 8, August 1981, pp. 3–4.
190. Sukhamoy Bhattacharya, *Bishay Janaswasthya*, op. cit.
191. Interview with Dr. Jnanabrata Sil, Former Secretary of Norma Bethune Janaswasthya Andolan, Age 81, Kolkata, March 2, 2019.
192. Jnanabrata Sil, "Sab Maran Nay Saman: Dr Norman Bethune", *Prokriti O Manush, Kalantar*, March 24, 2014, p. 3.
193. "Price War on Third World Drug Company", *New Scientist*, Vol. 93, No. 1291 Weekly, February 4, 1982, p. 293.

194. Low Cost Standard Therapeutics (LOCOST), *Impoverishing the Poor: Pharmaceuticals and Drug Pricing in India*, LOCOST/JSS Vadodara/ Bilaspur, 2004.
195. Sukhamoy Bhattacharya, Prasanga Oshudh, op. cit., pp. 40–41.
196. Punyabrata Goon, "The Struggle for Rational Drug Policy", *Rational Drug Bulletin*, Vol. 23, No. 1 Jan 2014, Kolkata: Community Development Medicinal Unit, p. 3.
197. Abhijit Hazra et al. (eds.), *Oshudh-Bishudh O Chikitsar Saranjam: Swasthyakarmider Nityasangi Hatiyar*, Kolkata: Community Development Medicinal Unit, 2007.
198. Shantanu Kumar Tripathi et al (eds.), *Oshudher Sangata Byabahar*, Kolkata: Community Development Medicinal Unit, 2007.
199. Community Development Medicinal Unit, http://cdmuindia.org/, retrieved on June 13, 2019.
200. *Rational Drug Bulletin*: ISSN 0972-3064.
201. Social Initiatives for Growth and Networking (SIGN), *Standard Treatment Guidelines: Primary Healthcare Facilities*, co-ordinated by Community Development Medical Unit (CDMU), Kolkata: CDMU, first edition 2012.
202. Krishnangshu Ray, "Foreword", in *Standard Treatment Guidelines: Primary Healthcare Facilities*, co-ordinated by Community Development Medical Unit (CDMU), Kolkata: CDMU, first edition 2012, 2019 (cited 3rd edition), pp. ix–x.
203. BODHI: 53258/94.
204. BODHI, Vol. 5, No. 3, July–August 1998.
205. Sandhya Srinivasan, "BODHI: Continuing Medical Education for Healthcare Workers", Info Change India, April 2006, http://www.infochangeindia.org/public-health/108-public-health/changemakers/43-bodhi-contuining-medical-education-for-healthcare-workers, retrieved on July 12, 2019.
206. *Asukh-Bisukh*: WBBEN/2001/7872; *Asukh-Bisukh*, Vol. 1, No. 1, May–June 2000.
207. "Asukh-Bisukh Para Jaruri—Kintu Keno?" (Editorial), *Asukh-Bisukh 69*, September–October 2011, p. 1.
208. Proceedings of National Seminar on Clinical Pharmacology held on May 23–24, 1996 at N.B. Medical College, Darjeeling organized by Department of Pharmacology, N.B. Medical College, Darjeeling.
209. Proceedings of National Seminar on Clinical Pharmacology held on November 2–3, 1998 at N.B. Medical College, Darjeeling organized by Department of Pharmacology, N.B. Medical College, Darjeeling.

210. Society for Social Pharmacology, *Social Pharmacology* (a collection of articles published in *Social Pharmacology Bulletin* No. 1–9), Hooghly: Society for Social Pharmacology, 2007, p. 24.
211. Swapan Kumar Jana et al. (eds.), *Prescription: Rogir Chikitsar Pratichchhabi*, Hooghly: Society for Social Pharmacology, 2013.
212. Punyabrata Goon, *Oshudhbishudh: Kichhu Darkari Katha*, Kolkata: Kathashilpa, 2017, pp. 84–86.
213. Complete list of 344 drugs banned by the Ministry of Health Family welfare, March 15, 2016, https://www.nhp.gov.in/Complete-list-of-344-drugs-banned-by-the-Ministry-of-Health-Family-welfare_pg, retrieved on July 16, 2019.
214. Jan Swasthya Abhiyan, *Access to Essential Medicines*, Delhi: National Coordination Committee, Jan Swasthya Abhiyan, 2007, pp. 44–52.
215. High Level Expert Group Report on Universal Health Coverage for India, Instituted by Planning Commission of India, Submitted to the Planning Commission of India, New Delhi, November 2011, pp. 131–135.
216. Tamil Nadu Medical Services Corporation Ltd., (TNMSC) was set up with the primary objective of ensuring ready availability of all essential drugs and medicines in the government medical institutions throughout the State by adopting a streamlined procedure for their procurement, storage and distribution. It was incorporated on July 1, 1994 and has commenced its functions of purchase, storage and distribution of drugs and medicines from January 1995. TNMSC aimed to make the drugs and materials available to the poorest of the poor and "Service to the Public". It later became a model for other states. Available at: https://tnmsc.tn.gov.in/html/aboutus.php, retrieved on June 16, 2022.
217. The *Mukhyamantri Nishulk Dave Yojana*, also called the *Chief Minister's Free Medicines Initiative*, was launched by the Government of Rajasthan in October 2011 and was developed in compliance with the state government's commitment to provide essential medicines free of cost to all patients visiting public health care facilities in Rajasthan. The scheme initially began with 240 medicines and later provided more than 600 medicines that were on the essential medicines list.

     World Health Organization, *Universal Access to Medicine in India: a Baseline Evaluation of the Rajasthan Free Medicine Scheme*, World Health Organization Country Office for India, 2014.
218. Government of West Bengal, No. HF/O/TDE/29/M-08/13, Dated January 9, 2013, TDE Branch, Department of Health and Family Welfare, Kolkata.
219. Parijat Bandyopadhyay, "Sarkari Haspatale Binamulye Nay Sab Oshudh", *Anandabazar Patrika*, October 29, 2017.

220. Government of West Bengal, *Establishment of Fair Price Outlet for Medicines, Consumables and Implants at selected Government Hospitals through Public Private Partnerships* (PPP), Kolkata: Health and Family Welfare Department, 2012, pp. 1–34.
221. Government of India, *Pradhan Mantri Bhartiya Janaushadhi Pariyojna*, New Delhi: Department of Pharmaceuticals, Ministry of Chemicals & Fertilizers. Available at: http://janaushadhi.gov.in/pmjy.aspx, retrieved on June 15, 2022.
222. Interview with Dr Jnanabrata Sil, July 17, 2019.
223. Arijita Dutta and Satarupa Bandyopadhyay, "Policy intervention for access to medicine: Does it work similarly for poor and non-poor?", *The International Journal of Health Planning and Management*, September 20, 2018, DOI: 10.1002/hpm.2671.

CHAPTER 6

Conclusion: Walking Toward a Better World

I

While historicizing the health movement (of the world including India) in general, and of West Bengal in particular, I have traced its origin. I have tried to diagnose the maladies of the health system by subjecting it to critical analysis. The efforts to heal the health system have been investigated. The probe has focused on the health policy and has revealed that the policy of the colonial government was followed in the formulation of the health policy of independent India. Thus, the Indian health policy has been focused on cure rather than prevention. To get immediate dividends, politicians emphasized treatment of disease rather than prevention. Consequently, the burden of disease within the country has increased. This study points out that it is necessary to pay attention to preventive medicine to build the health of the nation. The probe has also revealed that the common people were frequently deprived of government medical services. The colonial government provided very few medical facilities to people, and when they did so it was in service of their own interests. The expectations of the common people with regard to the government were very low. However, in independent India, the people had expectations from the ruler which were informed by the ideals of the welfare state. Medical service was one such arena where the expectations of people were high. The independent government did try to develop a health care

© The Author(s), under exclusive license to Springer Nature Switzerland AG 2025

N. Malakar, *Historicising the People's Health Movement in West Bengal, India*, https://doi.org/10.1007/978-3-032-02696-5_6

infrastructure. As the population of this country grew, so too did the demand for government health care services. Yet the government failed to meet the needs of the growing population. People's deprivation increased from the beginning of the 1990s when neo-liberal economic reforms were introduced into the country. The World Bank intervened in the formulation of India's health policy. As a result, user fees were introduced in government hospitals and the commercialization of health care began. The World Bank advised the governments of developing countries to move away from providing 'comprehensive health care services.' All of these developments violated people's 'right to health' and violated the principles of the Alma-Ata Declaration of 1978.

One may judge the impact of the health movement through analysing the situation in government hospitals. For that purpose, let us consider a serialized news-item on the issue. Here I will refer to two such reports: One from 1983 and the other from nearly four decades later, in 2022. In 1983, reporters from the *Anandabazar Patrika* visited five major government hospitals in Kolkata. Their report detailed how the institutions lacked life-saving drugs and oxygen cylinders, and that many X-ray and ECG machines were not in working condition. Jaydev Pathak, the vice-president of the *All Bengal Junior Doctors Federation* at Nil Ratan Sircar Medical College, stated that "there is no dearth of doctors. But there is a lack of medicines and other equipment. This happened almost a year ago. Two people died in this hospital in front of my eyes due to lack of injection."[1] Even four decades later, the situation had changed little. In 2022, the reporters for the *Anandabazar Patrika* visited four government hospitals in Kolkata. Patients complained that hospital trolleys were inadequate; that there was a shortage of essential medicines; that most medicines were bought from private outlets; that patients had to wait a long time for pathological tests; that people fell into the clutches of brokers, etc.[2]

These two newspaper surveys are simply snapshots of the overall situation. Not making any stray comment, this research has tried to reveal the entire picture. It shows, on the one hand, that government hospitals have deteriorated due to the reduction of government expenditure on the health sector, and, on the other hand, to fill the vacuum, that there has been an increase in the numbers of private health care providers. It has been found that before the outbreak of the COVID-19 pandemic, India's health care system was already broken down because 'over four-fifths of all the healthcare expenditure was private.' The pandemic has led to the highlighting of structural flaws in India's health system. Between 2011 and

2020, the population of India expanded by roughly 13.25 per cent, but combined spending on public health by the union and state governments grew by just 0.39 per cent in the same period.[3] During the first wave of the COVID-19 pandemic, the government's negligence led to significant hardships for migrant workers, resulting in numerous fatalities. During the second wave, the state also 'failed to protect the rights to life and health of its citizens.' Many hospitals turned away patients because of insufficient capacity and a number of hospitals asked patients to sign forms accepting the risk in case of death caused by shortages of oxygen. As a result of the government's failures, people were compelled to seek recourse in the courts.[4] The concept of 'social murder,' which Engels had coined in 1845 to explain how living and working conditions experienced by English workers led to premature death, might similarly be used to describe the failures of government policy in the domain of health care in India during the pandemic period.

The country's corporate hospitals had sprung up in the 1990s. Following that, private medical colleges started to emerge. The government has not only failed to fulfil its responsibilities, but also offered a degree of private capital in the health care sector. In the Liberalization, Privatization, Globalization (LPG) era, patients have become consumers in the open market. The government of India passed the *Consumer Protection Act of 1986* to protect consumers from cheating. That act gave consumers the opportunity to file litigation against fraudsters at low cost. But whether that law would be effective in the field of medical services had been the subject of debate for a considerable period. Ultimately, the Supreme Court settled the controversy and ruled that medical negligence can be prosecuted under that act.[5] In fact, action was required to be taken against the corruption found in corporate hospitals. Doctors protested strongly against that law. They argued that the act treats medical services as a commodity like other commodities, something to be bought and sold in the market; under a privatized scheme, the relationship between the doctors and the patients would become that of a buyer and a seller. The doctors said that if that law comes into force, doctors would lose the courage to take the necessary risks to treat patients. For example, the patient would be required to undergo a computed tomography (CT) scan for a mild headache. As a result, patients would suffer physically as well as financially. This is what had happened over the following decades. Doctors are forced to resort to more costly treatment.

Corporate power has been able to subjugate doctors. Which is why common people can't trust doctors. They think doctors are representatives of corporate power. A recent publication *Dissenting Diagnosis*,[6] shows how both corporate hospitals and drug companies exploit people. A proportion of doctors have become the assistants of corporate power. Because of the actions of those doctors, the medical professionals began to lose their social respect. In 2022, in a Supreme Court case, an association of medical representatives alleged that Micro Labs Limited, the manufacturer of *Dolo 650* (a paracetamol drug), had given bribes of Rs. 1000 crores to doctors to promote their product. A patient in Kolkata, expressing frustration with private hospitals, remarked: "What the hospitals are doing is not to say...Once the injection is pushed and the bill is made three times. But we have to come here despite knowing the fact." This statement indicates the way in which the ordinary people are being forced to accept the dominance of corporate hegemony. For many people, limitations of the public health system leave few options but to turn to private providers, despite knowing the risks of exploitation. However, as explored in earlier chapters, people-led health movements across India have challenged these very conditions—mobilizing against corporate excesses and advocating for accessible, equitable health care.

The era of so-called 'techno-medicine' witnessed the emergence of the specialist physician concept in place of the family physician concept. Before the use of modern technology in the field of medicine, doctors used to diagnose diseases clinically based on their experience or through inspection, palpation, percussion, and auscultation (IPPA). The doctor had to spend a long time talking to the patient. With the introduction of advanced technology-based healthcare, however, the need for doctor–patient interaction has diminished to a great extent. Manu Kothari and Lopa A. Mehta have opined that in modern medicine "the doctor sees neither the disease nor the patient. All he sees is some enemies that must be destroyed at all cost."[7] Expensive pathological tests became essential in this technology-based health care. This modern dependence on technology has taken medical treatment beyond the reach of financially backward people. This techno-medicine is the main profit-making tool of medical businessmen. Many people fall below the poverty line to meet their medical expenses.

Unnecessary treatment skyrocketed after the implementation of the Rashtriya Swasthya Bima Yojana (RSBY) health insurance scheme. A survey[8] conducted on more than 12,000 households in four blocks of Birbhum district of West Bengal in 2012 found that among the diseases which led people to be admitted in the hospital in the previous year, the main ones were fever, typhoid, stomach ailments, diarrhoea, and malaria. In 2013, however, an analysis of more than 400 patients in those homes who were hospitalized under the health insurance card found that 90 per cent of the patients were hospitalized for undergoing surgeries. Cataract surgery was predominant, followed by hysterectomy. Eighteen of the 57 women who underwent hysterectomy were under the age of forty. Notably, doctors do not want to perform hysterectomies on women under the age of 50. But that was done for the interest of the private hospitals so that they can get the amount allocated on the operation in the health insurance scheme. Other major surgeries include gall-bladder excision, hernia-hydrocele, hemorrhoids and appendix, respectively. The fact is that removal of the uterus, appendix, and gall-bladder does not cause major damage to human health. Thus, private hospitals made profits by performing such surgeries under the health insurance card.[9] The owner of a private hospital in Uluberia (Howrah, WB) stated that "the insurance company paying for treatment of malaria and diarrhoea cannot cover the cost of medicines," so they chose this path to make a profit.[10] The gynecologist Sanjeev Mukherjee stated that, "A doctor in Kandi (Murshidabad, WB) claims to have cut off the uterus of 45 women in one month. How is it possible? In a general sense, a doctor cannot perform 45 hysterectomies in his entire medical life."[11] Not only West Bengal, but also other states witnessed similarly unethical incidents. It has been reported that, from 2011 to 2013, there were 5503 cases of hysterectomy out of a total of 14651 cases covered by health insurance in Samastipur, Bihar.[12] In addition, as the money allotted by health insurance companies for the treatment of specific diseases was insufficient according to the demands of private hospitals, patients had to pay out of their pocket to receive medical care there.[13]

Seamus O'Mahony, a gastroenterologist at Cork University Hospital, argues that the period from the mid-1930s to the mid-1980s marked the 'golden years' of medicine. According to him, the medical profession has been corrupted by the 'medical-industrial complex' since the 1980s. His opinion is that "patients, doctors and society at large are the victims, dupes and slaves of this medical–industrial complex."[14] Bishan Basu, an activist doctor, asserts that the doctors who serve as the primary agents of the profit-seeking private health care system are themselves subjected to severe exploitation. While the stock prices of corporate lords continue to increase, the salaries of doctors remain stagnant. Typically, doctors receive only

10–15 per cent of the medical expenses incurred by patients; in the context of various so-called public welfare initiatives (health insurance), their rightful share diminishes to a mere 4–5 per cent. Furthermore, their financial stability and employment are precarious, and they possess limited authority over the management of hospital operations.[15]

The book has unearthed the unethical practices related to medicine and analysed the movement for essential and rational drugs in a detailed manner, which was a major part of the health movement. That movement succeeded in achieving its goal to a great extent which shows the tremendous potential of the movement.

To attempt to understand the attitudes of society towards the world of health and medicine one can consider the literature and films which reflect this world and its impact on various aspects of human life. The privatization of health has been depicted in contemporary Bangla literature and cinema. To give an example we may refer to a novel written by Suchitra Bhattacharya. In her novel *Aleek Sukh*, a character named Dr. Kingshuk Guha, a gynecologist, was portrayed as a greedy doctor. The story tells us that on one occasion Kavita, a female character, was admitted to a private hospital under the supervision of Dr. Guha. But she died due to medical negligence. As a result, the patient's family vandalized the hospital and even beat up the doctors. Actually, Dr. Guha was a busy man because he had to attend five chambers, conduct three operations, and attend fifty patients a day. He could not spend any more time with his patients. Forgetting his Hippocratic Oath, he became a money-making physician. To him, the patient was just a 'case' and the patient's relatives were the 'patient party.' Everything was a commercial transaction. Thus, a patient from a lower middle-class family like Kavita had to die. On the one hand, this novel visualizes the invisible wall between the doctor and the patient; on the other, it shows how consumerism can create a rift in relationships. A film based on that novel, *Aleek Sukh*, directed by Nandita Roy and Shiboprosad Mukherjee, was released in 2013. Another cinematic offering, the movie *Siddhanta* (2022), directed by Parthasarathi Joardar, shows that people's mistrust of doctors has been increasing. The doctor has become a villain to the people. People beat the doctors. Thus, doctors are forced to go abroad. In that movie, doctors and family members of the doctors in real life played their own role in 'reel life.'

One of the demands of the junior doctors' movement in the 1980s was that the government should recruit doctors according to need. But the government did not do this. At that time, many doctors did not get government jobs and so they began to do private practice. The number of corporate hospitals also increased in the 1990s, attracting large numbers of doctors. Government hospitals remained deficient in infrastructure compared to requirements and patients were repeatedly deprived. They blamed doctors for this situation because medical staff work on the front line of the hospital system. Hence there was a tendency among doctors not to accept government jobs. In the 1980s, junior doctors demanded that government jobs should be given to them. Today, the government is of the opinion that the doctors are reluctant to join the government hospitals. This is a half-truth, however.

Despite the absence of proper infrastructure, a few doctors did excel in their work. One of them is Dr. Dilip Mahalanabis, the pioneering figure in inventing the Oral Rehydration Solution (ORS). Actually, when cholera struck many countries together as an epidemic in the 1970s, the WHO attempted to combat the crisis by sending massive amounts of intravenous saline. Yet transporting saline was expensive and the procedure was complex. Skilled workers were needed to inject the saline into vein. At that time, Dr. Mahalanabis was in charge of a health center at Bangaon refugee camp on the India–Bangladesh border. He was working on the development of ORS as a staff member of the Johns Hopkins Center for Medical Research and Training, Kolkata. There was a shortage of health workers in refugee camps. Accordingly, he started to feed ORS to patients. Previously, it had been kept in a drum, from which he, along with his fellow workers, fed the patients. It was the duty of the health workers to refill the drum when it was empty. The death rate was 20–30 per cent in centers when dehydration was treated only with intravenous saline. In Dr. Mahalanbish's camp, however, the death rate was roughly 3 per cent. During the Liberation War of Bangladesh in 1971, the refugees took shelter in refugee camps in West Bengal. A lack of drinking water and poor sanitation led to cholera epidemics in the camps. ORS was effective in fighting the epidemic in those camps. The ORS technology of Dr. Mahalanbish crossed the boundaries of the Indian subcontinent and was later recognized globally. According to the *Lancet*, ORS is the greatest medical invention of the last century. This kind of 'silver-lining' is certainly one of the significant events in the history of health movements.

This kind of improvement can also be noticed in the arena of mental health. In this context, we may mention that an effort has been made on the part of the government to increase people's awareness about such conditions. In a significant move towards building up this kind of awareness, a mental health fair was organized in January 2020 by the Institute of Psychiatry, Kolkata and SSKM Hospital. A number of stalls were made to serve the purpose. There was an arrangement to test mental health. The doctors gave people a range of advice about ways to keep their minds in good condition. Prominent psychiatrists from Kolkata were also present. The aim of that four-day program was to bring the so-called mentally sick people back to a healthy life. Institutions such as AIIMS (Delhi), PGI-Chandigarh, Nimhans of Bengaluru, and JIPMAR of Pondicherry also participated in the fair, along with all of the mental hospitals and the psychiatry departments of the medical colleges based in the state. Significantly, in 2019 an effort was made by artists to introduce the inmates of the Pavlov Hospital to the world of creativity. A long workshop in this regard under the leadership of noted artist Srikanta Pal was a fruitful one. The so-called mental patients showed their creativity and the exhibition, which showcased their creative talent, was widely praised. It should also be noted that there was a sincere initiative to bring the cured mental patients into the mainstream of the society. In this regard, the initiative of the Election Commission of India deserved special mention. It permitted the cured mental patients to cast their votes in the parliamentary election of 2019.[16] These kinds of efforts are also part of the health movement.

Basically, the health movement is a right movement. It is the right of the people to get the health service as well as to have a living condition where physical, mental, and social wellbeing can be ensured. The health movement is working to make this dream a reality. Its aim is to march towards a better world. This notion of 'better world' means "where no one faces bankruptcy or poverty resulting from catastrophic illness or injury, where no impoverished person dies unnecessarily due to lack of care; a world in which patients and doctors make decisions about individual health care, not insurance companies, in which the decisions rest on medical necessity and medical appropriateness, not profits or spending limits."[17] It is the dream of a world where "the health care system supports comprehensive prevention services, from nutrition education to smoking cessation programmes to immunizations and much more, thus averting the onset of disease and preventing both untold human suffering and economic drain on the health care system and the economy overall."[18] Basically, the activists of the health movement work to fulfil this goal. In other words, these dreams inspire them to fight to achieve a world where everyone should be assured of their wellbeing.

The history of the health movement is not a chronicle of more failures and less success. It is a significant movement to ensure equity and equality. It can be termed as an important addition to the genre of new social movements. The history of the health movement, specifically in the area of West Bengal, has shown its tremendous potential, which has made this right movement a significant one. Despite its limitations, there are many success stories of the people's health movement. I would like to focus on some recent ones. The health movement, working as a pressure group, has forced the state to implement patient-oriented regulation. For example, the legal process, along with constant support from research and media advocacy led by civil society organizations like the All India Drug Action Network (AIDAN) and the Alliance of Doctors for Ethical Healthcare (ADEH), prompted the Department of Pharmaceuticals and the National Pharmaceutical Pricing Authority (NPPA) to regulate the prices of cardiac stents (February 2017).[19] Abhay Shukla et al. have pointed out that "the family of patient-victim Adya Singh, who tragically lost her life after treatment in a large corporate hospital accompanied by grossly inflated bills (September 2017), has started an organization called All India Patients' Right Group. Such voices are strengthening the impetus for regulation of the private health-care sector in India."[20] The health activists mobilized people to fight for the right to health and exposed abuses and corruption in the health sector, both public and private. In August 2024, after the brutal rape and murder of a female doctor (Abhaya) at the state-run R.G. Kar Medical College and Hospital in Kolkata, which exposes the failure of state to secure right to life and health of women in her 'secured' workplace, a movement for justice spread across the country, attracting people from different domains. *The West Bengal Junior Doctors' Front* (WBJDF) has been formed to address different issues such as inadequate infrastructure, patient care issues, and levels of security in state-run hospitals. 'Reclaim the Night' protests demanding 'Justice for Abhaya' and safety for women in the workplace hit the streets of West Bengal. The state government brought the 'Aparajita Bill' in the legislative assembly with the intention of enhancing security for women. However, this initiative has been met with criticism from women, who described it as being an 'ironic' measure. In October, an umbrella organization, called 'Abhaya Mancha,' was also formed with the combination of about 80 organizations from civil society. The slogan adopted by Abhaya Mancha was 'Long live the unity of doctors, health workers and people.' It has been found that the movement, which started as a doctors' protest, later turned into a mass movement. A press release from the WBJDF, dated 25 September 2024, stated that "'justice for Abhaya' is not just a movement of RG Kar Medical College or junior doctors; it has truly transformed into a comprehensive mass movement." Indeed, people protested and campaigned in an united fashion against medical malpractices, 'threat culture' in the health administration, and health syndicates. As a consequence, the government of West Bengal has been compelled to accept many of the demands raised by junior doctors. We may refer to this as a great success for the people's health movement. The recent movement in West Bengal advocating against injustice serves as a significant illustration of solidarity.

Paul Farmer has argued that structural violence, a type of violence which happens when people are deprived of basic rights due to social institutions or structures, limits the realization of civil rights; civil rights cannot be secured in the absence of protection of social and economic rights. According to him, new fields of health and human rights have emerged, in the wake of globalization, such as increasing inequality. In this new world-system people are deprived of the right to health. He argues: "it is time to take health rights as seriously as other human rights, and that intellectual recognition is only a necessary first step toward pragmatic solidarity, that is, toward taking a stand by the side of those who suffer most from an increasingly harsh 'new world order'."[21]

II

In the context of LPG, the journey towards a better world has been a major challenge for the health movement. Thus, it may appear that it is impossible for health activists to overcome the health crisis posed by the capitalist model and to continue to struggle against inequality and inequity. However, it should be borne in mind that, in the struggle for social and economic justice, the health movement does not stand alone. There are many social movements working with rights-based approaches at local, regional, national, and global levels. History shows that these movements criticized injustice, corruption, and 'predatory inequities of neoliberal globalization,' and forced the state to implement reforms. Departure from earlier Nehruvian welfarist commitments[22] by the post-liberalization Indian state signalled the "farewell to welfare state"[23] which necessitated the movement of the people. This kind of grassroots mobilization is seen particularly in the area of health, the focus of this book. So, we may try to bring out a systematic critical analysis of the various social movements operating in India. We may analyse social movements of other countries, where despite different ideological stands and lineages, movements came together to fight joint struggles against the larger forces of social, political and economic oppressions.

According to Paul Wilkinson, "A social movement is a deliberate collective endeavour to promote change in any direction and by any means, not excluding violence, illegality, revolution or withdrawal into 'utopian' community…A social movement must evince a minimal degree of organization, though this may range from a loose, informal or partial level of organization to the highly institutionalized and bureaucratized movement and the corporate group."[24] The term 'social movement' has been used in this context to refer to a formal and informal alliance of people, groups, and networks that adhere to a common set of objectives, theories, and commitments and who communicate and work together in different ways to accomplish those objectives. Our focus is on progressive social movements, which promote issues such as ecological sustainability, social, economic, and gender equity, and also combat discrimination.

We may begin with a discussion of what can retrospectively be understood as the human rights movement in India, which has a significant history. The *Indian Civil Liberties Union* (ICLU) was formed in Bombay in 1936. Its titular president was Rabindranath Tagore, and Sarojini Naidu served as the working president. As general secretary, K.B. Menon took charge. Within a short period of time, branches of the ICLU had been formed in Calcutta, Madras, and Punjab. The ICLU lodged protests against the oppression of people not only by the British Raj, but also by the rulers of the princely states.[25] Although the modern vocabulary of 'human rights' gained prominence after World War II, the ICLU's work reflected early articulations of rights-based claims and civil liberties. After India gained its independence, the people yearned that the state would fulfil all of their needs, including the basic ones of food, clothing, and shelter, as well as the rights and justice that had eluded them during the two centuries of colonial rule. But the post-colonial state persisted in violating these rights in a similar way to its colonial predecessor. As a result, movement also continued through various phases and under different regimes. To reorganize the civil rights movement, the Communists took the initiative. They were able to get the support of well-known intellectuals such as Meghnad Saha, K.P. Chattopadhyay, Sarat Bose, and N.C. Chatterjee. In order to protest against the state's persecution of Communists, the *Civil Liberties Committee* was established in West Bengal in 1948. In the same year, on 10 December, the *Universal Declaration of Human Rights* was adopted by United Nations General Assembly. Since the late 1960s, due to militant people's movements led by the Maoists (Naxalites), there had been great turmoil throughout the nation. As usual, the state responded by repressing its citizens. Additionally, during that time, the first civil rights organizations were founded in West Bengal and Andhra Pradesh, states where both militancy and repression were commonplace. Thus, in Calcutta, the *Association for the Protection of Democratic Rights* (APDR) was formed in 1972. Liberal intellectuals such as Kapil Bhattacharya, Amiya Bose, and Promode Sengupta were associated with the APDR. With the active participation of progressive writers like Sri Sri and Cherabandu Raju, the *Andhra Pradesh Civil Liberties Committee* (APCLC) was established in 1974.[26]

In 1972, J. P. Narayan, V. M. Tarkunde, a retired judge from the Bombay High Court, and others close to the Gandhian movement began to meet to discuss their worries about Prime Minister Indira Gandhi's centralized authority. They established groups in Delhi, Madras, Bombay, and Calcutta before coming together in Delhi in April 1974 to establish *Citizens for Democracy* (CFD), a nation-wide organization. On 25 June 1975, Indira Gandhi imposed national emergency and basic rights of Indian people were withdrawn, which gave momentum to the civil rights movement.[27] The declaration of a "Total Revolution" by Jayaprakash Narayan against the misrule in Bihar and the Union government played a leading role in building up the country's human rights movement.[28] Jayaprakash Narayan said that the people have the right to protest against any government if it fails to perform its duties. He placed a greater focus on the power of the people. According to him, people associated with the mass movement should not be associated with any political party.[29] The Naxalite movement and JP's movement shared many similarities. In 1976, the *People's Union for Civil Liberties and Democratic Rights* (PUCL & PUDR) was founded by Jayprakash Narayan. Branches of the organization were set up in different states of India. But it soon split into the two organizations, known as PUCL and PUDR. The main point of contention between the two bodies was ideological.[30]

The PUCL was not particularly active between March 1977 and July 1979, when the Janata government was in power. In 1980, Indira Gandhi returned to power and enacted potentially oppressive laws such as the *National Security Ordinance* (subsequently the *National Security Act* [NSA], reinstating preventive detention). At this point, Justice Tarkunde and others decided to revitalize the PUCL by turning it into a mass membership organization. As a result, on November 22–23, 1980, they held an All India Civil Liberties Conference in New Delhi.[31] Other regional organizations working on human rights since the 1980s were the *Committee for the Protection of Democratic Rights* (CPDR) (established in 1977) in Maharashtra, the Association for Democratic Rights (AFDR) (1978) in Punjab, the *Naga People's Movement for Human Rights* in Nagaland (1978), *Lok Adhikar Sangh* in Gujarat (1977), and *Citizens for Democracy* in Delhi, Mumbai, and other places.[32]

This people's right was an important issue in the environmental movements in India. One of the early and successful environmental movements was the Silent Valley movement, which aimed to save a subtropical forest in the Palakkad district of Kerala. In the 1970s, the government of Kerala took initiatives to construct a dam on Kunthipuzha River, also known as the Silent Valley Project, with the aim of generating hydroelectricity to expedite industrialization. The government argued that the Silent Valley Hydroelectric Project would create job opportunities and drive regional economic development. However, environmentalists drew people's attention to the adverse ecological impact on the Silent Valley. According to them, if the project was built, that evergreen subtropical forest would be harmed and several species of animals which had evolved over millions of years would become extinct. Thus, *Kerala Sasthra Sahithya Parishad* (KSSP), a 'science-for-the-people' organization, started the *Save Silent Valley Movement* in collaboration with wildlife conservationists.[33] A booklet, *The Silent Valley Movement Hydroelectric Project: A techno-economic and socio-political assessment*, was published by KSSP. In that project, however, there was no local people's involvement as there had been no displacement of people. The movement was fought primarily on environmental grounds, and mostly at the intellectual level.[34] Finally, the government was forced to abandon the project in 1983 under the pressure of the movement. The Silent Valley forests were declared a National Park in 1984.

Similarly, the *Chipko* movement was begun to protect the people's rights over natural resources. The Forest Department of the state government (Uttar Pradesh) auctioned hornbeam trees in the Garhwal region of the Himalayas to an Allahabad-based sport goods company, *Symonds*, for them to manufacture cricket bats and tennis rackets. This was an injustice for the rural people who depended on those forests for their subsistence. The people of Dasholi village stopped a group of loggers, who came on behalf of the company, from felling trees. Due to people's protest, laborers for the contractor were forced to go back. Those women saved a large number of trees. The subaltern people stood against the elite and state. After that, the government abandoned the contract system of felling and set up the *Uttar Pradesh Forest Corporation.*[35] Thus began the *Chipko* movement. This movement later spread to other parts of Garhwal region and India. Two well-known leaders of the *Chipko* movement were Chandiprsad Bhat and Sundarlal Bahuguna, who believed in nonviolent Gandhian methods of protest. Ramachandra Guha stated that "*Chipko* was representative of a wide spectrum of natural-resource conflicts that erupted in different parts of India in the 1970s and 1980s: conflicts over access to forests, fish and grazing resources; conflicts over the effects of industrial pollution and mining; and conflicts over the siting of large dams."[36]

Narmada Bachao Andolan (Movement to Save the Narmada) was formed against the building of a number of big dams along the Narmada River. The *Narmada Valley Development Project* included 30 large dams, 133 medium-sized dams, and 3000 small dams across the Narmada River. In 1979, the project plan appeared. One of the big dams of the project was the *Sardar Sarovar* dam in Bharuch district of Gujarat. The people living in its 'submergence zone' first came to know about the project when surveyors started arriving in the villages in 1985. In that year the *World Bank* sanctioned a loan of $450 million to build the *Sardar Sarovar* mega-dam. After getting information on the extent of displacement, the people opposed the displacement and questioned the projects' claim to 'public purpose'. "The Narmada Bachao Andolan (NBA), the first people movement to evict the World Bank, must fight not only for rights over economy, environment, and livelihood, but also for personhood, for humanity itself."[37] Arundhati Roy wrote "Big Dams are to a Nation's 'Development' what Nuclear Bombs are to its Military Arsenal. They are both weapons of mass destruction. They're both weapons Governments use to control their own people. Both Twentieth Century emblems that mark a point in time when human intelligence has outstripped its own instinct for survival."[38] Other organizations joined the NBA. In 1989, 50,000 people gathered at the Narmada Valley to protest against the project.[39] Under the leadership of Medha Patkar and Baba Amte, that movement became larger. The agitators demanded an appropriate resettlement and rehabilitation for the displaced people.

In 1984, the Bhopal disaster left thousands either dead or sick. Within the first week of the accident, about 30 people, with varying Leftist persuasions, gathered in two groups to form two organizations: the *Nagarik Rahat Aur Punarvas Committee* (NRPC) and the *Zahreeli Gas Kand Sangharsh Morcha* (ZGKSM).[40] In the wake of the Bhopal disaster, an environmental movement was formed across the nation under the banner of the *No More Bhopal Committee*, which emphasized the right of people to live in a pollution-free environment. Under pressure from that movement, the *Environment (Protection) Act, 1986* was enacted by the Indian parliament. It was an umbrella act under which all the different rules and regulations related to the environment were combined. Therefore, this act has become a crucial weapon of all environmental movements in the country. India has also witnessed a people's movement against the construction of nuclear power plants.[41]

I have tried to mention some major environmental movements which were formed by the people of different regions of India to protect the environment, their lives, and subsistence. They struggled for the rights to natural resources. In this ground, Indian environmental movements differed from those in the West. In India, these movements were linked to social justice. In their book[42] Madhav Gadgil and Ramachandra Guha divided the Indian population into three broad groups from socio-ecological point of view. These three groups were "omnivores, ecological refugees and ecosystem people." 'Omnivores' were elite people who reaped the benefits of all development policies. 'Ecological refugees' were displaced peasants and tribal peoples whose land was taken for development purposes. The last group, 'ecosystem people,' were those who depended on the natural environment for their livelihood. State policy negatively affected ecological refugees and ecosystem people. As a result, the movement for 'environmental equity' and 'environmental justice' was organized in India.

I have pointed out that the women were the important participants in the environmental movements of India. Their participation in those movements was no exception. Basically, the women's movement in India had been begun in the nineteenth century by mainly male reformers educated in Western education, where some exceptional women expressed their feelings through their writings. However, a new dimension was added when the women came to the forefront of the movement. In the last quarter of the twentieth century, India witnessed a real feminist movement, which is known as the contemporary women's movement.

From the late 1970s, women's organizations in India began to blame patriarchy for the plight of women, which led to an alignment of that movement with the global women's movement. By the late 1970s, India saw the emergence of independent women's organizations, which dealt with women's issues from a completely different perspective. After the state of emergency (1975–1977), various autonomous women's groups were set up all over the country, but mainly in the major cities. As Radha Kumar stated that "The distinguishing features of the new women's groups were that they declared themselves to be 'feminist' despite the fact that most of their members were drawn from the Left; that they insisted on being autonomous even though most of their members were affiliated with other political groups, generally of the far Left; and that they rapidly built networks among one another, ideological differences notwithstanding."[43]

According to Vibhuti Patel, the autonomous women's movement in India in the late 1970s and 1980s had three main characteristics. First, it was organized and run by the women and for the women. Second, those organizations worked to end the discrimination, exploitation, and oppression of women. Third, no political or social group or organization could command the autonomous women's movement to act in accordance with its decisions and necessities.[44] One such organization was *Saheli*,[45] founded in 1981 in New Delhi, which worked for women's rights and empowerment. *Saheli* launched campaigns against domestic violence, dowry, and so on.

The contemporary women's movement evolved from issue-based groups into distinct organizational identities. The women's health movement in India also began to grow in the 1980s. According to C. Sathyamala, there were two distinct streams of consciousness. One was the independent, non-partisan women's movement of the late 1970s, which was primarily made up of educated women from the middle class. The second one was the liberal stream from the voluntary health sector, which attempted to shed its missionary, white and colonial image to gain a secular pro-people foothold. The Western women's health movement, which was a subset of the larger women's liberation movement, had a distinct influence on both of these streams. While the Western and Indian women's movements shared a similar ideology, the Indian one developed its own unique understanding and, consequently, perspective on health issues concerning women of India.[46] Organizations like *Stree Shakti Sangathana* (formed in the late 1970s in Hyderabad) and *Saheli* began to work with women's health issues. They also continued their legal battles. The *Medico Friends' Circle* and the *Voluntary Health Association of India* worked closely with women's organizations in campaigns against harmful pregnancy testing, contraceptive drugs, and other health issues that affected women. There has also been a movement demanding justice for rape survivors. Organizations such as the Center for Enquiry into Health and Allied Themes (CEHAT) drew attention to the insensitive practices in the health sector. These groups, in particular, campaigned against the use of unscientific and anti-women practices within forensic medicine, such as the use of the two-finger test—which was wrongly used to determine a survivor's virginity status and assess her past sexual history.[47]

The queer and LGBT (Lesbian-gay-bisexual-transsexual) movement also started to take shape gradually in the 1990s.[48] A group striving towards a just, sustainable and egalitarian society formed *National Alliance of People's Movements* (NAPM) in 1992. It was an Indian coalition of progressive people's organizations and movements. The NAPM struggled against the hegemonic and exploitative policies associated with neo-liberalism.[49]

Another movement deserves special mention that is associated with the people's right to food. West Bengal witnessed two important food movements held in 1959 and 1966. Those were led by the Left parties against the then Congress-led West Bengal state government.[50] However, the Right to Food movement was started in 2001 on a national basis. *The Right to Food Campaign* (RFC), as its foundation statement states, is "an informal network of organisations and individuals committed to the realisation of the right to food in India."[51] The RFC formed a large network. It was composed of 16 national organizations, including women's organizations, labor unions, law networks representing minority communities, farmers' rights organizations, and other human rights organizations, as well as 16 subnational campaign representatives.[52] RFC asserted that "everyone has a fundamental right to be free from hunger and under-nutrition."[53]

The Right to Food Campaign in India began its journey in 2001. According to Vivek Srinivasan and Sudha Narayana, "It was a time of absurd paradox. Even as the food grain stocks held by the government rose to 50 million metric tons, several parts of the country were reeling from a third consecutive year of drought. The threat of severe hunger loomed large, yet efforts to address this threat were insufficient."[54] In this context, in April 2001a writ petition was filed in the Supreme Court of India by the *People's Union for Civil Liberties*, a civil society group based in the north Indian state of Rajasthan. The petition demanded that the country's huge food stocks should be used without delay to protect people from starvation.[55] It was commonly referred to as the 'Right to Food Case.' More than fifty orders were issued from time to time, including some of the most significant, such as universalizing school midday meals and the supplementary nutrition program for children under the age of six, pregnant and lactating mothers, and adolescent girls. Though some of those orders were ground-breaking in their content, it was quickly understood that putting them into action on the ground required people's pressure. As a result of the Supreme Court orders, various groups gathered together to set up the Right to Food campaign. Very quickly, the focus shifted from the Supreme Court case to the development of a larger public campaign for the right to food.[56]

The RFC was operated by a steering committee composed of representatives from national organizations and subnational activists. Among the steering committee members of the RFC were the *National Federation of Indian Women* (NFIW), the *Human Rights Law Network* (HRLN), the *People's Union for Civil Liberties* (PUCL), the *National Alliance of People's Movements* (NAPM), *Jan Swasthya Abhiyaan* (JSA), the *National Campaign for People's Right to Information* (NCPRI), *Bhartiya Gyan Vigyaan Samiti* (BGVS), the *National Campaign Committee for Unorganized Sector Workers* (NCC-USW), the *National Campaign for Dalit Human Rights* (NCDHR), the *National Confederation of Dalit Organisations* (NACDOR), the *New Trade Union Initiative* (NTUI), and the *Breastfeeding Promotion Network of India* (BPNI).[57] The first and second National Conventions on the 'Right to Food and Work' were held in Bhopal (Madhya Pradesh) (2004) and Kolkata (2005), respectively. The third was held in Bodhgaya (Bihar) on April 6–8, 2007, seeing participation from by over 800 people from 22 states, including representatives from national-level civil society organizations and networks, non-governmental organizations, village-level grassroots organizations, students, and other interested people. The Convention was attended by representatives from more than twenty states. During the three-day convention, a wide range of issues were discussed, including the *National Rural Employment Guarantee Act* (NREGA), the *Public Distribution System* (PDS), children's right to food, social exclusion, unorganized sector workers, deaths from hunger, the agrarian crisis, struggles for the right to food, and so on.[58]

RFC developed pamphlets, primers, and booklets for the grassroots organizations. It conducted field surveys on the status of hunger and starvation. RFC mobilized people for the struggle for subsistence rights. Funds were received from individual activists or participating organizations in the campaign. It did not accept funds from donor agencies.

RFC demanded a comprehensive law for food rights. In the election manifesto in 2009, the *Indian National Congress* promised to introduce a food security act. After coming to power, the Congress-led UPA government declared that the issue would be one of its priorities. Subsequently, a debate was continued about the bill on the streets and the floor of parliament. In an attempt to create pressure on the government, RFC also launched a number of protests and rallies in support of a comprehensive law. At the same time, several activists from RFC were offered membership in the *National Advisory Council*, which had been formed to monitor and develop the act. Finally, the *National Food Security Act* (NFSA) was enacted in 2013. This was the result of a long struggle against hunger and malnutrition. However, many demands of RFC were not met in the NFSA, particularly those concerning the "universalization of all entitlements, an independent grievance redressal mechanism, farmer's rights, agriculture, land, and water." But it is noteworthy that the RFC has been fighting for the right to food 'from the courts to the streets' for a long time.[59]

III

From India, let us move to the other parts of the globe. The Alternative Globalization Movement (AGM) and other very significant social movements in several countries emerged in the 1980s. The health movement may be best compared to a part of these AGMs, which, as a major collective force, emerged as a protest against the structural adjustment policies of the *World Bank* and the *International Monetary Fund* (IMF) within the developing world in the 1980s. The AGM is constituted by a vast network of groups and movements, including: indigenous peoples; human rights and ecology advocates; anarchists, socialists, and communists; NGO, interfaith and trade union activists; and many other left-leaning groups and individuals.[60] Its roots can be traced back to the 1970s' anti-IMF riots in Peru, Liberia, Ghana, Jamaica, and Egypt. The 'bread riots' were one such example. Bread is a major staple in the Egyptian diet; however, due to trade policies imposed by the U.S. and the IMF against food subsidies, the price of bread increased sharply. Therefore, Egyptians staged a protest.[61]

By the late 1990s, several Latin American countries were gripped by economic crises, which were accompanied by major corruption scandals. During that time, there was also an increase in social struggles and movements. These included the *Caracazo* of 1989, a protest movement against price hikes in Venezuela; the struggles in Cochabamba and El Alto in Bolivia against the privatization of water and gas; the Landless Workers' Movement in Brazil, which took over land from large plantation owners; the indigenous peasant uprising by the Zapatista National Liberation Army in Mexico; and large indigenous struggles in Ecuador.[62] In Chiapas, a state of Mexico, the Zapatistas' struggle started in 1994 against the *North Atlantic Free Trade Agreement* (NAFTA), which would adversely affect indigenous population. The Zapatista National Liberation Army (ZNLA) seized four areas of Chiapas. This people's movement was in favor of freedom, democracy, and justice. This social movement was a 'glocal' one to the neo-liberal world order.[63] These struggles spawned new political and social movements. Several progressive governments have replaced neo-liberal governments in Latin America since the turn of the millennium. In many of these countries, new forms of the 'welfare state,' based on social rights and citizenship, began to emerge.

Members of the Alternative Globalization Movement formed the *World Social Forum* (WSF) in 2001, asserting that 'another world is possible.'[64] The WSF provided a global platform for civil society organizations and people's movements to share their ideas and formulate alternatives to the dominant economic and development policies.[65] The WSF process is the most important manifestation of contemporary global justice movements (GJMs).[66] The first conference of the WSF was held in Brazil in 2001. The fourth conference of WSF was held in Mumbai, India, from January 16 to 21, 2004. The *Jan Swasthya Abhiyan* (JSA) took part in the proceedings. In January 2003, during the *Asian Social Forum* (ASF), held at Hyderabad, the constituent organizations of JSA conducted several workshops/seminars on key health issues with facilitation by JSA. ASF emerged out of WSF. Similarly, the *India Social Forum* (ISF), held in Delhi from November 9 to 13, 2006, was the Indian chapter of the WSF. The ISF was attended by thousands of people who discussed various subjects such as migratory labor, environment, displacement, women trafficking, children's rights, special economic zones, and issues of gender, sexuality, trans-sexuality, sex workers, and so on. More than 400 programs were held at the ISF, the majority of which were arranged by various organizations, with only 25 programs run directly by WSF India. A large number of participants from Africa, Asia, and South Asia were present at the ISF.[67]

Cassandra Mines' assets and mining concessions, in north-east Halkidiki, Greece, were sold to Hellas Gold S.A. Company in December 2003. The mining plan in the area was approved by the Greek state in July 2011. The selling of the mining concessions to Hellas Gold S.A. was a clear transfer of public assets for private profit. The proposed project would have extremely serious and far-reaching environmental consequences on local communities and have adverse impacts on the local economy. As a result, a popular and sustained struggle against the mining contract was developed in the region. Similar struggles against neoliberal economic projects and corporate exploitation emerged across the world in the following years. People in the area were mobilized in large numbers as a result of the conflict. Campaigns were launched to inform people about the impending threats created by the mining company. Several demonstrations occurred in regional cities and dwellings higher up in the mountains. The popular struggle in Halkidiki was constantly attacked by police. Three large protests in the Kakkavos Mountain in 2012 (in August, September, and October) were attacked with extreme violence by the police. The government attempted to use different strategies to curb the movement. In Halkidiki, the movement included peaceful people with various ideologies. Various parliamentary and non-parliamentary parties, political institutions, Canadian politicians, and European social and political organizations all supported that movement. The participation of thousands of people in demonstrations and other public activities evidenced the strength of the movement. Women played a crucial role in this social movement. They fought for the conservation of the environment, justice, and human rights.[68]

The above suggests that it is evident that a strong pro-democracy social movement was developed by civil society when an oppressive social, political, and economic environment emerged.

IV

These popular protests and resistances against the multipronged attacks of neo-liberalism have raised the possibility of undermining the power of rulers of the Indian state based on neo-liberalism. Therefore, the rulers have also undertaken some so-called social welfare schemes within neo-liberalism in order to pacify all of this resistance and protest, and also to hide the horrors of the system.[69] The application of such kinds of so-called welfare schemes in the sphere of health care (*Ayushman Bharat*, *Swasthya*

Sathi) has also been seen in recent times. But it is important to bear in mind that medical insurance schemes are not for the veritable welfare of the people. The government seeks to project its philanthropic image by launching such schemes. In other words, due to 'pressure from below,' the Indian government has been actively pursuing 'hegemonic,' 'dominant,' and 'market-oriented' policies while articulating community health discourses. Applying Polanyi's theory, state health policy might be described as a 'double movement,' According to him, a movement from [the] below to attenuate its seriously dislocating effects is compelled when the state attempts to construct a market-oriented society from [the] above. In short, the state veers between efforts to limit market expansion and countermovement to do so. According to Polanyi, a 'dual shift' in state policy, a combination of aggressive intervention to extend the play of market forces and expanded social protection, to relieve the hardship of those displaced by the market is necessary to create a market economy.[70]

It is true that the government of India has launched some limited welfare health programs. For example, the National Rural Health Mission (NRHM) offered financial support to states and union territories. It should be kept in mind, however, that the NRHM was launched in April 2005 to address significant criticism concerning the performance of the public health system in India. NRHM focused on community participation and action in the health system, following the *Mitanin* program launched in Chhattisgarh in 2002. *Mitanin* was a rights-based approach to health care. However, the renewed interest in health as public good and rights-based approaches to health care in India faced challenges due to the limits on public health financing, political neglect, and private sector dominance in health care. According to June Sekera, "public goods are goods and services that are supplied through non-market, public production. i.e., they are: a. created through collective choice, b. paid for collectively, and c. supplied without charge (or below cost) to recipients."[71] However, in 2018, Rajiv Kumar, the vice chairman of NITI Aayog, asserted that the National Health Protection Mission (Modicare) would expand private health care markets and promote the development of the private health sector, particularly in tier 3 and tier 4 towns, thereby making health care more affordable.[72] Health movement advocates for the detachment of health care from the marketplace, emphasizing that it should be regarded as a public good.

History tells us that youth played a rigorous role in the social movements. Youth-formed social movements were provoked by social deprivation and injustice. Sasha Costanza-Chock stated "young people are key actors in powerful social movements that transform the course of human history. Indeed, youth have been deeply important to every progressive social movement, including the *United States Civil Rights movement*, the transnational LGBTQ movement, successive waves of feminism, environmentalism and environmental justice, the labour, anti-war, and immigrant rights movements, and more."[73]

The youthfulness of the movement should also be mentioned. In the second and third decades of nineteenth-century Bengal, a group of youth, known as *Young Calcutta*, rebelled against the prevailing social orthodoxy. According to Binay Ghosh, it was not a student movement with specific demands for the students. It was, rather, a 'youth revolt' against the basic policy and structure of society. The rebellion of the *Young Calcutta* group was the first youth rebellion in modern India.[74] Young people have also made significant contributions to social service work. In this context, we can mention the works of *Red Volunteers* in West Bengal during 2020–2021, and the period of state-imposed lockdown caused by COVID-19. So, our argument is that, in the creation of a *more equitable, just, and caring world*, as declared at the Fourth People's Health Assembly (PHA 4) held in Savar, Bangladesh, in November 2018,[75] youth participation is crucial. As far as the health movement in West Bengal is concerned, it had been first organized by medical students and junior doctors, who believed in Left ideology.

Now the question arises, what are the future pathways of the health movement? To build a better world there was a need to develop a more effective and broad-based social movement, which was recognized by the third *People's Health Assembly* (PHA 3) held in Cape Town, South Africa, in 2012. To this end, the *People's Health Movement* committed, in a document titled *Cape Town Call to Action*, "to building alliances with others who seek progressive and transformative change, including movements of informal and formal sector workers, the landless, indigenous peoples, women and youth, those struggling against big dams, nuclear power plants, dangerous mining and hazardous working conditions."[76] Thus, solidarity should be the main focus of the health movement. We may state, in the words of noted Indian poet Shankha Ghosh,

Aay Aaro Haate Haat Rekhe
Aay Aaro Bendhe Bendhe Thaaki[77]

(Let us hold more hands on hand, let us live a little closer, tied together).

Notes

1. Sudeb Raychaudhuri, "Hal Eki, Oshudher Abhab, X-ray ECG Jantra Achal", *Anandabazar Patrika*, Kolkata, July 5, 1983.
2. Nilotpal Biswas, "Trolley Nei, Kole Chepei Outdoorer Pathe Rogi", *Anandabazar Patrika*, Kolkata, July 19, 2022, p. 12; Aryabhatta Khan, "Hearter Rogir ECG-r Tarikh Pete Der Mas!", *Anandabazar Patrika*, Kolkata, July 20, 2022, p. 10; Chandan Biswas, "Purano Rog Niyei Rutan N.R.Se", *Anandabazar Patrika*, Kolkata, July 21, 2022, p. 10; Nijaswa Sangbaddata, "Chikitsak Aar Oshudher Ghatti Niye Chalchhe Medical", *Anandabazar Patrika*, Kolkata, July 22, 2022, p. 11.
3. Purendra Prasad, "State and Health Markets in the Time of Pandemic", *Economic and Political Weekly*, Vol. LVII, No. 23, June 4, 2022, p. 42.
4. https://www.icj.org/indian-government-fails-to-protect-right-to-life-and-health-in-second-wave-of-covid-19-pandemic/#:~:text=Since%2015%20April%20India%20has,mask%20wearing%20and%20social%20distancing., retrieved on November 5, 2024.
5. Sujit Kumar Das, *Daktar Banam Rogi: Bhokta Suraksha Aain 1986*, Kolkata: Drug Action Forum, 1995, pp. 1–12.
6. Arun Gadre and Abhay Shukla, *Dissenting Diagnosis*, Gurgaon: Penguin Random House, 2016.
7. Manu L. Kothari and Lopa A. Mehta, "Violence in Modern Medicine", in Ashis Nandy (ed.), *Science, Hegemony and Violence: A Requiem for Modernity,* New Delhi: Oxford University Press, 1990, pp. 167–210.
8. Paper presented by Sumit Majumder and Anamitra Barik at a workshop on People's Health and Public Policy at Institute of Development Studies Kolkata on July 17–18, 2014.
9. Swati Bhattacharya, "Ekhane Sastay Jarayu Bad Deoya Hay", *Anandabazar Patrika*, September 4, 2014, p. 4. (This article has also been incorporated in Abhijit Vinayak Bandyopadhyay and Swati Bhattacharya, *Bikalpa Biplab: Jebhabe Daridra Kamano Sambhab*, Kolkata: Ananda Publishers, 2019, pp. 69–70.)
10. Ibid., p. 71.
11. Ibid.
12. Ibid.
13. Speech of Biswajit Mitra in a panel discussion on pros and cons of health insurance organized by Doctors' Dialogue and Pranati Publishers at Subarna Banik Samaj Hall, Kolkata on February 21, 2022.
14. Seamus O'Mahony, *Can Medicine Be Cured?*, London: Head of Zeus, 2019, p. 14.
15. Bishan Basu, *Kine Ana Swasthya*, Kolkata: Dhansere, 2020.

16. Shiv Sahay Singh, "Raising Their Spirits with Hard-Won Voter id Cards", in *The Hindu*, February 16, 2019, https://www.thehindu.com/news/national/other-states/raising-their-spirits-with-hard-won-voter-id-cards/article26292535.ece, retrieved on August 28, 2022.
17. Jennifer Prah Ruger, *Health and Social Justice*, Oxford: Oxford University Press, 2009, p. x.
18. Ibid.
19. Abhay Shukla, "Healthcare Corruption: Responses from People's Health Movements", in Samiran Nundy et al. (eds.), *Healer or Predators?: Healthcare Corruption in India*, New Delhi: Oxford University Press, pp. 479–498.
20. Abhay Shukla et al., "People's over Profits: Reshaping India's Private Health Care", in Ritu Priya and Syeda Hameed (eds.), *Dreams of a Healthy India*, Gurugram: Penguin, 2023, pp. 175–192.
21. Paul Farmer, *Pathologies of Power*, Berkeley/Los Angeles/London: University of California Press, 2003, p. 246.
22. Aditya Mukherjee, *Nehru's India: Past, Present and Future*, New Delhi: Penguin Books India PVT, Limited, 2024.
23. S. Mohammed Irshad, *Farewell to Welfare State: NITI Aayog, Demonetisation and GST*, Kolkata: Setu Prakashani, 2019.
24. Paul Wilkinson, *Social Movement*, London: Pall Mall Press Ltd, 1971, p. 27.
25. Nilanjan Dutta, "From Subject to Citizen: Towards a History of the Indian Civil Rights Movement", in Michael R. Anderson and Sumit Guha (eds.), *Changing Concepts of Rights and Justice in South Asia*, Delhi: Oxford University Press, 1998, pp. 275–288.
26. Sabyasachi Chatterjee, "Nobel Peace Prize 2022: Fight for Rights is Awarded", *Science and Culture*, Vol. 88, No. 11–12, November–December, 2022, pp. 441–442.
27. Barnett R. Rubin, "The Civil Liberties Movement in India: New Approaches to the State and Social Change", *Asian Survey*, Vol. 27, No. 3, March 1987, pp. 373–374.
28. Gouri Shankar Nag, "Manabadhikar Andolan—Prasangik Vabna", in Sajal Basu (ed.), *Bharote Samajik Andolan*, Kolkata: Bookpost Publishers, 2016, pp. 198–204.
29. Jayaprakash Narayan, "Gano-andolan Lokashakti", in Sajal Basu (ed.), op. cit., pp. 249–257.
30. Ghanshyam Shah, *Social Movements in India: A Review of Literature*, New Delhi: Sage Publications India Pvt Ltd, cited second edition 2004, pp. 242–249.
31. Barnett R. Rubin, op. cit.
32. Ghanshyam Shah, op. cit.

33. P.P. Karan, "Environmental Movements in India", *Geographical Review*, Vol. 84, No. 1, Jan., 1994, pp. 32–41.
34. V. Ratan Reddy, "Environmental Movements in India: Some Reflections", *Journal of Indian School of Political Economy*, October–December 1998, p. 688.
35. Vandana Shiva and J. Bandyopadhyay, "The Evolution, Structure, and Impact of the Chipko Movement", *Mountain Research and Development*, Vol. 6, No. 2, May 1986, pp. 133–142; Jayanta Bandyopadhyay, "Chipko Movement: Of Floated Myths and Flouted Realities", *Economic and Political Weekly*, Vol. 34, No. 15, April 10–16, 1999, pp. 880–882; Ramachandra Guha, *Environmentalism: A Global History*, New York: Longman, 2000, pp. 115–119.
36. Ramachandra Guha, op. cit. p. 16.
37. L. S. Aravinda, "Globalisation and Narmada People's Struggle", *Economic and Political Weekly*, Vol. 35, No. 46, November 11–17, 2000, pp. 4002–4005.
38. Arundhati Roy, "The Greater Common Good", *Frontline*, Vol. 16, No. 11, May 22–June 4, 1999, p. 29.
39. People's Health Movement, *Global Health Watch 2: An Alternative World Health Report*, London/New York: Zed Books, 2008, p. 366.
40. Satinath Sarangi, "The Movement in Bhopal and its Lessons", *Social Justice*, Vol. 23, No. 4, Environmental Victims (Winter 1996), pp. 100–108.
41. Varigonda Kesava Chandra, *Society, Resistance and Civil Nuclear Policy in India: Nuclearising the State*, London/New York: Routledge, 2021.
42. Madhav Gadgil and Ramachandra Guha, *Ecology and Equity: The Use and Abuse of Nature in Contemporary India*, London/New York: Routledge, 1995.
43. Radha Kumar, "From Chipko to Sati: The Contemporary Indian Women's Movement", in Nivedita Menon (ed.), *Gender and Politics in India*, New Delhi: Oxford University Press, 1999, pp. 347–348.
44. Ranjana Kakkar, *Issues of Concern in the Women's Movement in India* (1970–1990), an unpublished PhD thesis, Department of Medieval and Modern History, University of Allahabad, Allahabad, 2002, pp. 26–30.
45. https://sites.google.com/site/saheliorgsite/, retrieved on March 31, 2023.
46. C. Sathyamala, "Women's Health Movement in Independent India", in Amiya Kumar Bagchi and Krishna Soman (eds.), *Maladies, Perspectives and Curatives: Debates in Public Health in India*, New Delhi: Tulika Books, 2005, pp. 96–108.
47. Padma Bhate-Deosthali et al., *The Aftermath of Rape: Survivors Speak*, London/New York: Routledge, 2022.

48. Apurba Ghosh, *Queer Identities in Bengal: A Study on Alternative Sexuality and Gender*, Unpublished MPhil. Dissertation, Department of History, University of Kalyani, 2021, pp. 158–169.
49. Yogesh Snehi, "National Alliance of People's Movements", in Arnold P Kaminsky and Roger D Long (eds.), *India Today: An Encyclopedia of Life in the Republic*, England: ABC-CLIO, 2011, pp. 495–496.
50. Suranjan Das and Premansu Kumar Bandyopadhyay (eds.), *Food Movement of 1959: Documenting a Turning Point in the History of West Bengal*, Kolkata: K.P. Bagchi & Company, 2004.
51. Foundation Statement, Right to Food Campaign, http://www.righttofoodcampaign.in/about/foundation-statement, retrieved on March 29, 2023.
52. Preethi Krishnan and Mangala Subramaniam, "Understanding the State: Right to Food Campaign in India", *The Global South*, Vol. 8, No. 2, The Global South and/in the Global North: Interdisciplinary Investigations (Fall 2014), pp. 101–118.
53. Foundation Statement, Right to Food Campaign, op. cit.
54. Vivek Srinivasan and Sudha Narayana, "Food Policy and Social Movements: Reflections on the Right to Food Campaign in India", Case Study 11-1 of the Program: "Food Policy for Developing Countries: The Role of Government in the Global Food System", 2007, edited by Per Pinstrup Andersen and Fuzhi Cheng, Cornell University.
55. *People's Union for Civil Liberties vs. Union of India and Others*, Writ Petition [Civil] 196 of 2001.
56. People's Health Movement, *Global Health Watch 4: An Alternative World Health Report*, London/New York: Zed Books, 2014, pp. 388–394.
57. http://www.righttofoodcampaign.in/about/collective-statement, retrieved on March 29, 2023.
58. Ibid.
59. Dipa Sinha and Biraj Patnaik, "National Food Security Act 2013: Moving From Exclusion to Inclusion", *Oxfam India Policy Brief*, No. 18, April 2016.
60. Heather Gautney, *Protest and Organization in the Alternative Globalization Era: NGOs, Social Movements, and Political Parties*, New York: Palgrave Macmillan, 2010, p. 39.
61. Ibid.
62. People's Health Movement, *Global Health Watch 4: An Alternative World Health Report*, London/New York: Zed Books, 2014, pp. 59–60.
63. Richard Stahler-Sholk, "The Zapatista Social Movement: Innovation and Sustainability", *Alternatives: Global, Local, Political*, Vol. 35, No. 3, Indigenous Politics: Migration, Citizenship, Cyberspace, July–September 2010, pp. 269–290.

64. Thomas Ponniah and William F. Fisher, "The World Social Forum and the Reinvention of Democracy", in William F. Fisher and Thomas Ponniah (eds.), *Another World is Possible: World Social Forum Proposals for An Alternative Globalization*, London: Zed Books, reprint 2015 (first published 2003), pp. 1–20.
65. Jose T. Bravo, "Dispatches from the World Social Forum", *Race, Poverty & the Environment*, Vol. 11, No. 1, Reclaiming our Resources: Imperialism & Environmental Justice (Summer 2004), pp. 56–60.
66. Dieter Rucht, "Social Forums as Public Stage and Infrastructure of Global Justice Movements", in Jackie Smith, Scott Byrd, Ellen Reese, and Elizabeth Smythe (eds.), *Handbook on World Social Forum Activism*, London: Paradigm Publishers, 2012, pp. 11–28.
67. Mukul Sharma & Charu Gupta, "Search for Answers at India Social Forum", *Economic and Political Weekly*, Vol. 41, No. 48, December 2–8, 2006, pp. 4937–4939; R. Venkatesan and Ravi Narayan, "Challenges for Health as a Social Movement", in SOCHARA Team, *Social Justice in Health*, Bangalore: SOCHARA, 2014, p. 154.
68. People's Health Movement, *Global Health Watch 4: An Alternative World Health Report*, London/New York: Zed Books, 2014, pp. 382–387.
69. "Editorial", in Shovanlal Duttagupta (ed.), *Naya Udarnitibader Abhighat O Bartaman Bharat*, Kolkata: Bahuswar, 2023, pp. iii–iv.
70. Purendra Prasad, op. cit.; Stuart et al., "India's Transforming Political Economy", in Sanjay Ruparelia et al. (eds.), *Understanding India's New Political Economy*, London/New York: Routledge, 2011, p. 2; Karl Polanyi, *The Great Transformation: The Political and Economic Origins of Our Time*, Boston: Beacon Press, 2001.
71. June Sekera, "Re-thinking the Definition of "Public Goods", March 30, 2018, https://rwer.wordpress.com/2014/07/09/re-thinking-the-definition-of-public-goods/#_ftnref19, retrieved on October 31, 2024.
72. "Modicare will expand private healthcare market: NITI Aayog VC", https://www.livemint.com/Politics/Aw6b1LV0uPZxsJ7z63FjUK/Modicare-will-expand-private-healthcare-market-NITI-Aayog-V.html, retrieved on October 31, 2024.
73. Sasha Costanza-Chock, *Youth and Social Movements: Key Lessons for Allies*, The Kinder and Braver World Project: Research Series (danah boyd, John Palfrey, and Dena Sacco, editors), Harvard University, December 17, 2012, available at: https://cyber.harvard.edu/sites/cyber.harvard.edu/files/KBWYouthandSocialMovements2012_0.pdf
74. Binay Ghosh, *Metropolitana Mon Madhyabitta Bidroha*, Kolkata: Orient Longman Ltd, 1960, pp. 94–105. In his article Ghosh cited the theory of Shmuel Noah Eisenstadt. Eisenstadt opined that the intellectual development among the youth is high in such a country where motion of eco-

nomic development and social development are not equal...The youth of this country consider the society to be conservative and crude in many ways. Therefore, their rebellion is primarily intellectual and has an emphasis on society. Shmuel Noah Eisenstadt, *From Generation to Generation: Age Groups and Social Structure*, New York: The Free Press, 1956.

75. The Struggle for Health is the Struggle for a More Equitable, Just and Caring World Declaration of the Fourth People's Health Assembly—PHA4 Savar, Bangladesh, November 15–19, 2018, https://phmovement.org/wp-content/uploads/2019/05/PHA4-Declaration_FINAL_EN.pdf, retrieved on March 30, 2023.
76. David Sanders, Wim De Ceukelaire and Barbara Hutton, *The Struggle for Health: Medicine and the Politics of Underdevelopment*, Oxford: Oxford University Press, 2023, p. 317.
77. *A Selection of Poems by Shankha Ghosh*, Kolkata: Dey's Publishing, 2008, p. 191.

Bibliography

Primary Sources

Government Sources

Documents of the Government of India
Policy Papers

- *National Health Policy, 2017*, New Delhi: Ministry of Health and Family Welfare.
- *National Health Policy*, New Delhi: Ministry of Health and Family Welfare, 1983.
- *National Health Policy-2002*, New Delhi: Ministry of Health and Family Welfare, 2003.
- *National Rural Health Mission (2005–2012)*, Mission document, New Delhi: Ministry of Health & Family Welfare.
- *Pharmaceutical Policy 2002*, New Delhi: Department of Pharmaceuticals, Ministry of Chemicals and Fertilizers.
- *Pradhan Mantri Bhartiya Janaushadhi Pariyojna*, New Delhi: Department of Pharmaceuticals, Ministry of Chemicals & Fertilizers, 2008.

© The Author(s), under exclusive license to Springer Nature Switzerland AG 2025
N. Malakar, *Historicising the People's Health Movement in West Bengal, India*, https://doi.org/10.1007/978-3-032-02696-5

Reports

- F. Norman White, *A Preliminary Report on the Influenza Pandemic of 1918 in India*, Simla, 1919.
- *Annual Report of the Public Health Commissioner with the Govt. of India*, Delhi, 1933.
- *Health in India, National Sample Survey (NSS) 71st Round*, January–June 2014, Report No. 574 (71/25.0), Government of India, New Delhi, 2016.
- *High Level Expert Group Report on Universal Health Coverage for India*, Planning Commission of India, New Delhi, 2011.
- *National Health Profile 2018*, Central Bureau of Health Intelligence, Ministry of Family Welfare, Government of India, New Delhi, 2018.
- *Report of the Committee on Drugs and Pharmaceutical Industries* (Hathi Committee Report), Ministry of Petroleum & Chemicals, Government of India, New Delhi, April 1975.
- *Report of the Health Survey and Development Committee* (Bhore Committee), Volumes I to IV, Delhi, 1946.
- *Report of the National Commission on Macroeconomics and Health*, Ministry of Health & Family Welfare, Government of India, New Delhi, 2005.
- *Report of the Working Group on Health for All by 2000 A.D.*, Ministry of Health and Family Welfare, Government of India, New Delhi, 1981.
- *Health for All: an Alternative strategy*, report of a study group set up jointly by Indian Council of Social Science Research (ICSSR) & Indian Council of Medical Research (ICMR), Indian Institute of Education, Pune, 1981.

Five-Year Plans

- *Ninth Five-Year Plan (1997–2002)*, Vol. II, Planning Commission.
- *Twelfth Five-Year Plan (2012–2017)*, Social Sectors, Volume III, Planning Commission.

Report of the Planning Committee

- K.T. Shah (ed.), *Report of Sub-committee on National Health* (Sokhey Committee), National Planning Committee, Bombay: Vora & Co, 1948.

Acts/Rules

- Government of India, *Patents Rules, 1972*, the Gazette of India, vide S.O. 301(E) dated 20th April, 1972 in Part II, Section 3, sub-section (ii).
- *The Consumer Protection Act, 1986*, Government of India.
- *The Drugs and Cosmetics Rules, 1945* (As amended up to August 15, 2013), Ministry of Health and Family Welfare, Government of India.
- *The Patents Act, 1970* (No. 39 of 1970), the Gazette of India, Extraordinary, Part II—Section i dated September 21, 1970.
- *The Patents (Amendment) Act, 2005*, No. 15 of 2005, the Gazette of India, April 5, 2005.

Lok Sabha Debates

- *Lok Sabha Debates*, Fifteenth Series, Vol. XXX, Twelfth Session, 2012/1934 (Saka), No. 11, Friday, December 7, 2012/Agrahayana 16, 1934 (Saka).
- *Lok Sabha Debates*, Fifteenth Series, Vol. XXX, Twelfth Session, 2012/1934 (Saka) No. 16, Monday, December 14, 2012/ Agrahayana 23, 1934 (Saka)
- *Lok Sabha Debates*, Fifteenth Series, Vol. XXX, Twelfth Session, 2012/1934 (Saka), No. 17, Monday, December 17, 2012/ Agrahayana 26, 1934 (Saka)
- *Lok Sabha Debates*, Fifteenth Series, Vol. XXXIII, Thirteenth Session, 2013/1935 (Saka), No. 23, Tuesday, April 23, 2013/Vaisakha 3, 1935 (Saka).

Notifications

- *Drugs (Prices Control) Order, 1979*, Department of Pharmaceuticals.
- *Complete list of 344 drugs banned by the Ministry of Health & Family Welfare*, Government of India, March 15, 2016.
- *Notification (Drug and Cosmetic (Ninth Amendment) Rules)*, New Delhi: Ministry of Health & Family Welfare, in the Gazette of India, April 3, 2017.
- *Memorandum No Z15025/83/2017/DIR/CGHS, Dated 8th September 2017*, Ministry of Health and Family Welfare, Government of India.

Documents of the West Bengal State Government

Policy Papers

- *Concept Paper cum Suggestion Solicitation Paper for Health Care Infrastructure builds up in Public Private Participation (PPP) Mode*, Department of Health and Family Welfare, 2011.
- *Department of Health, The Health Service (Cadre, Pay and Allowance) Rule 1958, with Some Important Government Orders, Corrected up to 1st September 1966*, 1967.
- *Establishing Diagnostic Services in Block Primary Health Centres/ Rural Hospitals through Public Private Partnerships*, Department of Health and Family Welfare, January 2010.
- Government of West Bengal, *Establishment of Fair Price Outlet for Medicines, Consumables and Implants at selected Government Hospitals through Public Private Partnerships (PPP)*, Health and Family Welfare Department, 2012.
- *Policy for Public Private Partnerships in the Health Sector*, Department of Health and Family Welfare, January 2006.
- *West Bengal Human Development Report-2004*, Development and Planning Department, 2004.

West Bengal Legislative Assembly Proceedings

- *Assembly Proceedings*, West Bengal Legislative Assembly
- Vol. 2, No. 1, Second Session, from 10 February to 30 March 1948.
- Vol. 54, No. 3, Fifty-Fourth Session, from 9 February to 10 May 1973.
- Vol. 56, No. 2, Fifty-Sixth Session, from February to May 1974.
- Vol. 58, No. 1, Fifty-Eighth Session, February–May 1975.
- Vol. 62, Sixty Second Session, 11 October to 19 October 1976.
- Vol. 66, No. 5, Sixty-Sixth Session, August to October 1977.
- Vol. 70, No. 2, Seventieth Session, February to April, 1979.
- Vol. 78, No. 2, Seventy-Eighth Session, from 1 September 1982 to 8 October 1982.
- Vol. 79, No. 3, Seventy-Ninth Session, from 11 April 1983 to 23 April 1983.
- Vol. 81, No. 4, Eighty-First session, from 16th April to 27th April 1984.
- Vol. 83, No. 3, Eighty-Third session, from 11th March to 10th May 1985.
- Vol. 88, No. 2, Eighty-Eighth session, from May to June 1987.

- Vol. 92, No. 4, 1989, Ninety-Second session, from February to May 1989.
- Vol. 95, No. 1, Ninety-Fifth Session, from March to May 1990.
- Vol. 106, No. 4, Hundred and Sixth Session, from March to August, 1995.

Acts

- *The West Bengal Clinical Establishments (Registration, Regulation and Transparency) Act, 2017*, the Kolkata Gazette, March 17, 2017.
- *West Bengal Act VII of 1990, The West Bengal State Health Service Act, 1990*, the Calcutta Gazette, Extraordinary, May 16, 1990.

West Bengal State Government Reports & Other Publications

- *Annual Report on the Health of the Population of West Bengal: For the Year 1950* (by B.C. Das Gupta Director of Health Services, West Bengal), 1953.
- *Annual Report on the Health of the Population of West Bengal: For the Year 1951* (by B.C. Das Gupta, Director of Health Services, West Bengal), 1954.
- *Report of Administrative Reforms Committee*, Home (Personnel and Administrative Reforms) Department, 1983.

Health on the March (A Government of West Bengal Publication)

- State Bureau of Health Intelligence, Directorate of Health Service, Vols. 1980, 1986, 1987, 1991, 2005–06, 2011–2012, 2015–16, 2016–18. Government of West Bengal.

Economic Review (A Government of West Bengal Publication)

- Vol. 1988–89 (Statistical Appendix), 2008–2009, 2010–2011 (Statistical Appendix), 2011–2012, 2012–2013, 2014–2015.

Budget Statements

- Budget Statement by Asim Kumar Dasgupta, Minister-in-charge, Finance, Government of West Bengal, June 2, 2001.
- Budget Statement by Dr Asim Kumar Dasgupta, Minister in Charge, Finance, Government of West Bengal, 2004.

Non-government Sources

World Bank Documents

- *Financing Health Services in Developing Countries: An Agenda for Reform* (A World Bank Policy Study), Washington, DC: World Bank, 1987.
- *World Development Report 1993: Investing in Health*, Washington DC: World Bank, 1993.
- *India Health Systems Project II*, Report No. 15106-IN, Washington DC: World Bank, 1996.

Memorandum, Rules and Regulations & Annual Reports of Different Health-Related Organizations

- Drug Action Forum, West Bengal, Memorandum & Rules (1/S/52867), 1987.
- Memorandum of Association and Rules & Regulation, Norman Bethune Janaswasthaya Andolan (Registration No S/56685 of 1987–88).
- Press release of Medical College Unit, ABJDF, September 11, 1991.
- Proceedings of the meeting of the executive committee of the Norman Bethune Janaswasthya Andolan, held on October 2, 1999, Chairman of the meeting was Dr Jnanabrata Sil.
- Programmes and Constitution of Forum for People's Health (Adopted in Third Conference of Forum for People's Health on May 31, 2009.
- West Bengal Voluntary Health Association (WBVHA), Memorandum and Rules & Regulation, Registration No: S/14704 of 1974.

Election Manifestos

- Election Manifesto of the Left Front, West Bengal Assembly Election 1982.
- Election Manifesto of the Left Front, West Bengal Assembly Elections 2001.
- Manifesto of Trinamool Congress, West Bengal Assembly Election Manifesto 2011.
- Election Manifesto Communist Party of India (Marxist), 17th Lok Sabha Election, 2019.

Interviews

- Interview with Dr. Jnanabrata Sil, Former Secretary of Norman Bethune Janaswasthya Andolan, Kolkata, February 3, 2019.
- Interview with Srijan Sen, Activist of Dr. Dwarkanath Kotnis Memorial Committee, Kolkata, dated April 3, 2019.
- Interview with Dr. Sankar Kumar Nath, Doctor and Historian of Science & Medicine, November 30 2019.
- Interview with Binay Bsau Mallick, Joint Secretary of Janaswasthya Committee, dated January 31, 2020.
- Interview with Dr. Punyabrata Goon, Health Activist, Kolkata, dated January 31, 2020.
- Interview with Dr. Hiralal Konar, a former secretary of the Health Service Association, Kolkata, February 13, 2020.
- Interview with Dr. Smarajit Jana (1952–2021), Health Activist, Kolkata, February 14, 2020.
- Interview with Bimal Sarkar, President of Rakhi Humanist Society, October 6, 2021.

Memoirs

English

- Arthur Newsholme & John Adams Kingsbury, *Red Medicine: Socialized Health in Soviet Russia*, London: William Heinemann (Medical Books) Ltd, 1934.
- Clifford Whittingham Beers, *A Mind That Found Itself*, New York: Longmans, Green, and Co, 1908.
- Ilina Sen, *Inside Chhattisgarh: A Political Memoir*, India: Penguin Books Ltd, 2014.
- Surendranath Banerjea, *A Nation in Making, Bombay*, Calcutta, Madras: Oxford University Press, 1925.

Bengali

- Aniruddha Sengupta, *Ek Ganyer Daktarer Galpo*, Kolkata: Gurchandali Publication, 2019.
- Punyabrata Goon, *Pa Miliye Path Chala*, Kolkata: Katha Shilpa, 2018.
- Punyabrata Goon, *Shankar Guha Niyogir Sange Koyek Bochhor: Ek Sohojoddhar Protibedon*, Kolkata: Book Mar (Setu Prakashani), not dated.
- Sthabir Dasgupta, *Swapner Sottor: Maya Rahiya Gelo*, Kolkata: Dhansere, 2018.

Letters

- Letter from David Werner to Dr Sujit Kumar Das dated November 28, 1986, reprinted in the Souvenir of the third annual convention of *Drug Action Forum* on the National Drug Policy, WB, Kolkata, February 1987, p. 3.
- Letter from the Joint Platform of Doctors, West Bengal to the Director of Health Services, Government of West Bengal, December 27, 2017.
- Letter of Comrade Dinesh Singh (Dr Jnanabrata Sil) to Comrade Haridas Malakar, West Bengal State Control Committee, dated August 14, 1987.
- Letter of Dinesh Singh (Dr Jnanabrata Sil) to the State Secretary of CPI (M), dated May 9, 1986.
- Letter of Gauripada Dutta to Comrade Dinesh Singh dated September 24, 1987.

English Newspapers & Periodicals

- BODHI.
- *British Medical Journal.*
- *Bulletin of the History of Medicine.*
- *Current Science.*
- *Drug Disease Doctor.*
- *Economic & Political Weekly.*
- *The Economic Times.*
- *Frontier.*
- *Health Promotion International.*
- *Health Spectra.*
- *India Today.*
- *Indian Journal of Medical Research.*
- *Indian Journal of Public health.*
- *International Journal of Health Services.*
- *Journal of Indian Medical Association.*
- *Journal of Public Health Policy.*
- *Journal of the Asiatic Society.*
- *Medico Friend Circle Bulletin.*
- *New Scientist.*
- *Proletarian Era.*
- *Rational Drug Bulletin.*
- *The Hindu.*

- *The Hindustan Times.*
- *The Lancet.*
- *The Marxist*
- *The Modern Review.*
- *The National Medical Journal of India.*
- *The Statesman.*
- *The Telegraph.*
- *The Times of India.*

Bengali Newspapers & Periodicals

- *Aajkaal.*
- *Anandabazar Patrik.*
- *Ankure Shuru.*
- *Anubikshan.*
- *Anyakatha.*
- *Bartaman.*
- *Bijnan O Bijnankarmi.*
- *Bikshan.*
- *Chaturanga.*
- *Chikitsa O Sarkar.*
- *Chikitsak o Samalochak.*
- *Doctors' Dialogue.*
- *Ei Samay.*
- *Ganashakti.*
- *Janaswasthya Katha.*
- *Jugantar.*
- *Kalantar.*
- *Paribesh O Janaswasthya.*
- *Paschimbanga.*
- *Sangbad Pratidin*
- *Shramajibi Swasthya.*
- *Swasthya Bikshan.*
- *Swasthya Deepika.*
- *Swasthya O Paribesh.*
- *Swasthya Samachar.*
- *Swasthyer Britte.*
- *Utsa Manush.*

Unpublished Thesis

- Amrita Bagchi, *Health Care in Crisis: the Changing Pattern of Private Health Care in Post-independence Kolkata*, unpublished PhD thesis, Department of History, Jadavpur University, 2010.
- Bijoya Roy, *Private Investment in Public Sector Medical Care Institutions: A Study of Processes in Tertiary and Secondary Level Care in Six Districts of West Bengal*, unpublished PhD thesis, Centre of Social Medicine and Community Health, School of Social Sciences, Jawaharlal Nehru University, 2007.
- Indranil Mukhopadhyay, *Public Health Care Expenditure in India a Study of Kerala, Tamil Nadu and West Bengal*, an unpublished PhD thesis, Centre of Social Medicine and Community Health, Jawaharlal Nehru University, New Delhi, 2011.
- Poonam Bala, *State and Indigenous Medicine in Nineteenth and Twentieth-Century Bengal: 1800–19*, unpublished thesis, University of Edinburgh, 1987.
- Rama Vaidyanathan Baru, *Some Aspects of the Private Sector in Medical Care and Its Inter-relationship with the Public Sector: A Study of Hyderabad-Secunderabad*, unpublished PhD thesis, Centre of Social Medicine and Community Health School of Social Sciences, Jawaharlal Nehru University, New Delhi, 1992.
- Sabyasachi Chatterjee, *A Historical Study of the Science Movements in West Bengal 1947–1997*, unpublished PhD thesis, Department of History, Jadavpur University, 2004.

Secondary Sources

Monographs and Edited Volumes

- A. Venkat Raman and James Warner Björkman, *Public–Private Partnerships in Health Care in India: Lessons for Developing Countries*, London/New York: Routledge, 2009.
- Abhay Bang and Ashvin J. Patel (eds.), *Health Care Which Way to Go?: Examination of Issues and Alternatives*, New Delhi: Medico Friend Circle, first published 1982, cited edition 1985.
- Achintya Kumar Dutta, *Trauma in Public Health: Tuberculosis in Twentieth-century India*, Kolkata: K P Bagchi & Company, 2018.
- Adam Gaffney, *To Heal Humankind: the Right to Health in History*, New York: Routledge, 2018.

- Alex Vadakumthala (ed.), *Reproductive Health: Catholic Ethics and Praxis in India*, New Delhi: Health Commission, Catholic Bishops' Conference of India, 2007.
- Alfred Crosby, *Ecological Imperialism: The Biological Expansion of Europe, 900–1900,* Cambridge: Cambridge University Press, 1993.
- Allan Nevins, *A Pocket History of the United States*, New York: Pocket Books, 1990.
- Amar Jesani et al. (ed.), *Market, Medicine and Malpractice*, Mumbai: CEHAT & SPHAA, 1997.
- Amar Jesani, *Laws and Health Care Providers: A Study of Legislation and Legal Aspects of Health Care Delivery*, Mumbai: CEHAT, 1996.
- Amar Jesani, Manisha Gupte and Ravi Duggal, *NGOs in Rural Health Care* (Volume One: An Overview), Bombay: The Foundation for Research in Community Health, 1986.
- Amartya Sen, *Development as Freedom*, New York: Alfred A. Knopf, 2000.
- Amit Sengupta et al., *Economic Constraints to Access to Essential Medicines in India*, New Delhi: Society for Economic and Social Studies & Centre for Trade and Development, 2009.
- Amiya Kumar Bagchi and Krishna Soman (eds.), *Maladies, Preventives and Curatives: Debates in Public Health in India*, New Delhi: Tulika, 2005.
- Amiya Kumar Hati, *Medicine and Pharmacology (Series: History of Science in India, Volume-II)*, Kolkata: The Ramakrishna Mission Institute Culture, 2014.
- Amrita Bagchi, *Healthcare in Post-Independence India: Kolkata and the Crisis of Private Healthcare Services*, New York & London: Routledge, 2023.
- Anant Phadke, *Drug Supply and Use: Towards a Rational Policy in India,* New Delhi: SAGE Publications Pvt., 1998.
- Anil Kumar, *Medicine and the Raj: British Medical Policy In India, 1835–1911,* New Delhi: Sage Publications, 1998.
- Anil Kumar, *Medicine and the Raj: British Medical Policy in India, 1835–1911*, London/New Delhi: SAGE Publications, 1998.
- Ann F. La Berge, *Mission and Method The early Nineteenth-century French Public Health Movement*, Cambridge: Cambridge University Press, first published 1992, first paperback edition 2002.
- Ann Taket, *Health Equity, Social Justice and Human Rights*, New York/London: Routledge, 2012.

- Anuj Kapilashrami and Rama V. Baru (eds.), *Global Health Governance and Commercialisation of Public Health in India: Actors, Institutions and the Dialectics of Global and Local*, London/New York: Routledge Taylor and Francis Group, 2018.
- Arabinda Samanta, *Living with Epidemics in Colonial Bengal*, New York/London: Routledge, 2018.
- Arabinda Samanta, *Malarial Fever in Colonial Bengal, 1820–1939: Social History of an Epidemic*, Kolkata: Firma KLM, 2002.
- Archana Prasad (ed.), *Environment, Development and Society in Contemporary India: An Introduction*, Delhi/Kolkata: Macmillan, 2008.
- Arthur Leslie Morton, *A People's History of England*, London: Victor Gollancz Ltd., 1938.
- Arun Gadre and Abhay Shukla (ed.), *Dissenting Diagnosis*, Gurgaon, Haryana: Penguin Books, 2016.
- Ashis Nandy (ed.), *Science, Hegemony and Violence: A Requiem for Modernity*, Delhi: Oxford University Press, India, 1990.
- Ashvin J. Patel (ed.), *In Search of Diagnosis: Analysis of Present System of Health Care*, New Delhi: Medico Friend Circle, first edition 1977, cited edition 1985.
- Bidyut Chakrabarty, *Left Radicalism in India*, London & New York: Routledge, 2014.
- Biplab Dasgupta, *Globalisation: India's Adjustment Experience*, New Delhi: Sage Publications India Pvt. Ltd., first edition 2005, cited edition 2006.
- Biswamoy Pati and Mark Harrison (ed.), *Society, Medicine and Politics in Colonial India*, New York: Routledge, 2018.
- Biswamoy Pati and Mark Harrison (eds.), *Health, Medicine and Empire: Perspectives on Colonial India*, India: Orient Longman, 2001.
- Biswamoy Pati and Mark Harrison (eds.), *The Social History of Health and Medicine in Colonial India*, London/New York: Routledge, 2009.
- Byasdeb Dasgupta, Archita Ghosh, and Bishakha Ghosh (eds.), *Neoliberalism in the Emerging Economy of India: The Political Economy of International Trade, Investment and Finance*, London, New York: Routledge, 2021.
- Chamsy el-Ojeili and Patrick Hayden, *Critical Theories of Globalization*, New York: Palgrave Macmillan, 2006.
- Chittabrata Palit and Achintya Dutta (eds.), *History of Medicine in India: The Medical Encounter*, New Delhi: Kalpaz Publications, 2004.

- Chittabrata Palit and Amit Bhattacharyya, *Science, Technology, Medicine and Environment in India: Historical Perspective*, Calcutta: Bibhasa, 1998.
- Christian Aspalter, Kenny Teguh Pribadi and Robin Gauld, *Health Care Systems in Developing Countries in Asia*, New York and London: Routledge, 2017.
- Christopher Hamlin, *Public Health and Social Justice in the Age of Chadwick: Britain, 1800–1854*, Cambridge: Cambridge University Press, 1998.
- Claudio Schuftan, *Health and Human Rights Readers*, Mumbai: CEHAT, 2003.
- David Arnold, *Colonizing the Body: State Medicine and Epidemic Disease in Nineteenth-Century India*, Berkeley/London: University of California Press, 1993.
- David Garland, *The Welfare State: A Very Short Introduction*, Oxford: Oxford University Press, 2016.
- David Hardiman and Projit Bihari Mukharji (eds.), *Medical Marginality in South Asia: Situating Subaltern Therapeutics*, New York & London: Routledge, 2012.
- David Hardiman, *Missionaries and Their Medicine: A Christian Modernity for Tribal India*, Manchester: Manchester University Press, 2008.
- David Werner, *Where There is No Doctor*, Berkeley: Hesperian Health Guides, 1977.
- David Werner, *People's Struggle for Health and Liberation in Latin America: A Historical Perspective*, Cuenca, Ecuador: Health Wrights, 2013.
- Debasis Bose, Sankar Kumar Nath and Jayanta K. Das (ed.), *175 Years of Medical College—Commemorative Volume*, Kolkata: Medical College Ex-Students' Association, 2009.
- Debraj Bhattacharya, *Exploring Marxist Bengal c.1971–2011*, Kolkata: K P Bagchi & Company, 2016.
- Deepak Kumar (ed.), *Disease & Medicine in India: A Historical Overview*, New Delhi: Tulika, first published 2001, reprint 2012.
- Deepak Kumar (ed.), *Science and Empire: Essays in Indian Context (1700–1947)*, New Delhi: Anamika Prakashan, 1991.
- Dianna Melrose, *Bitter Pills Medicines and the Third World Poor*, Oxford: OXFAM, 1987.

- Dorothy Porter, *Health, Civilization and the State: A History of Public Health from Ancient to Modern Times*, London and New York: Routledge, 1999.
- Edward Blunt (ed.), *Social Service in India*, London: His Majesty's Stationery Office, reprinted 1946 (first edition 1939).
- F. B Smith, *The People's Health, 1830–1910*, New York: Holmes and Meier, 1979.
- Fiona Dias Saxena and Gracy Andrew, *Barefoot Counseling: A Manual for Community Workers*, Goa: Sangath, 2002.
- Fran Collyer (ed.), *The Palgrave Handbook of Social Theory in Health, Illness and Medicine*, London: Palgrave Macmillan, 2015.
- Frederick Engels, *The Condition of the Working Class in England in 1944* (translated by Florence Kelley Wiscunewetzky), New York: John W. Lovell Company, 1887.
- Gabriella Wass (ed.), *Corporate Activity and Human Rights in India*, New Delhi: Human Rights Law Network, 2011.
- George Rosen, *A History of Public Health*, Baltimore: Johns Hopkins University Press, 1958.
- Ghanshyam Shah, *Social Movements in India: A Review of Literature*, New Delhi: SAGE Publications India, 2004.
- Glenn Laverack, *Health Activism: Foundations and Strategies*, London/New Delhi/Singapore: SAGE Publications, 2013.
- Gonoshasthaya Kendra, *From Battlefront to Community: Story of Gonoshasthaya Kendra*, Dhaka: Gonoprakashani, 2003.
- Gordon Wolstenholme and Maeve O'Connor (eds.), *Health of Mankind*, London: J. & A. Churchill Ltd., 1967.
- Gouri Pada Dutta, *Health Care in India: An Appraisal*, Kolkata: P.K. Choudhuri, 1987.
- Gouripada Dutta, *Promised but Not Implemented: Treatise of Health Policy*, Kolkata: Asok Kumar Pal, 2003.
- Gouripada Dutta, *Social Issue of Health*, Kolkata: Pratyaya, 2003.
- Henry E. Sigerist, *Medicine and Health in Soviet Union*, Bombay: Jaico Publishing House, 1947.
- Henry E. Sigerist, *Socialised Medicine in the Soviet Union*, London: Victor Gollaucz, Ltd., 1937.
- Howard Waitzkin, *Medicine and Public Health at the End of Empire*, New York: Routledge, 2011.

- Imrana Qadeer (ed.), *India: Social Development Report 2014: Challenges of Public Health*, New Delhi: Oxford University Press, 2015.
- Imrana Qadeer et al (eds.) *Public Health and The Poverty of Reforms: The South Asian Predicament*, New Delhi: Sage Publications, 2001.
- Imrana Qadeer, K. B. Saxena and P. M. Arathi (eds.), *Universalising Healthcare in India: From Care to Coverage*, Delhi: Aakar Books, 2021.
- Imrana Qadeer, *Public Health in India: Critical Reflection*, Delhi: Danish Book, 2011.
- Irfan Habib, *Man and Environment: The Ecological History of India*, Delhi: Tulika Books, 2010.
- Ishita Pande, *Medicine, Race and Liberalism in British Bengal: Symptoms of Empire*, New York: Routledge, 2010.
- Ivan Illich, *Medical Nemesis: The Expropriation of Health*, New York: Pantheon Books, 1976.
- Jack Belden, *China Shakes the World*, London: Monthly Review Press, 1970.
- James Le Fanu, *The Rise and Fall of Modern Medicine*, London: Hachette, 2011.
- Jasodhara Bagchi (ed.), *The Changing Status of Women in West Bengal, 1970–2000: The Challenge Ahead*, New Delhi: Sage Publications India Pvt Ltd, 2005.
- Jean Drèze and Amartya Sen, *An Uncertain Glory: India and Its Contradictions*, London: Penguin Books Limited, 2013.
- Jennifer Prah Ruger, *Health and Social Justice*, Oxford: Oxford University Press, 2009.
- Jill Stewart (ed.), *Pioneers in Public Health: Lesson from History*, London/New York: Routledge, 2017.
- Jim Downns, *Maladies of Empire: How Colonialism, Slavery, and War Transformed Medicine*, London: Belknap Press of Harvard University Press, 2021.
- John Coggon, *What Makes Health Public: A Critical Evaluation of Moral, Legal, and Political Claims in Public Health*, Cambridge: Cambridge University Press, 2012.
- Jonathan Glover, *Causing Death and Saving Lives*, London: Penguin, 1977.
- Jude Howell (ed.), *Non-Governmental Public Action and Social Justice*, London: Palgrave Macmillan, 2013.

- Jyoti Basu (ed.), *Documents of the Communist Movement in India 1994–96*, Vol. 25, Kolkata: National Book Agency, 1998.
- Jyoti Basu et al (eds.), *People's Power in Practice: 20 Years of Left Front in West Bengal*, Kolkata: National Book Agency, 1997.
- K.N. Reddy and V. Selvaraju, *Health Care Expenditure by Government in India: 1974–75 to 1990–91*, New Delhi: National Institute of Public Finance & Policy, 1994.
- K. Park, *Park's Book of Preventive & Social Medicine,* Jabalpur: Bhanot Publishers, 2015.
- K. Srinath Reddy, *Make Health in India: Reaching a Billion Plus,* Hyderabad: Orient BlackSwan, 2019.
- K. Sujatha Rao, *Do We Care?: India's Health System*, New Delhi: Oxford University Press, 2017.
- Kabita Roy, *History of Public Health: Colonial Bengal 1921–1947*, Kolkata: K.P. Bagchi, 1998.
- Kamala S. Jayarao and Ashvin J. Patel (eds.), *Under the Lens: Health and Medicine*, New Delhi: Medico Friend Circle, 1986.
- Karl Marx and Frederick Engels, *Communist Manifesto*, Chicago: Charles H. Kerr & Company, 1906.
- Kunal Sarkar, *The Sickness of Health: Journy of Indias's Healthcare from Colonial Era to Corona*, Kolkata: BEE Books, 2021.
- Lawrence O. Gostin and Lindsay F. Wiley, *Public Health Law: Power, Duty, Restraint*, Oakland, CA: University of California Press, 2016.
- Leela Visaria and Rajani R. Ved, *India's Family Planning Programme Policies, Practices and Challenges,* New York/London: Routledge, 2016.
- Leena V. Gangolli et al. (ed.), *Review of Healthcare in India*, Mumbai: Centre for Enquiry into Health and Allied Themes, 2005.
- Low Cost Standard Therapeutics (LOCOST), *Impoverishing the Poor: Pharmaceuticals and Drug Pricing in India*, Vadodara/ Bilaspur: LOCOST/JSS 2004.
- M. Govinda Rao and Mita Choudhury, *Inter-State Equalisation of Health Expenditures in Indian Union*, New Delhi: National Institute of Public Finance and Policy, 2008.
- M.N. Rao and K.K. Radhalaxmi, *History of Public Health in India*, Kolkata: Navana Printing Works, Private Ltd, 1960.
- Madhuri Sharma, *Indigenous and Western Medicine in Colonial India*, New Delhi: Cambridge University Press India Pvt. Ltd., under the imprint of Foundation Books, 2012.

- Madison Powers and Ruth Faden, *Social Justice: The Moral Foundations of Public Health and Health Policy*, New York: Oxford University Press, 2008.
- Manfred Berg and Geoffrey Cocks (eds.), *Medicine and Modernity: Public Health and Medical Care in Nineteenth- and Twentieth-Century Germany*, Cambridge: Cambridge University Press, 2002.
- Marjorie Mayo, *Community-based Learning and Social Movements*, Bristol: Policy Press, 2020.
- Mark Harrison, *Disease and Modern World: 1500 to the Present Day*, Cambridge: Polity Press, 2004.
- Mark Harrison, *Public Health in British India: Anglo-Indian Preventive Medicine 1859–1914*, Cambridge History of Medicine Series, Cambridge: Cambridge University Press, 1994.
- Martin Donohoe (ed.), *Public Health and Social Justice*, San Francisco: Jossey-Bass, 2013.
- Mary P. Sutphen and Bridie Andrews (eds.), *Medicine and Colonial Identity*, New York/London: Routledge, 2003.
- Mary-Jane Schneider, *Introduction to Public Health*, United States of America: Jones & Bartlett Learning, Fifth edition 2017.
- Meera Chatterjee, *Implementing Health Policy*, New Delhi: Manohar, 1988.
- Meredith Fort, Mary Anne Mercer, and Oscar Gish (eds.), *Sickness and Wealth the Corporate Assault on Global Health*, Cambridge/ Massachusetts: South End Press, 2004.
- Michael Marmot, *The Health Gap: The Challenge of an Unequal World*, London: Bloomsbury Publishing, 2015.
- Michel Foucault, *Discipline and Punish: The Birth of the Prison*, New York: Vintage Books, Second edition 1995.
- Mihir Desai, Kamayani Bali Mahabal (ed.), *Health Care Case Law in India*, Mumbai: CEHAT and ICHRL, 2007.
- Mikko Mattila, Lauri Rapeli, Hanna Wass and Peter Söderlund, *Health and Political Engagement*, New York/London: Routledge, 2017.
- Murphy Halliburton, *India and the Patent Wars: Pharmaceuticals in the New Intellectual Property Regime*, New York: Cornell University Press, 2017.
- Myron Wiener, *State Politics in India*, New Jersey: Princeton University Press, 2015.

- Nilanjan Dutta, *Rights and the 'Left': West Bengal 1977–2011*, Kolkata: Setu Prakashani, 2015.
- Nitish Sengupta, *Builders of Modern India*, New Delhi: Publication Division, Government of India, 2016.
- Noshir Antia et al., *Developing an Alternative Strategy for Achieving Health for All*, Pune/Mumbai: Foundation for Research in Community Health, 2004.
- Nupur Dasgupta and Amit Bhattacharya (ed.), *Essays in History of Science Technology and Medicine*, Kolkata: Setu Prakashani, 2014.
- O.P. Jaggi, *History of Science, Medicine in India: Modern Period* (General Editor: D.P. Chattopadhyay, Philosophy and Culture in Indian Civilization, Volume IX, Part 1), New Delhi: Oxford University Press, 2011.
- Omana George and Sanjiv Pandita (eds.), *Invisible Victims of Development: Workers' Health and Safety in Asia*, Hong Kong: Asia Monitor Resource Centre, 2012.
- P.M. Arathi (ed.), *Public Health in India: Policy Shifts and Trends* (Series Editor: Manoranjan Mohanty, Social Change in Contemporary India, Volume VI), New Delhi: SAGE Publications India Pvt Ltd, 2022.
- P.K Sanyal, *A Story of Medicine and Pharmacy in India*, Kolkata: B. Pharm, 1960.
- Partha Sarathi, *Left Politics in West Bengal: Examining the 'Marxists' and 'Maoists'*, Kolkata: Purbalok Publication, 2016.
- Paul Farmer, *Pathologies of Power: Health, Human Rights, and the New War on the Poor*, Berkeley/Los Angeles/London: University of California Press, 2002.
- Paul Weindling (ed.), *Healthcare in Private and Public from the Early Modern Period to 2000*, New York: Routledge, 2015.
- Philip D. Jordan, *The People's Health: A History of Public Health in Minnesota to 1948*, Minnesota: Minnesota Historical Society, 1953.
- Poonam Bala (ed.), *Medicine and Colonialism: Historical Perspectives in India and South Africa*, London: Routledge, 2014.
- Poonam Bala, *Imperialism and Medicine in Bengal: A Socio-Historical Perspective*, New Delhi: SAGE Publications, 1991.
- Pradip Kumar Bose (ed.), *Health and Society in Bengal: A Selection from Late 19th-Century Bengali Periodicals*, New Delhi: SAGE Publications India Pvt Ltd, 2006, p. 277.

- Projit Bihari Mukharji, *Nationalizing the Body: The Medical Market, Print and Daktari Medicine*, London/New York, Delhi: Anthem Press, 2009.
- Purendra Prasad and Amar Jesani (eds.), *Equity and Access: Health Care Studies in India*, New Delhi: Oxford University Press, 2018.
- R. A. Lewis, *Edwin Chadwick and Public Health Movement 1832–1854*, London: Longmans, Green and Co., 1952.
- R. Biswas-Diener and E. Diener (eds.), *Noba Textbook Series: Psychology*, Milwaukie: DEF Publishers, 2013.
- R. Maria Saleth, S. Galab and E. Revathi (eds.), *Issues and Challenges of Inclusive Development: Essays in Honor of Prof. R. Radhakrishna*, Singapore: Springer Nature Singapore Pte Ltd., 2020.
- Radha Holla (ed.), *Fast Furious and Flexible: The Story of Health Action International (HAI) 1981–2006*, Colombo: Health Action International Asia Pacific, 2006.
- Rakhahari Chatterji and Partha Pratim Basu (ed.), *West Bengal under the Left 1977–2011*, London/New York: Routledge, 2020.
- Rama V Baru, *Private Health Care in India: Social Characteristics and Trends*, India: SAGE Publications, 1998.
- Ravi Duggal et al., *Appropriate Role for the Private Sector in Health Care of India: Political Economy of Private Healthcare*, Independent Commission on Development & Health in India and VHAI, 2013.
- Ross Mallick, *Development Policy of a Communist Government: West Bengal Since 1977*, New York: Cambridge University Press, 1993.
- Roy Porter, *London: A Social History*, Cambridge, MA: Harvard University Press, first paperback edition 1998, cited edition 2001.
- Ruth Sidel and Victor W Sidel, *The Health of China*, Boston: Beacon Press, 1982.
- S Bhattacharya (ed.), *Interaction of Health & Social Sciences*, Calcutta: Health and Social Sciences Seminar Committee, University College of Medicine, Calcutta University, 1991.
- Samiran Nundy et al. (eds.), *Healers or Predators?: Healthcare Corruption in India*, New Delhi: Oxford University Press, 2018.
- Sandeep Sinha, *Public Health Policy and the Indian Public Bengal, 1850–1920*, Kolkata: Vision Publications, 1998.
- Sandra Morgen, *Into Our Own Hands: The Women's Health Movement in the United States, 1969–1990*, New Jersey/London: Rutgers University Press, 2002.

- Sougata Talukdar, *Right to Health in India: Law, Policy and Practice*, New Delhi: SAGE Publications India Pvt Ltd, 2022.
- Sridhar Venkatapuram, *Health Justice: An Argument from the Capabilities Approach*, Cambridge: Polity, 2011.
- Srikanta Ghosh, *The Indian Mafia*, New Delhi: Ashish Publishing House, 1991.
- Sujata Mukherjee, *Gender, Medicine, and Society in Colonial India: Women's Health Care in Nineteenth- and Early Twentieth-century Bengal*, New Delhi: Oxford University Press, 2017.
- Sumit Sarkar, *Modern India, 1885–1947*, New Delhi: Macmillan India Limited, 1959.
- Sunil Nandraj et al, *Private Health Sector in India*, Mumbai: CEHAT, 2011.
- Sunil S. Amrith, *Decolonizing International Health India and Southeast Asia, 1930–65*, New York: Palgrave Macmillan, 2006.
- Suvankar Dey (ed.), *Health Has a History*, Kolkata: K P Bagchi & Company, 2021.
- Suvobrata Sarkar (ed.), *History of Science, Technology, Environment, and Medicine in India*, New York/London: Routledge, 2022.
- Sydney Gordon and Ted Allan, *The Scalpel, the Sword: The Story of Dr. Norman Bethune*, New York and London: Monthly Review Press, revised edition 1973.
- Theodore H. Tulchinsky and Elena A. Varavikova, *The New Public Health*, Amsterdam: Elsevier, 2014 (third edition).
- Upinder Singh, *A History of Ancient and Early Medieval India: From the Stone Age to the 12th Century*, Delhi: Pearson, second impression 2012.
- V. Berridge, D.A. Christie and E.M. Tansey (eds.), *Public Health in the 1980s and 1990s: Decline and Rise?*, London: Wellcome Trust Centre, 2006.
- V. Gordon Childe, *Man Makes Himself*, New York: New American Library, 1951.
- Vani Kant Borooah, *Health and Well-Being in India*, London: Palgrave Macmillan, 2018.
- Vincent Tucker (ed.), *Cultural Perspective on Development*, London: Frank Cass, reprinted version 2002 (first published 1997).
- Vivek Neelakantan, *Tracing Human Rights in Health*, Mumbai: CEHAT, 2006.

- W.F Bynun and Roy Porter (eds.), *Companion Encylopedia of the History of Medicine*, volume 1 & 2, London/New York: Routledge, 1994.
- William Bynum, *The History of Medicine: A Very Short Introduction*, New York: Oxford University Press, 2008.
- William F. Fisher and Thomas Ponniah (eds.), *Another World is Possible: World Social Forum Proposals for An Alternative Globalization*, London: Zed Books, reprint 2015 (first published 2003).
- Zafrullah Chowdhury, *The Politics of Essential Drugs—The Makings of a Successful Health Strategy: Lessons from Bangladesh*, Dhaka, Bangladesh: The University Press Limited, 1996.
- Zhou Xun, *The People's Health: Health Intervention and Delivery in Mao's China, 1949–1983*, Montreal & Kingston, London, Chicago: McGill-Queen's University Press, 2020.

Articles

- Achin Chakraborty and Subrata Mukherjee, "Health Care in West Bengal: What Is Happening?", *Economic & Political Weekly*, Vol. 38, No. 48, November 29–December 5. 2003, pp. 5021–5023.
- Amit Sengupta, "New Drug Policy: Prescription for Mortgaging Drug Industry", *Economic & Political Weekly*, Vol. 29, No. 39, September 24, 1994, pp. 2526–2532.
- Amiya Kumar Bagchi, "Neo-Liberal Reforms with Cosmetic Changes?", *Economic & Political Weekly*, Vol. 39, No. 32, August 7–13, 2004, pp. 3572–3574.
- Amor Benyoussef & Barbara Christian, "Health Care in Developing Countries", *Social Science and Medicine,* Vol. 11, No. 6–7, 1977, pp. 399–408.
- Anant Phadke, "All India Drug Action Network: Report of The All-India Meeting on 30th & 31st January, 1985", *Medico Friend Circle Bulletin 111*, March 1985, pp. 12–13.
- Anant Phadke, "All India Drug Action Network", *Medico Friend Circle Bulletin 105*, September 1984, pp. 10–13.
- Anant Phadke, "Regulation of Doctors and Private Hospitals in India", *Economic & Political Weekly*, Vol. 51, No. 6, February 6, 2016, pp. 46–55.

- Anil Kumar, "The Indian Drug Industry under the Raj, 1860–1920", in Biswamoy Pati and Mark Harrison (ed.), *Health, Medicine and Empire: Perspective of Colonial India*, India: Orient Longman, 2001.
- Anwar Jaffry et al., "Towards a People's Science Movement", *Economic & Political Weekly*, Vol. 18, No. 11, March 12, 1983, pp. 372–376.
- Arun Bal, "Distortions in Drug Policy: Who is to be Blamed?", *Economic & Political Weekly*, Vol. 21, No. 23, June 7, 1986, pp. 1029–1032.
- Barbara Starfield, "Is US Health Really the Best in the World?", *Journal of American Medical Association*, Vol. 284, No. 4, 26 July 2000, pp. 483–485.
- Bijoya Roy and Siddharta Gupta, "Public–Private Partnership and User Fees in Healthcare: Evidence from West Bengal", *Economic & Political Weekly*, Vol. XLVI, No 38, September 17, 2011, pp. 74–78.
- Bijoya Roy, "Why Public–Private Collaboration is Bad News For Healthcare in India", *The Wire*, March 20, 2017.
- Bipul Malakar and Madhumita Deb, "Childcare and Reproductive Health in West Bengal: A Picture of Steady March", in Ajitava Raychaudhuri and Tuhin K. Das (eds.), *West Bengal Economy: Some Contemporary Issues*, Kolkata: Allied Publishers, 2005, pp. 291–333.
- Biren Roy, "Doctors, Left Front and Health Services", *Economic & Political Weekly*, Vol. 18, No, 44, October 29, 1983, pp. 1867–1868.
- Bruno Jobert, "Populism and Health Policy: The Case of Community Health Volunteers in India", *Social Science & Medicine*, Volume 20, Issue 1, 1985, pp. 1–25.
- C. Niranjan Rao, "Patents and Pharmaceuticals in India", *Economic & Political Weekly*, Vol. 41, No. 20, May 20–26, 2006, pp. 1975–1977.
- C.S Pichamuthu, "People's Health and State's Responsibilities", *Current Science*, Vol. 15, No. 10, October 1946, pp. 269–272.
- Charu C. Garg and Anup K. Karan, "Reducing Out-of-Pocket Expenditures to Reduce Poverty: A Disaggregated Analysis at Rural–Urban and State Level in India", *Health Policy and Planning*, Volume 24, No. 2, March 2009, pp. 116–128.
- Chittabrata Palit and Tinni Goswami, "Sanitation, Empire, Environment: Bengal (1980–1920)", *Proceedings of the Indian History Congress*, Vol. 68, Part One, 2007, pp. 731–744.

- David Arnold, "Death and the Modern Empire: The 1918–19 Influenza Epidemic in India", *Transactions of the Royal Historical Society*, Vol. 29, 2019, pp. 181–200.
- David Arnold, "The Rise of Western Medicine in India", *Lancet*, Vol. 348, October, 1996, pp. 1075–1078.
- David Arnold, "Touching the Body: Perspectives on the Indian Plague, 1896–1900", in Ranajit Guha (ed.), *Subaltern Studies V*, Delhi: Oxford University Press, 1987, pp. 55–90.
- David I. Macht, "A Drug or Poison?", *The Scientific Monthly*, Vol. 47, No. 1, July 1938, pp. 34–40.
- David L. Rabin & Patricia J. Bush, "The Use of Medicines: Historical Trends and International Comparisons", *International Journal of Health Services*, Vol. 4, No. 1, Winter 1974, pp. 61–87.
- David Werner, "Rising up in Latin America", *World Nutrition*, Volume 5, Number 4, April 2014, pp. 344–345.
- Debabar Banerji, "A Simplistic Approach to Health Policy Analysis: The World Bank Team on the Indian Health Sector", *International Journal of Health Services*, Vol. 24, No. 1, 1994, pp. 151–159.
- Debabar Banerji, "The Battle for Total Health Care", in *India International Centre Quarterly*, Vol. 14, No. 3, India, 1987, pp. 119–128.
- Debabar Banerji, "The People and Health Service Development in India: A Brief Overview", *International Journal of Health Services*, Volume 34, Number 1, 2004, pp. 123–142.
- Drimi Chaudhuri, "Bengal's public healthcare needs to be rescued from Apathy", *DNA India*, February 28, 2018.
- Edgar Sydenstricker, "The Changing Concept of Public Health", *The Milbank Memorial Fund Quarterly*, Vol. 13, No. 4, October, 1935, pp. 301–310.
- Ernest M. Gruenberg, "Public Health and the People's Health", *Public Health Reports (1896–1970)*, Vol. 72, No. 1, January 1957, pp. 47–50.
- G.C. Malhotra, "Parliamentary Committee with Special Reference to Departmentally Related Standing Committee", *The Journal of Parliamentary Information*, Vol. XLIV, No. 3, September, 1998, pp. 236–264.
- Ganapati Mudur, "Doctors in India defy guidelines on generic drugs", *British Medical Journal*, 1 July 2013, Vol. 347.

- Gavin Mooney, "Neoliberalism is Bad for Our Health", *International Journal of Health Services*, Vol. 42, No. 3, 2012, pp. 383–401.
- George Rosen "Approaches to a Concept of Social Medicine: A Historical Survey", *The Milbank Memorial Fund Quarterly*, Vol. 26, No. 1, January, 1948, pp. 7–21.
- George Rosen, "Hospitals, Medical Care and Social Policy in the French Revolution", *Bulletin of the History of Medicine*, Vol. 30, No. 2, March–April, 1956, pp. 124–149.
- Gerard Porter et al., "Over-the-counter sales of antibiotics for human use in India: The challenges and opportunities for regulation", *Medical Law International*, Vol. 21, No. 2, 2021, pp. 149–150.
- Halfdan Mahler, "The Meaning of Health For All by the Year 2000", in *World Health Forum*, Vol. 2, No. 1, WHO, 1981, pp. 5–22.
- Harsh Sethi, "Alternative Development Strategies: A Look at Some Micro Experiments", *Economic & Political Weekly*, Vol. 13, No. 31/33, Special Number, August 1978, pp. 1307–1316.
- Henry E. Sigerist, "From Bismarck to Beveridge: Developments and Trends in Social Security Legislation", *Journal of Public Health Policy*, Vol. 20, No. 4, 1999, pp. 474–496.
- Howard Waitzkin, "The Social Origins of Illness: A Neglected History", *International Journal of Health Services*, Vol. 11, No. 1, 1981, pp. 77–103.
- Imrana Qadeer and Indira Chakravarthi, "The Neo-liberal Interpretation of Health", *Social Scientist*, Vol. 38, No. 5/6, May–June 2010, pp. 49–61.
- Indranil Banerjee, "Deadly Bacteria *Shigella Dysenteriae* sweeps through West Bengal, Leaves Hundreds Dead", *India Today*, May 15, 1984.
- Indranil Banerjie, "14 villages get affected by poisonous gas emitted from Kesoram Rayon Factory at Tribeni", *India Today*, June 30, 1984.
- Isaiah Azariah, "Dr. Ida Scudder and The Revolution in Indian Medical Education", *Journal of Third World Studies* (University Press of Florida), Vol. 7, No. 1, Historical and Contemporary Third World Problems and Issues, Spring 1990, pp. 133–143.
- J.C. Hume. "Colonialism and Sanitary Medicine: The Development of Preventive Health Policy in the Punjab, 1860–1900", *Modern Asian Studies*, Vol. 20, No. 4, 1986, pp. 703–724.
- Jackie Range, "India's Poor Get Health Care in a Card", *The Wall Street Journal*, August 26, 2008.

- Jayanta Kumar Ray, "Organising Villagers for Self-reliance: A Study of Gonoshasthya Kendra in Bangladesh", *The Calcutta Historical Journal*, Vol. V, No. 1, July–December, 1980.
- John Ashton, Paula Grey and Keith Barnard, "Healthy cities—WHO's New Public Health Initiative", *Health Promotion International*, Vol. 1, No. 3, 1986, pp. 319–324.
- John Chalker, "The International Network for Rational Use of Drugs (INRUD)", *The Politics of Medicines* (e-Encyclopaedia), 2012.
- John Coggon and Lawrence O. Gostin, "The Two Most Important Questions for Ethical Public Health", *Journal of Public Health*, Vol. 42, No. 1, pp. 198–202.
- K. Sujatha Rao, "The Government's Previous Health Insurance Schemes Failed. Why Should the New One Work?", *The Wire*, February 5, 2018.
- Kalpana Sharma, "Viewing Health as an Inalienable Right", *India Together*, October 7, 2005.
- Karthikeyan K. Kumarasamy et al., "Emergence of a new antibiotic resistance mechanism in India, Pakistan, and the UK: a molecular, biological, and epidemiological study", *The Lancet*, Vol. 10, No. 9, September, 2010, pp. 597–602.
- Kenneth J. Arrow, "Uncertainty and Welfare Economics of Medical Care", *The American Economic Review*, Vol. 53, Issue 5, December, 1963, pp. 941–973.
- Krishna Soman and Subharanjan Dasgupta, "Public Health: Historical Experience", *Economic & Political Weekly*, Vol. 38, No. 47, November 22–28, 2003, pp. 4942–4944.
- Leda Machado, "The Participation of Women in the Health Movement of Jardim Nordeste, in the Eastern Zone of São Paulo, Brazil: 1976–1985", *Bulletin of Latin American Research*, Vol. 7, No. 1, 1988, pp. 47–63.
- Lois Gibb, "Citizen Activism for Environmental Health: The Growth of a Powerful New Grassroots Health Movement", in *The Annals of the American Academy of Political and Social Science,* November, 2002, Vol. 584, Health and the Environment (November, 2002), pp. 97–109.
- Mahua Sarkar, "Pollution, Public Health and the People of Calcutta: The Nineteenth Century", *Journal of the Asiatic Society*, Vol. LXII No. 4, 2020, pp. 85–120.

- Mampi Bose, "Bengal's Healthcare Has Become Dysfunctional: Here's How We Can Fix It", *The Wire*, June 27, 2019.
- Manoj Sharma and Gayatri Bhatia, "The Voluntary Health Movement in India: A Strengths, Weaknesses, Opportunities, and Threats (SWOT) Analysis", *Journal of Community Health*, Vol. 21, No. 6, December 1996, pp. 453–464.
- Margaret Whitehead et al., "Equity and health sector reforms: can low-income countries escape the medical poverty trap?" *The Lancet*, Vol. 358, September 8, 2001, pp. 833–836.
- María Hamlin Zúniga, "The International People's Health Council", *Development in Practice*, Vol. 3, No. 1, February, 1993, pp. 59–61.
- Mark Harrison, "Quarantine, Pilgrimage, and Colonial Trade: India 1866–1900", *Indian Economic and Social History Review*, Vol. 29, No. 2, 1992, pp. 117–144.
- Mark Heywood, "South Africa's Treatment Action Campaign: Combining Law and Social Mobilization to Realize the Right to Health", *Journal of Human Rights Practice*, Vol.1, No. 1, March 2009, pp. 14–36.
- Mark Nichter, "Community Health Worker Scheme: A Plan for Democratisation", *Economic & Political Weekly*, Vol. 15, No. 1, January 5, 1980, pp. 37–43.
- Milton Terris, "Epidemiology and the Public Health Movement", *Journal of Public Health Policy*, Autumn, 1987, Vol. 8, No. 3, pp. 315–329.
- Moni Nag, "Political Awareness as a Factor in Accessibility of Health Services: A Case Study of Rural Kerala and West Bengal", *Economic & Political Weekly*, Vol. 24, No. 8, February 25, 1989, pp. 417–426.
- Montu Bose and Arijita Dutta, "Health Financing Strategies to Reduce Out of-Pocket Burden in India: a Comparative Study of Three States", *BMC Health Services Research*, Vol. 18, November 2018.
- Moumita Chakraborti, "Tracing Medicine and Politics in Colonial Bengal, c.1920– c.1940", *Journal of the Asiatic Society*, Vol. LX, No. 2, 2018, Kolkata, pp. 49–68.
- Partha Chatterjee, "The Coming Crisis in West Bengal", *Economic & Political Weekly*, Vol. 44, No. 9, February 28, 2009, pp. 42–45.
- Partha Dutta, "Health and Healing in Colonial Bengal: The Christian Missionaries and the Imperial Impact", *Vidyasagar University Journal of History*, Vol. VI, 2017–2018, pp. 87–95.

- Partha Sarathi Banerjee, "Power and Political Violence in West Bengal", *Economic & Political Weekly*, Vol. 46, No. 6, February 5–11, 2011, pp. 16–18.
- Patralekha Chatterjee, "Seeing Health Care as a Human Right in India", *The Lancet*, Vol. 377, No. 9761, January 15, 2011, pp. 195–196.
- Punyabrata Goon, "The Journey of Shramajibi Swasthya Udyog (Working Class Health Project)", *Sanhati*, September 17, 2012.
- Punyabrata Goon, "The Struggle for Rational Drug Policy", *Rational Drug Bulletin*, Vol. 23, No. 1 Jan 2014, p. 3.
- R.S. Arole, "Comprehensive Rural Health Project, Jamkhed", *Medico Friend Circle Bulletin 49*, January 1980, pp. 1–6.
- Rama V. Baru, "A Limiting Perspective on Universal Coverage", *Economic & Political Weekly*, Vol. 47, No. 8, February 25, 2012, pp. 64–66.
- Rama V. Baru, "Privatisation of Health Services: A South Asian Perspective", *Economic & Political Weekly*, Vol. 38, No. 42, October 18–24, 2003, pp. 4433–4437.
- Rama V. Baru and Madhurima Nundy, "Blurring of Boundaries: Public–Private Partnerships in Health Services in India", *Economic & Political Weekly*, Vol. 43, No. 4, January 26–February 1, 2008, pp. 62–71.
- Ramesh Bhat, "Issues in Health: Public–Private Partnership", *Economic & Political Weekly*, Vol. 35, No. 52/53, December 30, 2000–January 5, 2001, pp. 4706–4716.
- Ravi Narayan et al, "A People's Charter for Health and Beyond", *The National Medical Journal of India*, Vol. 14, No. 2, 2001, pp. 67–70.
- Ravi Narayan et al., "The People's Health Movement", *Oxford Research Encyclopedia of Global Public Health,* May 29, 2020.
- S Srinivasan, "'Medicines for All', the Pharma Industry and the Indian State", *Economic & Political Weekly*, Vol. 46, No. 24, June 11–17, 2011, pp. 43–50.
- S. Srinivasan, "A Network for the Rational and Ethical Use of Drugs", *Indian Journal of Medical Ethics*, Vol. 1, January–March 2004, pp. 13–14.
- Sabyasachi Bhattacharya, "History from Below", *Social Scientist*, Vol. 11, No. 4, April 1983, pp. 3–20.

- S.K. Jana et al., "A Historical Perspective on the Rational Use of Drugs (RUD) in India", *Indian Journal of Pharmacology*, Vol. 38, No. 5, October 2006, pp. 374–375.
- Smita Chakraburtty, "The Fire at AMRI: Need for Legislation on Corporate Culpability", *Economic & Political Weekly*, Vol. 52, No. 34, August 26, 2017, pp. 15–17.
- Solomon R. Benatar et al., "A Shared Statement of Ethical Principles for Those Who Shape and Give Health Care", *British Medical Journal,* Vol. 318, No. 7178, January 23, 1999.
- Soumitra Ghosh and Nabanita Datta Gupta, "Targeting and Effects of Rashtriya Swasthya Bima Yojana on Access to Care and Financial Protection", *Economic & Political Weekly*, Vol. 52, No. 4, January 28, 2017, pp. 61–70.
- Sreenivasa Raju, "The Good and The Bad about 'Master Health Check-Up' in India", *The Times of India*, September 10, 2012.
- Sujit K. Das "Left Front's Scheme for Modernising Health Care: Ill-Conceived", *Economic & Political Weekly*, Vol. 23, No. 14/15, April 2–9, 1988, pp. 690–691.
- Sujit K. Das, "Humbling the Mighty: A Small Beginning", *Economic & Political Weekly*, Vol. 24, No. 37, 16 September 1989, pp. 2057–2058.
- Sujit K. Das, "Trouble on the Health Front", *Economic & Political Weekly*, Vol. 22, No. 15, April 11, 1987, pp. 629–630.
- Sujit K. Das, "Left Front's Health Circus", *Economic & Political Weekly*, Vol. 23, No, 21, May 21, 1988, pp. 1056–1058.
- Sujit K. Das, "Public Health: A Question of Entitlements", *Economic & Political Weekly*, Vol. 27, No. 39, September 26, 1992, pp. 2095–2096.
- Sumanta Banerjee, "West Bengal's Next Quinquennium, and the Future of the Indian Left", *Economic & Political Weekly*, Vol. 46, Issue No. 23, June 4, 2011, pp. 14–19.
- Sumanta Roy, "Marxists vs Paternalists vs Liberals: Where healthcare stands in India", *Down to Earth*, June 29, 2020.
- Sumanta Sen, "Massive breakdown of medical services in Calcutta due to protest by junior doctors", *India Today*, October 31, 1983.
- Susanne MacGregor, "Welfare, Neo-Liberalism and New Paternalism: Three Ways for Social Policy in Late Capitalist Societies", *Capital & Class*, Vol. 23, No. 1, Spring 1999, pp. 91–118.

- Swadhin Mondal et al., "Catastrophic out-of-pocket payment for health care and its impact on households: Experience from West Bengal, India", *Economics Bulletin*, Vol. 34, No. 2, 2014, pp. 1303–1316.
- T. Sundararaman, "Opinion: Modicare is more an election gimmick than a real solution to India's health needs", *Scroll*, February 5, 2018.
- Veeranarayana Kethineni, "Political Economy of State Intervention in Health Care", *Economic & Political Weekly*, Vol. 26, No. 42, October 19, 1991, pp. 2427–2433.
- Vikas Bajpai, "National Health Policy, 2017: Revealing Public Health Chicanery", *Economic & Political Weekly*, Vol. 53, No. 28, July 14, 2018.

Index[1]

A

[1] Note: Page numbers followed by 'n' refer to notes.

© The Author(s), under exclusive license to Springer Nature Switzerland AG 2025
N. Malakar, *Historicising the People's Health Movement in West Bengal, India*, https://doi.org/10.1007/978-3-032-02696-5

P

Q

R

S

T

U

FSC
www.fsc.org
MIX
Papier | Fördert gute Waldnutzung
FSC® C083411

Kolibri 360 GmbH
Ferdinand-Jühlke-Straße 7
99095 Erfurt, Deutschland
produktsicherheit@kolibri360.de